CONTROLLING CHOLESTEROL

Despite the "negative press" we hear about cholesterol, it's important to understand that the substance isn't all bad. In fact, as it travels about in the bloodstream, cholesterol often performs essential work in our bodies. For example, it promotes synthesis of the cells' vital membranes and is a component of many of the key hormones produced in the body. It also aids digestion as an ingredient in the bile acids.

Unfortunately, however, not all cholesterol get processed in beneficial ways—and that's where the danger begins. To put it bluntly, *an elevated level of blood cholesterol is a major cause of the epidemic of coronary heart disease.*

But death or debilitation isn't inevitable! Preventive medicine *does* have an answer to this problem. Armed with sufficient knowledge and know-how, you can protect yourself from the deadly work of killer cholesterol. So I've written this book to let you know the latest, most important information and techniques available to help you fight this disease.

—Dr. Kenneth H. Cooper, from *Controlling Cholesterol*

DR. KENNETH H. COOPER'S
PREVENTIVE MEDICINE PROGRAM

Controlling Cholesterol

Kenneth H. Cooper, M.D., M.P.H.

Dad,

Because I love you and want you to have a long & happy retirement.

Paul

BANTAM BOOKS
NEW YORK · TORONTO · LONDON · SYDNEY · AUCKLAND

NOTE

Fitness, diet, and health are matters which necessarily vary from individual to individual. Readers should speak with their own doctor about their individual needs before starting any diet program. Consulting one's physician is especially important if one is on any medication or is already under medical care for any illness.

CONTROLLING CHOLESTEROL
A Bantam Book

PRINTING HISTORY

*Bantam hardcover edition / February 1988
8 printings through April 1988
Bantam paperback edition / February 1989*

Library of Congress Cataloging-in-Publication Data

Cooper, Kenneth H.
   Controlling cholesterol.

   Includes index.
   1. Low-cholesterol diet—Recipes.   2. Exercise therapy.
I. Title.
RM237.75.C66   1988   616.1'0654   87-19530
ISBN 0-553-27775-8

Published simultaneously in the United States and Canada

Bantam Books are published by Bantam Books, a division of Bantam Doubleday Dell Publishing Group, Inc. Its trademark, consisting of the words "Bantam Books" and the portrayal of a rooster, is Registered in U.S. Patent and Trademark Office and in other countries. Marca Registrada, Bantam Books, 666 Fifth Avenue, New York, New York 10103.

PRINTED IN THE UNITED STATES OF AMERICA

0   0 9 8 7 6 5

To those people who are keenly
interested in improving the quality and
the quantity of their lives by
adhering closely to the concepts of
modern preventive medicine.

ACKNOWLEDGMENTS

To prepare a book so detailed and complicated as one dealing with the ever-changing subject of cholesterol, I have required the assistance and cooperation of many people. To adequately acknowledge all would be impossible, but several are more than worthy of attention.

Scott M. Grundy, M.D., Ph.D., Director, Center for Human Nutrition, University of Texas Health Science Center at Dallas, was my professional consultant and adviser throughout the book, from its inception to publication.

William Proctor was invaluable with his editorial advice and contributions. Without Bill's help, this book probably would never have been written. Bruce Peschel provided artistic help.

My good friend and literary agent, Herb Katz, was extremely helpful in expediting the business arrangements for this book and in offering significant editorial suggestions. My editor at Bantam, Coleen O'Shea, provided guidance which greatly enhanced the practical value of the manuscript.

Dan Leizman, a Summer Intern at the Aerobics Center and a full-time medical student at Ohio State University Medical School, spent innumerable hours in the library conducting research into the scientific literature. Wayne Loney, my very able clinical assistant, also helped with the collection of research materials.

Marianne Fazen, laboratory technologist at the Cooper Clinic, helped immensely in preparing charts, cross-checking data, and determining the availability and practicality of national blood testing.

Georgia Kostas, M.P.H., R.D., Director of Clinical Nutrition at the Cooper Clinic, was the major contributor to the dietary sections.

The transcriptionists at the Cooper Clinic typed and retyped most of the material in this book many, many times.

Under the direction of their supervisor, Barbara Bartolomeo, that task was accomplished accurately and efficiently.

My executive secretary, Harriet Guthrie, helped immeasurably in organizing and obtaining materials for this book. Not only did Harriet help with the preparation of the book, she kept my clinic and administrative requirements under control, giving me the time necessary to prepare the book.

Last but not least, I want to thank all those people and Cooper Clinic patients who allowed me to tell their stories, which have helped emphasize and clarify various points in this book. Permission to identify some of them as individuals, and not only as case histories, gives the book a more human and personal touch.

Once again, many thanks to all of you who helped make this book a reality.

CONTENTS

INTRODUCTION

Developing a
Preventive Program

The key to good health and long life is *prevention*. By taking measures now to prevent the development of various diseases and health problems, you can greatly enhance your chances to enjoy an energetic existence well into the future.

In this book and those to follow in the *Preventive Medicine's Answer* series, my objective has been to give you the practical tools you need to develop your own personal preventive medicine program. By following the suggested guidelines, you'll find yourself in a much stronger position to control your health and improve your way of life.

It's appropriate that this first book in our series goes, quite literally, to the very heart of the matter, for in it we confront our greatest killer: heart disease. I became deeply involved in studying the link between cholesterol and heart disease in the early 1970s, when I first established the Aerobics Center in Dallas.

My objective at that time was to provide the best information and treatment that preventive medicine could offer in all medical fields. Soon it became apparent that a major part of our work at the Center focused on the cholesterol issue. In fact, the Aerobics Center is now engaged in a wide variety of cholesterol-related work, such as:

• Serving as a testing site for a possible breakthrough cholesterol-lowering drug produced by a major pharmaceutical company

• Hosting an international conference on "Cholesterol Issues of the '80s" for many of the world's leading experts on cholesterol

• Establishing a Lipid Problems Clinic to help patients who don't respond to the normal preventive medicine approach

• Conducting ongoing research into the work of deadly cholesterol based on our extensive data repositories of patients

In short, our work is demonstrating that if you lower your total cholesterol level and otherwise control the various fats in your blood, you'll be taking one of the most significant preventive steps available to protect your heart. Fortunately, increasing numbers of Americans seem to be learning this important lesson.

In September 1985, the American Health Foundation attempted to publicize the relation between high cholesterol in the blood and heart disease by sponsoring a five-day "health fair" in New York City. To highlight the health problem, the organization offered free tests of blood cholesterol. At the most, the promoters of the event expected 2,000 to 3,000 people to respond. They were shocked when nearly 30,000 individuals showed up, some waiting as long as three hours to take the free test. Overwhelmed, the organizers made arrangements for additional personnel and equipment to be flown in; still, more than 15,000 people had to be turned away.

Such incidents suggest that, finally, Americans are beginning to realize that there is a relationship between high blood cholesterol and heart disease. Furthermore, they know that if the problem is identified and corrected early, heart attacks may be prevented or at least delayed. Because an estimated 1.5 million people in the United States have heart attacks each year, this is a topic worthy of everyone's interest.

Even though increasing numbers of Americans seem to be aware of this deadly relationship, there is still a question about cholesterol in the minds of many, including some physicians. For example, a national survey conducted in 1983 revealed that 80 percent of American physicians who were questioned felt there was a correlation between high blood pressure and heart disease. Also, 80 percent felt that cigarette smoking was a major coronary risk factor. Yet, only 39 percent felt that there was enough scientific evidence to document a relationship between high blood cholesterol and heart disease. By 1986, that percentage had increased to 64 percent.*

Why was there such a dramatic change among physicians in such a short period of time? Perhaps it was because of the growing number of scientific studies being published in the medical literature documenting this relationship.

Until the results of the Lipid Research Clinics Coronary Primary Prevention Trials were released in early 1984, there was always a question about whether cholesterol was actually the cause of heart disease or was merely guilty by association. But in this study at 12 clinics around the country of 3,806 men with markedly elevated cholesterol, a reduction in cholesterol levels was achieved by using a medication known as Questran, or cholestyramine. Associated with this reduction in cholesterol was a highly significant decrease in heart attacks and sudden death. Every 1 percent decrease in the blood cholesterol level was accompanied by a 2 to 3 percent decrease in the incidence of heart attacks and sudden deaths. Other studies have documented comparable results. With the publication of these facts, particularly in the nonscientific literature, national interest in this subject has soared.

Despite these trends, there's still an appalling lack of knowledge about cholesterol, its relationship to heart disease, and the ways it can be controlled. But efforts are continuing to spread the word about cholesterol and push back the frontiers of our knowledge. For example, the pharmaceutical firm Merck and Company recently launched a $100 million development program to educate the public, conduct scientific research, and promote their new product, Lovastatin. This prescription drug, not yet approved for public use, has been shown to be extremely effective in lowering the blood cholesterol in patients with high cholesterol levels.

Fortunately, however, the majority of people who have an elevated blood cholesterol do not have to resort to extensive and expensive drug-related measures. With the proper utilization of sound preventive medicine principles, high cholesterol levels usually can be controlled without medication. The purpose of this book is to explain how you can apply those principles in your own health care.

But before you initiate any type of preventive program, it's

*Cholesterol Awareness Surveys 1983, 1986, National Heart, Lung and Blood Institute.

necessary to know some basic facts about how cholesterol works, the way it's produced and disposed of, and how it's affected by diet and exercise. Also, any successful education and prevention program must be accompanied by regular evaluations. To this end, specific details are provided in this book about how you can get your cholesterol checked. Physicians and laboratories all over the country are willing to collaborate in this effort to make all Americans more knowledgeable about their cholesterol.

I encourage you first to study this book in detail and then have your blood cholesterol measured to determine whether you have a problem. If you do have a problem, you should follow the preventive medicine guidelines described in this book. Should all else fail, then resort to the use of medications known to lower cholesterol. In any case, it's mandatory that you keep in touch with your physician, dietician, or medical consultant in order to achieve optimum results.

I'm hopeful that there will be at least as great a decrease in deaths from heart attacks in the next decade as there has been in the past ten years. Today, the most common first symptom of severe heart disease is sudden death. Tomorrow, with a proper preventive program at work, that doesn't have to be so. Long life, rather than sudden death, should become the byword for our future.

PART I

What Is Cholesterol— And Why Is It a Problem?

ONE

How to Use This Book

The word *cholesterol* has become almost as familiar as your next-door neighbor. You see it on many food labels in the local grocery store. The term often jumps out from newspaper headlines and advertisements. And increasingly you find friends and acquaintances saying, "This food has too much cholesterol," or "My cholesterol level is a little too high."

But even though many of us talk glibly about cholesterol, we often don't understand exactly what it is and how it relates to our health and well-being. For example, many people think that if they have a certain cholesterol level in their blood, they can assume that they're automatically safe from heart disease. Usually, this is a correct assumption. But, as we'll see later, it *is* possible to have *low* blood cholesterol and still die from atherosclerosis, heart disease that takes the form of hardening of the arteries.

Also, when we talk of "hardening of the arteries," many people just assume that's a normal part of aging. But in fact, to say that you suffer from hardening of the arteries may be just another way of saying that you have serious problems with one or more risk factors for atherosclerosis of the coronary arteries. These risk factors may include cigarette smoking, high blood pressure, diabetes, or high cholesterol levels—yet, for most people, all these risk factors can be eliminated or at least controlled.

Of course, it's not surprising that there's a considerable amount of confusion about cholesterol. Of several Nobel Prizes awarded for research into cholesterol in this century, one was a mistake! The scientist who received the award in 1928 described a chemical structure for cholesterol which was later proved to be incorrect. So you shouldn't be disturbed if you don't understand everything about the subject, because the way cholesterol works in your body isn't so easy a concept to grasp.

On the other hand, it's absolutely essential, both for your safety and for the healthy hearts and arteries of your family members, that you understand more about the implications of cholesterol for human health. To be sure, this substance, which is both manufactured by your body and introduced through your diet, is absolutely essential to your health. Among other things, you need cholesterol for membrane synthesis in your cells. Without it, the cells of the body couldn't function; indeed, you couldn't even stay alive. But when cholesterol isn't handled properly, your life is in serious danger.

Cholesterol bears a large part of the responsibility for the sad and sickly condition of our arteries and hearts. Atherosclerosis of the coronary arteries and its consequence, coronary heart disease, is responsible for more than 550,000 deaths in the United States each year, according to the National Institutes of Health. That's more deaths than are caused by all forms of cancer combined.

But death is only the last step in a disease process which affects millions of us. Specifically, more than 5.4 million Americans have symptoms of coronary heart disease, and a large but undetermined number of others harbor undiagnosed atherosclerotic disease.

Cholesterol—ordinarily an odorless, white, powdery, fatty substance—when dissolved in the blood, plays a major role in this terrifying scenario. It's our partner in this dance of death. To put it bluntly, *an elevated level of blood cholesterol is a major cause of the epidemic of coronary heart disease.*

But death or debilitation isn't inevitable! Preventive medicine *does* have an answer to this problem. Armed with sufficient knowledge and know-how, you can protect yourself from the deadly work of killer cholesterol. So I've written this book to let you know the latest, most important information and techniques available to help you fight this disease.

Specifically, you'll learn:

• The current thinking on what's the best range for your blood cholesterol

• How to evaluate the important forms in which cholesterol is carried in your blood

• How to distinguish between "good" and "bad" cholesterol

• The predictive value of the "cholesterol ratio"—and how you can compute it from your own blood values

• Why up-to-date research suggests that triglycerides may be more important than scientists previously thought

• How to set up the best diet to lower your cholesterol

• New findings on the use of vitamin and drug treatments in lowering blood cholesterol

• Some practical suggestions for including nutrients like fish oils and olive oil in your diet to lower your cholesterol

• Why a seemingly slight imbalance in the fatty components in your blood may substantially increase your coronary risk

• The latest thinking on the use of soluble fibers, such as oat bran, in controlling cholesterol

• Information you need to have about the link between inherited family traits and cholesterol

• The evidence that the deadly process of atherosclerosis—or hardening of the arteries—can be reversed

• How to calculate your personal "cholesterol coronary risk"

• New findings on the link between stress and cholesterol

Also, we'll explore how you can make the best use of medical support systems as you move to put your cholesterol in balance. For example, you'll learn how to cut through medical red tape and get no-hassle, relatively inexpensive blood tests. You need to have these blood tests, of course, to determine and monitor the cholesterol levels in your blood. In addition, there will be tips and suggested techniques for talking to your family doctor about how to achieve a proper balance of cholesterol in your body.

Despite all the "negative press" we hear about cholesterol, it's important to understand that the substance isn't all bad. In fact, as it travels about in the bloodstream, cholesterol often performs essential work in our bodies. For example, it promotes synthesis of the cells' vital membranes and is a component of many of the key hormones produced in the body. It also aids digestion as an ingredient in the bile acids.

Unfortunately, however, not all the cholesterol gets processed in beneficial ways—and that's where the danger begins. Excess cholesterol continues to circulate in the blood and may eventually be deposited in the walls of the arteries. Over a period of years, this excess cholesterol contributes to formation of a plaque on the interior walls of your arteries. As a result, your arteries become narrower and narrower, much like what happens with the sludge deposits in an old water pipe.

This clogging process is known in popular parlance as "hardening of the arteries," or, in a more technical, medical sense, as atherosclerosis (or arteriosclerosis). In fact, the danger lies more in the narrowing than in the hardening of the arteries. You can get narrowing of the arteries at any age, by the way, whether you're 30, 40, 50, or older. Youth provides no insurance against this disease. When one or more of the coronary arteries which feed blood to your heart become narrowed and roughened, a blood clot may form on the plaque and block the flow of the life-giving fluid. The result will be a heart attack: the tissues in the part of the heart supplied by the blocked artery will die; and, in some cases, *you* may die.

But this ominous series of events is not inevitable. An internal time bomb doesn't have to explode in your system or in those of your loved ones—because there's something you can do about it. You can act to *prevent* this attack on your health and your life. It's just a matter of learning the facts about the causes of heart attacks, and using those facts in protecting your health and that of your family.

A very important part of preventing heart attacks is *controlling* your cholesterol—not eliminating it altogether. As I've mentioned, cholesterol is essential to life. Without it, you couldn't function as a normal, healthy human being. On the other hand, if too much of it is present in your blood, you're looking down the barrel of a cocked and loaded weapon—which is pointed directly at your heart.

So what can you do to strengthen your defenses against this killer?

You need two key things to mount an effective counterattack against out-of-control cholesterol: (1) sufficient knowledge about the deadly work of the substance; and (2) the means and motivation to *act* on that knowledge. In other words, you first must know something about the problem and about practical ways to apply your knowledge. Then, you'll be more likely to *do* something about it to improve your prospects of a long and healthy life.

Consider first the issue of knowledge. How much do you really know about cholesterol? To test your basic understanding, I'd suggest that you take the following quiz.* When I've put these questions to medical professionals, I've found that many of them don't do too well. So don't worry if you don't have all the answers at your fingertips. This little test should serve as a helpful introduction to the subject of proper nutrition. Even more important, it will give you a feel for steps you may want to take to improve your health—such as reducing the amount of cholesterol in your diet.

A Quick Nutrition and Cholesterol Quiz

1. The cholesterol in our bodies comes from _____.
   (a) all types of fats we eat
   (b) mostly animal fats
   (c) our own bodies and all types of fats we eat
   (d) our own bodies and mostly animal fats

2. About _____% of the calories in the average American diet comes from fat.
   (a) 25   (b) 30   (c) 40   (d) 50   (e) 55

3. About _____% of the calories in the average American diet *should* come from fat.
   (a) 10–15   (b) 15–20   (c) 25–30   (d) 35–40   (e) 50

*Sources for this questionnaire include our own studies at the Aerobics Center in Dallas; the work of Dr. Scott M. Grundy, Director, Center for Human Nutrition, University of Texas Health Science Center at Dallas; and *Patient Care* (January 30, 1986).

4. The Senate Select Committee on Nutrition and Human Needs recommends that _____% of calories in the diet come from protein.
   (a) 5–10 (b) 10–15 (c) 15–30

5. The Senate Select Committee on Nutrition and Human Needs recommends that carbohydrates provide about _____% of energy intake.
   (a) 30 (b) 40 (c) 50 (d) 60 (e) 70

6. A person of average weight should limit daily dietary cholesterol intake to _____ mg.*
   (a) 100 (b) 200 (c) 300 (d) 400 (e) 500 (f) 600

7. The average American gets _____ mg. of dietary cholesterol.
   (a) 150 (b) 300 (c) 450 (d) 600 (e) 800 (f) 1,000

8. True or false: I'm exactly at my optimum body weight, so I couldn't possibly have a cholesterol problem.

9. True or false: There's no point in anyone having a cholesterol check before about age 30.

10. Which of the following tests is best at predicting the risk of coronary artery disease?
    (a) triglyceride levels
    (b) total cholesterol level
    (c) high-density lipoprotein (HDL) cholesterol level
    (d) low-density lipoprotein (LDL) cholesterol level

11. Which of the following combinations of tests is best at predicting the risk of coronary heart disease?
    (a) total cholesterol level and HDL cholesterol level
    (b) LDL cholesterol level, total cholesterol level, and triglyceride levels
    (c) HDL cholesterol level, total cholesterol level, and LDL cholesterol level
    (d) HDL cholesterol level, total cholesterol level, and triglyceride levels

12. Scientific studies show cancer to be more strongly correlated with intake of _____ than with other elements of diet.
    (a) protein (b) fat and calories (c) carbohydrates (d) alcohol

*Cholesterol in the blood is most commonly measured in terms of mg/dl or milligrams per deciliter. Dietary intake is measured in terms of milligrams (mg.).

13. The most desirable range for the average person's blood cholesterol is _____ mg/dl.
    (a) 180–190   (b) 190–200   (c) 200–210   (d) 210–220
    (e) 220–230

Quiz Answers

This test will provide some idea about whether you have the beginnings of an understanding about the cholesterol issue. Here are the suggested answers to the questions, with a few explanatory comments:

1. (d) Our own bodies and mostly animal fats. Although a significant amount of the cholesterol in our blood and body tissues comes from our diets, liver cells in the body produce cholesterol independently of any dietary intake.

2. (c) About *40%* of the calories in the average American diet comes from fat.

3. (c) According to government researchers at the Senate Select Committee on Nutrition and Human Needs as well as many preventive medicine specialists, no more than *30%* of the calories in the average American diet *should* come from fat.

4. (b) The Senate Select Committee on Nutrition and Human Needs recommends that *10–15%* of calories in the diet come from protein.

5. (d) The Senate Select Committee on Nutrition and Human Needs recommends that carbohydrates provide about *60%* of energy intake.

6. (c) The Senate Select Committee on Nutrition and Human Needs recommends limiting dietary cholesterol intake to less than 100 mg. per 1,000 calories, not to exceed *300 mg.* per day. But those with a need to lower their cholesterol counts may have to achieve lower limits—even 100 mg. or less.

7. (c) The average American now gets *450 mg.* of dietary cholesterol per day.*

*My answer differs from the one in *Patient Care,* which is 600 mg., because current data indicate that Americans have now decreased their cholesterol intake to this level.

8. False. You *could* have a cholesterol problem. Although your cholesterol levels may go up as your body weight goes up, many factors other than the fat content of your body determine your cholesterol levels. The only way to know for sure is to get a proper blood test.

9. False. Proper preventive medicine requires that even young children have their cholesterol levels checked. It's important to be sure youngsters haven't inherited a high level of cholesterol in their blood, which could lead to an early coronary heart disease problem. The American Heart Association recommends that regular testing for cholesterol levels begin by age 20.

10. (c) Of the tests listed, the *high-density lipoprotein (HDL) cholesterol level* is probably the best at predicting the risk of coronary artery disease. The HDLs seem to provide major protection against the development of atherosclerosis. But as more evidence comes in, *all four* of the listed factors are emerging as important risk indicators.

11. (c) According to the latest findings, the combination of *HDL cholesterol* level, *total cholesterol* level, and *LDL cholesterol* level is best at predicting the risk of coronary heart disease.*

12. (b) Epidemiologic studies show cancer to be more strongly correlated with intake of *fat and calories* than with other elements of diet.

13. (a) Many experts and studies recommend that a person's cholesterol should be kept below 200, and in my opinion, readings in the 180–190 range or even lower are best.

Note: The numerical differences between "right" and "wrong" answers in these questions may not seem too great. But in fact, as we'll see, scientific studies have shown that there may be a *big* difference in coronary risk between, say, a total cholesterol level of 200 and a level of 220.

How did you do on this test? Many people, including physicians, answer more than half of the questions incorrectly.

*My answer here is different from the one given in *Patient Care:* They chose answer (d). But as you'll see after we get farther into this book, current thinking in preventive medicine indicates that the three factors mentioned in choice (c) are the best predictive tool.

But, no matter how you scored, there's much more to learn about cholesterol and the impact it can have on your body's systems and your health.

Your first objective should be to understand exactly what's going on with the cholesterol in your blood and arteries. Next, you should become aware of how you can improve the condition of your blood vessels through changes in your diet and lifestyle. Then, you'll be much more likely to take constructive steps to improve your health and possibly save your life.

I've already mentioned some of the key topics we'll be discussing, but there are many more we'll consider as well. These include:

• The precise way cholesterol does its deadly work

• How to achieve the "normal" or "safe" ranges for cholesterol

• The difference between "good" and "bad" cholesterol

• The latest findings on the link between low cholesterol and cancer

• The pros and cons of using alcohol to affect your cholesterol

• How aerobic exercise can improve your cholesterol balance

• When to use drug therapy

• When to use niacin or nicotinic acid, one of the B-complex vitamins which works like a drug

• Coffee and the cholesterol question

• Some lessons about healthy diet and lifestyle from Indians and Eskimos with low rates of coronary heart disease

• How obesity can upset blood chemistry

• A potential problem that exists with birth control pills

• The connection between age and cholesterol

• The difference in cholesterol levels in men and women

• The controversy over polyunsaturated fats

• The problem with smoking

• Why you should monitor cholesterol consumption in your children's diets

But sufficient knowledge is only the first step in preventive medicine. It's also important to *stay* motivated and incorporate certain eating, exercise, and lifestyle changes *permanently* in your life. Otherwise, your cholesterol may careen out of control at some later point.

So how can you achieve an ongoing transformation of your cholesterol levels? One way is to get *personal* about your approach to cholesterol. By this I mean always to keep in mind how the facts you read apply to you as an individual.

To this end, I've attempted to organize this book so that it can be used quickly and effectively by anyone who wants to apply the basic knowledge about cholesterol. In chapter 9 you'll find low-cholesterol menus which are easy to prepare; simple explanations of medical and scientific concepts; and clear, unequivocal "action principles" under each topic.

The book is divided into short chapters, with all the key points and issues included in a comprehensive index at the back of the book. In addition, in Appendices I and II you'll find the most comprehensive list available of the cholesterol values of various foods. This will help you choose those dishes that tend to be lowest in cholesterol and fat.

The goal has been to give you a practical reference work, which is the next best thing to having a knowledgeable physician at your side. As much as possible, *I* want to lead you personally, step by step, toward formulating an effective defense against the cholesterol menace.

It's extremely important for you to establish a relationship with local medical experts who understand how the latest research on cholesterol can be applied to improve your health. To get the maximum benefits, you should have your cholesterol levels checked and evaluated at regular intervals. That means finding the right medical laboratory, as well as the right physician, to help you determine your status and monitor your progress.

Various studies have shown that people who are involved in face-to-face counseling—or even in counseling conducted through mail or by telephone—are most successful in lowering their cholesterol levels. So, take steps to get your physician, a medical laboratory, a supportive network of family and friends—

and this book—working for you. Then, you'll be more likely to keep your blood components in proper balance.

With cholesterol, then, knowledge is truly power. Conversely, as Thomas Mann wrote, "the actual enemy is the unknown." By inference, it's been noted that you have to know your enemy well if you hope to defeat him. So, as a first step in understanding how to combat the excess cholesterol that may be lurking inside you, let's examine the "personal history" of the killer.

TWO

The Personal History of a Killer

Like many mass killers, cholesterol was born into the world under rather innocent, unpretentious circumstances. The earliest known scientific investigation into this substance, which would later be identified as one of the deadliest forces in our bodies, dates back to 1733. In that year, a French scientist by the name of Antonio Vallisnieri discovered that gallstones were soluble in alcohol.

It shouldn't be particularly surprising that this researcher was fascinated by gallstones: These hard, rocklike sources of pain—which are produced by the gallbladder and may vary in size from a little seed to a hefty plum—were popular playthings at many of the social functions of eighteenth-century French aristocrats.

But what exactly do gallstones have to do with cholesterol?

Just this: What we know today as cholesterol is a major component of most gallstones. Still, like a mischievous child whose criminal nature has not yet surfaced for all to see, the substance remained covered up for decades, secreted behind the protective skirts of the gallstone.

It wasn't until 1769 that cholesterol was actually extracted from gallstones in the form of powdery white flakes. The chemist who achieved this feat was another Frenchman, Poulletier de la Salle.

De la Salle conducted his experiments in the political climate that preceded the mass killings of the French Revolution. But as he prepared the first pure cholesterol by crystallizing a gallstone in an alcohol solution, the researcher was unaware that he was confronting a lethal force in his own laboratory. Still, the orderly processes of research continued as another scientist confirmed de la Salle's findings in 1775.

Despite these breakthroughs, the killer continued to do its deadly work completely under cover for the next forty years. To be sure, heart trouble abounded in the Western world during this period. But the major cause of coronary disease didn't as yet even have a name.

Then, Michel Chevreul, a French chemist, took some crucial steps, beginning in 1815, to lift the shroud of secrecy. First, he succeeded in differentiating the white flakes from other waxes. Specifically, he discovered that the gallstone-related substance was *"unsaponfiable"*—or incapable of being transformed, as are many other fats, into soap.

Chevreul, who apparently didn't have an inkling about the connection between his research and heart disease, continued with his investigations throughout the next decade. By 1824, he had discovered the fascinating white substance in both human and animal bile—the yellow fluid produced by the liver, which helps with digestion of fatty foods in the intestine.

Perhaps just as important, at the beginning of this period of fruitful discovery Chevreul gave the great enemy of the healthy heart a name: "cholesterine." Appropriately enough, the word was derived from the Greek *chole,* meaning "bile," and *stereos,* meaning "solid."

"Je nummerai cholesterine, de . . . bile, et . . . solid, la substance cristallisee des calculs biliaires humains!" Chevreul declared exuberantly to his colleagues.

During the next twenty-five years, scientists from many nations identified cholesterine in brain tissue, the human blood, tumors, and hens' eggs. Also, as part of this discovery process, researchers showed that cholesterines from eggs, gallstones, and bile were identical. Most significant of all, the substance was found in arteries which had been ravaged by atherosclerosis. As yet, however, this process of fatty buildup in the arteries was not called "atherosclerosis."

In a related development in 1856—one which was destined to converge with cholesterol research about fifty years later— Rudolf Virchow, a prominent German pathologist, kicked off the study of atherosclerosis. Specifically, Virchow observed that significant changes occur in artery walls during the "hardening" process, as plaque builds up and clogging of the blood vessels occurs.

As the nineteenth century moved on and scientific techniques improved, scientists discovered that cholesterine contained alcohollike molecules. So, the name of the substance was changed to "cholesterol." The great killer had finally been given its true name.

With the advent of the twentieth century, the scientific findings on atherosclerosis, or hardening of the arteries, and cholesterol came together. Up to this point, the study of cholesterol had been primarily a matter of abstract scientific interest. Despite some indications that cholesterol was present in clogged arteries, no one had yet made the connection between the substance in the blood system and coronary artery disease. But then the ominous features of the killer began to emerge in more frightening detail.

In 1904, the name "atherosclerosis" was first used to describe the infiltration of fats into artery walls which causes a buildup of plaque in the circulatory system. At the same time, scientists proposed that the fats, or lipids as they are known technically, came directly from the blood to the artery wall. There, they produced streaks of fatty deposits, which later turned into full-fledged clogging.

At almost the same time, in 1905, a German graduate student named Adolf Windaus began trying to determine the chemical structure of cholesterol. Working at the Institute of Chemistry, at the University of Freiburg in Germany, he made such tremendous strides in his research that he was eventually awarded the Nobel Prize in 1928. Unfortunately, later investigation showed that his description of the structure of the cholesterol molecule was in error.

The Nobel committee let him keep his prize, however, and he went back to his laboratory to try to work out the correct solution. But it wasn't until more than two decades later that other scientists finally discovered the true chemical structure of cholesterol.

Still, despite his mistakes, Windaus was a towering figure in the early twentieth-century work on cholesterol. He participated in major research in 1910 with two other scientists, which began to bring together the loose threads in the cholesterol mystery: they found that heart tissue damaged by atherosclerosis had a much higher content of cholesterol than normal tissue.

In many respects, this was one of those "Eurekas!" that scientists are always looking for. Suspicions had been growing about the seemingly benign—and even rather pretty—white substance which had titillated the French in their drawing rooms and laboratories in the eighteenth century. There were worries that cholesterol might actually be a kind of wolf in disguise.

Now, however, the evidence was mounting for a direct connection between cholesterol and atherosclerosis—that vessel disease which could literally strangle the life out of a human heart. In Germany, Windaus continued his research into the cholesterol content of atherosclerosis. Significant dietary research also began under the direction of the Russian scientist Nikolai Anitschkow. The scientific community took serious notice when he fed cholesterol to rabbits and succeeded in producing fatty buildups, or lesions, in their arteries.

Scientists began to get the killer in their sights. Over a period of nearly two centuries, they had identified it, named it, and begun to get a record of its "fingerprints" and other significant characteristics. But the connection between cholesterol and coronary heart disease had been tenuous at best. With Anitschkow's experiments, however, the connection between cholesterol-laden foods and hardening of the arteries began to be much clearer.

As the scientific activity accelerated, researchers found that the animal body gets cholesterol in two ways: (1) through the diet, but (2) primarily through the internal production of the substance in the body's cells. One study of albino rats found that their blood cholesterol levels *increased* by one-third during a period when they were consuming a cholesterol-free diet!

During the next fifty years, up to the late 1960s, the world's scientists, acting like an international legion of fine homicide detectives, began to put together the missing pieces in the cholesterol story. Among other things, they found that cholesterol is formed in the body by the progressive buildup of small molecules. Also, they studied in more detail how cholesterol is produced and disposed of in the liver. And they took steps to fine-tune their understanding of exactly how the fatty "garbage" begins to build up on diseased artery walls.

In a development that was to have important implications for preventive medicine, a number of researchers suggested that a breakdown of the *components* of cholesterol might be extremely helpful in linking cholesterol and hardening of the arteries. Specifically, they began to explore how the "lipoprotein" components—including the now-famous "good" high-density lipoprotein (HDL) and "bad" low-density lipoprotein (LDL)—might be involved in the process of artery disease. Lipoproteins, by the way, are substances in the blood made up of protein and fat, including cholesterol.*

From the 1940s through the 1960s, the precise work of the killer started to become quite clear. Medical researchers established an association between atherosclerosis and hypertension and also atherosclerosis and diabetes. Then, Ancel Keys of the University of Minnesota—one of the foremost pioneers in the field of cardiovascular research—proposed that atherosclerosis might not be just an inevitable result of the aging process. Rather, he said, the disease might be related to environmental factors.

Soon afterward, tests were launched which showed that levels of blood cholesterol—which now had been linked directly to atherosclerosis—could be decreased through changing the diets of animals. Also, researchers in Framingham, Massachusetts, launched the now-famous long-term Framingham Study on Heart Disease. This study has clearly shown that as the blood cholesterol decreases, the incidence of heart attacks and sudden death also decreases.

Finally, the research, which would lead to the indictment and conviction of perhaps the greatest mass killer in world history, was in the home stretch. By the late 1960s the circumstantial evidence against cholesterol was sufficiently solid that many scientific fingers were pointing directly at it. It seemed hard to believe that the white substance had been regarded as just a harmless, fascinating oddity in the eighteenth century! Exactly two hundred years had passed since Poulletier de la Salle had started it all by discovering that those then-unnamed white flakes were a major component of gallstones.

But still, the scientific prosecutors were not quite satisfied enough to go to court. The results of some of the major studies in which people were followed for many years were just beginning to come in, but the conclusions weren't yet definitive. Cautious researchers preferred, quite properly, to wait until all the evidence was collected before they brought charges and pushed hard for a guilty verdict.

*John Gofman discovered lipoproteins in 1949 and 1950.

They didn't have long to wait. Between 1970 and now, we have finally managed to put it together. Now we're ready to answer the big question: "What do we finally understand about cholesterol?"

THREE

What Do We Finally Understand About Cholesterol?

During the past decade or so, scientific research on the killer profile of cholesterol has produced some dramatic new insights. These breakthroughs—which have tremendous implications for your personal health—have occurred on two major fronts.

First, scientists have been probing deep into the body's biochemistry to try to determine exactly what goes on in the bloodstream. Among other things, these researchers have been asking, "What produces that deadly clogging of the arteries that we know as atherosclerosis?"

Second, medical investigators have been following broad populations of people over long periods of time in what are known as "longitudinal studies." These studies have focused, in part, on the role that cholesterol and saturated fats in the diet and in the bloodstream play in the development of heart disease.

Both of these approaches to the cholesterol problem have handed up a solid indictment against cholesterol. But these are two separate stories—the first of which will be told here,* and the second in the following chapter.

Let's take a look deep inside your body's fabulously complex circulatory system. The action of cholesterol, as it moves about in the microscopic world of your body's molecules and

*The basic information about the role of cholesterol in the body as presented in this chapter comes largely from conversations with Dr. Scott M. Grundy, Director of the Center for Human Nutrition at the University of Texas Health Science Center at Dallas.

blood particles, can best be understood as a piece of real-life biological theater—a story of dangerous adventure on the high seas of your body's blood flow.

Imagine, if you will, that you can shrink to one one-thousandth of your present size and become an observer of exactly what's going on inside your cell tissues and blood vessels. The first thing you'll encounter is a cast of characters and seaworthy vessels. These, quite literally, are engaged in a life-or-death naval action throughout the recesses of your veins and arteries. Some of the major players include:

The powerful shipbuilder and shipping magnate.	— The liver.
A supply ship which is built in the liver and which travels through the bloodstream. This vessel also carries a kind of destructive "Trojan Horse."	— Very low-density lipo-protein (also known as "VLDL").
The innocent victim.	— Your circulatory system, including the artery walls and the heart.
The villain—and "Trojan Horse"—transported from the liver by the VLDL.	— Apolipoprotein B (aka "Apo B").
A fatty "orphan" in the blood, which is produced in the liver and becomes the unwitting tool of the villain.	— Low-density lipoprotein (aka "LDL"), which escorts a potentially dangerous "passenger," cholesterol.
The accomplice in crime and "passenger" accompanying the LDL.	— Cholesterol.
Possible hero.	— High-density lipoprotein (aka "HDL").
Hero and "booster" in the bloodstream.	— Apolipoprotein E (aka "Apo E").
A "dock worker" which helps unload the VLDL "ship."	— Apolipoprotein C (aka "Apo C").

High-energy passenger on VLDL "ship."	— Triglycerides.
Rescue team.	— Receptors, situated on the surface of the body's cells, which "pull in" free LDLs for beneficial use by the body.
Supporting characters.	— Various other bodily tissues and chemicals.

The plot of this little drama, in which these various characters play important roles, revolves around a couple of key questions: Will the "victims"—the circulatory system, and especially the artery walls and the heart—be attacked and destroyed by three VLDL passengers: the "villain" apolipoprotein B; its accomplice cholesterol; and their unwitting tool, the low-density lipoproteins? Or will the various heroes in the scenario, such as the HDLs and Apo Es, be able to step in and ward off the deadly attack?

These are not merely some intellectual queries, which are of little practical interest. Rather, they are questions each of us *must* ask as we consider this disturbing—and extremely real— plot which is unfolding in our bodies.

The action begins with the liver, which serves as a kind of powerful "shipbuilder" and "shipping magnate," as it orchestrates the entire cholesterol metabolism in the body. As it takes in and sends out cholesterol in various lipoproteins, the liver has a number of important tools at its disposal. One of the most important of these is an enzyme—known by the tongue-twisting title "HMG-CoA-Reductase"—which controls the amount of cholesterol being produced by the liver. The levels of this reductase catalyst in your blood are a direct indication of how much cholesterol is being produced by your liver. The role of the reductase catalyst is especially important because almost 75 percent of the cholesterol in our bodies is manufactured by the liver—*not* introduced through the food we eat.

In addition to secreting this all-important reductase enzyme, the liver produces or metabolizes many of the other actors in the cholesterol drama. For example, since cholesterol is a fat, it is not soluble in water (or blood). So, to be transported throughout the body, cholesterol from dietary sources must be changed into a water-soluble form. This is accomplished in the liver, which places a blanket of protein around the cholesterol; the new molecules which are thus produced are called lipoproteins. When dissolved in the blood, they carry cholesterol and other products to all parts of the body. Finally, excess fatty products are returned via the bloodstream to the liver, where they are broken down and disposed of through the intestines.

In addition to this "inside job" done by the liver in producing and regulating the cholesterol, there's another way that cholesterol may get into your system. A small amount of cholesterol and a large amount of another fatty substance, triglycerides, enter your body every day in your diet in the form of the largest lipoproteins, called chylomicrons. These lipids in your food move through the intestines, into the circulatory system and finally, to the bodily tissues. Adequate aerobic exercise and sufficient amounts of certain enzymes in your body can clear away the chylomicrons and their remnants from your system rather rapidly. But if your body fails to clear away these lipids, your cholesterol and triglyceride levels may rise, and you may be at a greater risk of developing atherosclerosis. Also, sometimes the transport of various fatty substances in and out of the liver doesn't work the way it's supposed to. In short, there may be tragic flaws in the system. But let me offer one word of caution here: It's important, as we follow this plot to its climax, that we not make hasty judgments about where the blame for cholesterol problems should be laid. For example, if you find that you have a problem with your cholesterol level, you may automatically conclude that there's something seriously wrong with your liver. You may even assume you've got some sort of liver disease. But in fact there's probably nothing wrong with your liver—except perhaps that a few types of molecules, out of the millions in the liver, aren't working properly. The problem most likely lies only in the way these abnormal molecules handle your cholesterol and fats, not in the overall function of the organ.

Before we get more deeply into the details of the cholesterol drama, it's also helpful to understand that there are two types of people who have a problem with cholesterol: (1) those who lack the means to get LDL and its cholesterol out of their blood properly; and (2) those who produce too many lipoproteins, which carry the cholesterol. In either case, too much cholesterol gets left unused in the blood. That excess tends to accumulate on the artery walls and may eventually clog up the vessels to dangerous or even lethal levels.

This, then, is an overview of the action. Now let's take a closer look at exactly what may be happening on the high seas of your circulatory system.

The liver, acting in its capacity as "shipping magnate," first begins to direct the work and movements of the cholesterol. The cholesterol, as I've already explained, may be produced by your body in amounts determined by the HMG-CoA-Reductase, or it may come from animal products or be encouraged by saturated fats consumed in your diet. As part of its preliminary preparations, the liver fits out a kind of cholesterol-carrying "ship"—called "very low-density lipoprotein," or VLDL. Other "passengers" on the ship VLDL include various other fatty substances such as triglycerides, and also proteins called "apolipoproteins."* Once it's loaded up, the VLDL is then sent out from the liver into the blood. (Figure 1.)

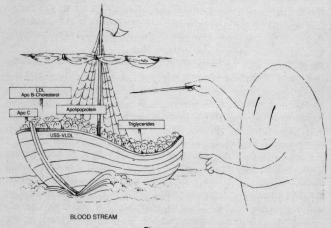

LDL
Apo B-Cholesterol

Apo C

Apolipoprotein

Triglycerides

USS-VLDL

BLOOD STREAM

Figure 1

As the VLDLs circulate, they "unload" their triglycerides, which are then used as energy by the tissues or stored as fat.

*Phospholipids, another type of fat, are a relatively stable component of all lipoproteins, so they will not be included in this discussion.

The VLDL loses its triglycerides in two stages. In the first step, when the VLDL has lost much of its triglycerides, it is called a VLDL remnant. In the second step, most of the remaining triglycerides are lost from the VLDL remnant. The result is the triglyceride-poor LDL. In other words, when VLDL gets rid of the triglycerides, it does not lose its cholesterol. As a result, LDLs are very rich in cholesterol.

Much of the cholesterol in the bloodstream resides in these LDLs, and this cholesterol can be used in essential ways by various body tissues. For example, some of the LDLs are pulled out of the blood by "receptors" on the body's cells. The cholesterol in these LDLs then proceeds to play a vital role in the cells' membranes. In addition, LDL cholesterol is used in the production of steroid hormones in the adrenal glands and the sex organs, and it participates in the formation of bile acids in the liver.

But, as we'll see, this is not the whole story behind LDL cholesterol—not by a long shot. Like the wily Greeks in Homer's ancient classic *The Iliad,* the VLDL "ship," and its product LDL, carries a kind of "Trojan Horse." This gift horse is a special protein, known as "apolipoprotein B" or "Apo B," which wraps itself around the cholesterol to produce a deadly combination within the LDL particle.

To be sure, LDLs *do* perform functions that are important to the continuation of life in the body's tissues. But sometimes, when the cells' receptors don't pick them up, LDLs get lost, almost like molecular orphans, in the bloodstream. When this happens, instead of doing good work in the body, the cholesterol of the LDL, guided by the villain Apo B, becomes a menacing presence, one that can ultimately terminate life.

But we're getting ahead of our story. Let's go back to the liver, where the VLDL "ship" has just been assembled and loaded. (Figure 1.) The VLDL comes shooting out of the liver into the bloodstream and heads for various tissues in the body, where it unloads its passengers and cargo for the body's use.

When the VLDL ship lands in the various organs, it encounters an enzyme known as "lipoprotein lipase." (Figure 2.) This enzyme, which is in the capillaries or tiny blood vessels on the tissue surfaces of all body organs, then triggers the passenger-unloading process.

First, the enzyme contacts a substance called apolipoprotein C, or "Apo C" for short. I like to think of Apo C as a kind of

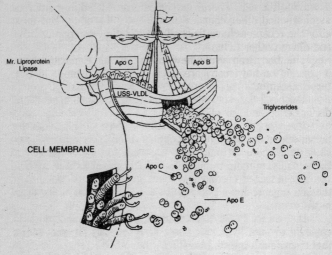

Figure 2

"dock worker," because of what happens when it interacts with lipoprotein lipase. Specifically, the interaction causes the VLDL to begin to unload its triglycerides, which provide the body with energy. Also, the VLDL leaves behind the LDL cholesterol and its Apo B partner.

One of the most important things that takes place at this point is the work of a kind of "rescue team" of protein strands, which scientists have called "receptors." These reach out to the LDLs, with their circulating Apo B and accompanying cholesterol, and haul them into the body's cells. About 80 percent of the LDL receptors in the body are found in the liver, and another 20 percent are found in other tissues.

As a matter of fact, an understanding of the work of these receptors is at the cutting edge of current cholesterol research. The subject is so important that the 1985 Nobel Prize for medicine was awarded to Dr. Michael S. Brown and Dr. Joseph L. Goldstein of the University of Texas Health Science Center at Dallas for their research into the role of these receptors.

One of the major things that Goldstein and Brown discovered is that there is a constant recycling of the receptor "rescue teams." First, they'll reach up, grab the LDL, and pull it down into the cell. There, its cholesterol is used in membrane synthesis and other chemical functions of the body. But then, after the receptors have finished this job, they can pop up again and drag in other LDLs.

The body can grow new receptors or eliminate them, depending on how many are needed at a given time. In fact, these receptors—which consist of a single strand of protein wound in a fragile, exquisite configuration—can appear and disappear in a matter of seconds.

The work of the receptors has important implications for the development of hardening of the arteries, or atherosclerosis, in your body. If your receptors work properly and if you have enough of them to take all the LDL into your body's cells, you should have no problem with atherosclerosis. When everything in your body and diet is in order, a sufficient number of receptors will be produced in response to the cells' need for cholesterol. Also, the liver must have enough receptors to enable it to "catch" and dispose of the excess LDL cholesterol that comes back into the liver.

But now, enter the villains.

A major problem arises when there are too few receptors for the number of LDLs floating around in the bloodstream. Suppose you eat too many foods high in cholesterol or in saturated fats, or your body produces too much cholesterol. In such a case, excessive numbers of LDLs may arrive at the various cell receptor sites.

As the plot begins to thicken, a couple of disturbing questions arise: Will there be enough receptors to pick up the extra LDLs? Or will these LDLs become free-floating—and potentially dangerous—"orphans" in the circulatory system?

A big source of the impending danger is the LDL's partner, Apo B. The Apo B starts off operating just as it's supposed to do: it serves as a kind of "key" that connects with the cell receptors and "locks" the LDL into the cell for its work there. That was the very purpose that the master shipbuilder, the liver, had in mind when it sent the Apo B off on this voyage!

As long as the Apo B does this job and attaches the LDL properly to a receptor, all is fine. The LDL is then pulled into the cell and broken down there for use. But sometimes there are too few receptors available. In that case, excess LDL, with its Apo B and cholesterol, may accumulate in the bloodstream. This is where the life-threatening problems may begin.

Some people have a serious genetic problem with their LDL. In other words, they may have inherited certain genetic defects which make it impossible for them to process properly the LDL in their blood.

Here's the way the difficulty may arise: LDL receptors are produced by specific genes. Normally, you must inherit two genes which make LDL receptors, one from each parent. This provides the genetic background to supply an adequate number of LDL receptors to keep the blood cholesterol low.

People who inherit one nonfunctioning gene and therefore have only one normal gene don't make enough LDL receptors. Frequently, they have cholesterol levels ranging from 300 to 500 mg/dl. (In contrast, safe cholesterol levels for both men and women should generally be below 200.) Where there's one nonfunctioning gene, the excess LDL makes its way into an artery wall to produce the deadly atherosclerosis. In such cases, severe atherosclerosis often develops by the time a person is in his thirties. Fortunately, this condition isn't too common: It affects only about 1 in 500 people.

Even less common is the situation where a person inherits abnormal genes from *both* parents. Under these circumstances, there will be *no* functioning LDL receptors. As a result, cholesterol levels may reach 700 to 1,000 mg/dl, and atherosclerosis may strike when the person is a young child or teenager. If this condition goes untreated, these people usually die of heart attacks before age 20.

One case in point is that of a six-year-old girl who in September 1983 was found to have a total cholesterol level of 1,079 mg/dl. Further studies on her at the University of Texas Health Science Center at Dallas revealed that one of her LDL receptor genes wasn't functioning at all, and the other was badly defective.

Shortly after this examination, she suffered a heart attack and had to undergo two coronary bypass operations. Also, one of her heart valves had to be replaced.

But even this lifesaving surgery didn't control her problem. She had to undergo combined heart and liver transplant operations at the University of Pittsburgh Health Center in February 1984.

After these transplant operations, the girl's cholesterol dropped dramatically to a count of 301. Because this figure was still high, she was placed on a cholesterol-restricted diet and also a medication.* As a result of this treatment, her cholesterol declined to 171 mg/dl, a normal value for her age.

Two years later, the child was alive and doing quite well, with a normal cholesterol count. Also, she had no further symptoms of severe atherosclerosis.

Obviously, cases like this are rare. But don't get too comfortable—at least not yet. Even if you have the proper genes and the normal number of LDL receptors, a diet rich in cholesterol or saturated fats will cause your body to make fewer receptors for LDL. Why is this? The reason is fairly simple: In effect, the extra cholesterol and saturated fats in your diet cause your blood to become overloaded with LDL cholesterol. In other words, the body doesn't need all the available LDL cholesterol. So, excess amounts of LDL, accompanied by cholesterol and its Apo B partner, tend to float loose in the bloodstream.

In effect, the LDL becomes a kind of "orphan," with no home to go to. When this happens, the LDL may find a new home in an artery wall, and the result will be atherosclerosis.

To put it another way, after the VLDL ship has docked and made the delivery of its triglyceride cargo to the body's cells, there's still a great deal of cholesterol and protein "garbage" left over, which needs to be swept out of the bloodstream. Many of the remnants of the VLDL become transformed into the dangerous LDL. To keep your circulatory system in healthy balance, the remnants of the VLDL and the leftover LDL must be shipped back to the liver for final disposal.

But how exactly does this garbage get picked up and delivered back to the liver?

One way is through the action of Apo E, one of the "heroes" in this internal drama that's going on at every moment inside your body. The Apo E is one of the passengers on the ship VLDL. After the VLDL has unloaded its cargo, the Apo E still stays "on board," as part of the VLDL remnant.

This Apo E serves as a sort of "booster system" to take the remnants of the VLDL out of the blood and back to the liver. The reason that the Apo E is so efficient as a cleanup force is that it has an exceptional ability to "hook up" with

---

*The medication used in this case was Lovastatin. It lowers the production of cholesterol in the liver by interacting with the enzyme HMG-CoA-Reductase, and also increases the LDL receptor activity.

receptors which get the VLDL remnants out of the blood-stream. If this booster system didn't exist, many more VLDL remnants would be converted to LDLs, and the level of LDLs in your bloodstream would be much higher. But fortunately, the Apo E acts so quickly that many of the remnants of the VLDL are picked up and whisked away to the liver before they even have a chance to be broken down into LDLs!

Another very important player at this cleanup stage of the cholesterol plot is the high-density lipoprotein, or HDL. These cholesterol-carrying lipoproteins probably are produced in the liver, intestines, or other parts of the body. They are made up of 20 percent cholesterol, surrounded by an Apo A lipoprotein blanket. HDL cholesterol is called "good" cholesterol because high levels in your blood are associated with a lower risk of atherosclerosis and coronary heart disease. Scientific research has also shown that a low level of HDL cholesterol is associated with a high risk of coronary heart disease. (Figure 3.)

But are HDLs really the good guys in the cholesterol scenario? Is their fine reputation really warranted?

I like to refer to HDLs as *possible* heroes in this developing cholesterol drama because their exact role hasn't quite been nailed down. In fact, there are two theories about the role of HDLs: Some scientists believe that the HDLs can pick up excess cholesterol out of the arteries and actually carry it back to the liver and dump it there. If so, the HDLs may even be able to remove cholesterol that has started to accumulate as plaque on the walls of the blood vessels.

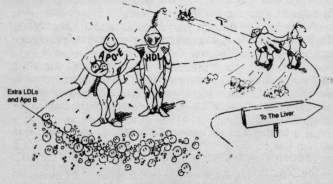

Figure 3

In other words, the HDLs may act as sort of white-knight "garbagemen" to clean up excess cholesterol. In this way, they could prevent—and perhaps even reverse—the buildup of cholesterol in the arteries.

But there's another theory which doesn't give the HDLs quite so much credit. According to this belief, low levels of HDLs merely *accompany* high levels of other lipoproteins. They simply serve as a *signal* of higher coronary risk.

Specifically, this theory says that the level of HDLs in your blood may just indicate the amount of concentration of the VLDL remnants after the VLDL ship has unloaded its cargo—and after it has broken up on the shoals and reefs of your body's cells. If the Apo E "booster system" is working properly, the Apo E will then take the VLDL remnants back to the liver. Otherwise, these VLDL remnants, which include LDLs, may enter the artery walls and produce atherosclerosis. So, if your HDL level is low, this may just reflect the fact that too many remnants are circulating, that they're not being removed, and that the danger has increased that they will produce atherosclerosis.

Probably there's truth in both these theories. In other words, HDLs most likely play both (1) an active role in removing LDL garbage, and (2) a passive role, signaling that other components of the blood are working or not working to help remove the waste materials. In any case, one thing is certain: When HDLs are present in large quantities in your blood, your risk of heart disease is low. Conversely, when HDLs are present in low quantities, your risk of atherosclerosis is higher. In men and women over 50 years of age, the level of the HDL cholesterol may be the best predictor of future coronary events. Total cholesterol and LDL cholesterol are the best lipid predictors of heart disease in men under age 50.

Now, to return to our story: Unused LDLs, with their excess Apo B and its cholesterol partner, are floating around in the bloodstream. They have become "orphans," no longer functioning in their intended manner. This is where the main problems start.

Up to this point in our unfolding drama, the Apo B has stayed with the LDL as a helpful guide and facilitator. You'll recall that it's the Apo B which provides the key to bind the LDL to the "rescuer" receptors. This action enables the LDL cholesterol to be pulled into the body's tissues for productive work.

But now, with the LDL "orphaned" in the bloodstream, its Apo B turns into a villain. The Apo B is a tough, insoluble substance which tends to adhere to artery walls, as well as to receptors. As a result, as the LDL and its accompanying Apo B bounce around in your bloodstream, they'll eventually penetrate a blood vessel wall. Because of the Apo B, they get stuck on the wall. Gradually, the Apo B and its accompanying cholesterol tend to accumulate and build up to form a material known as "plaque."

In short, the formation of a plaque is started by LDL cholesterol *and* its protein partner Apo B. And make no mistake about it: the development of plaque is one of the most dangerous, unhealthy things that can happen to your body. As more plaque develops, a significant degree of clogging of blood vessels may occur. That's what hardening of the arteries, or atherosclerosis, is all about.

You can see why LDL cholesterol is often referred to as "bad" cholesterol—although that accusation isn't entirely correct. As we've already discussed, the LDL can play a vital role in providing cells with needed cholesterol. Yet, when the LDLs get "orphaned" in your bloodstream, they penetrate arterial walls and their cholesterol begins to build up there.

In some ways, then, the LDL cholesterol in your blood is a kind of innocent bystander or victim. It's a tool of the more active, villainous agent, the Apo B. Once the Apo B gets into an artery wall, it won't let go. As a result, the LDL and its cholesterol become trapped on the wall. When this occurs, the LDL cholesterol itself becomes a major factor in the clogging process.

Suppose, then, you are going to put the components of your blood system on trial for their "crimes on the high seas" of your circulatory system. You might charge the Apo B as the principal perpetrator and mastermind in your hardening of the arteries. But the LDL cholesterol would certainly have to be indicted as an accomplice or accessory to the crime!

As the plaque builds up more and more, your arteries get narrower and narrower. Now the internal biological drama that's being played out in your system turns toward the tragic. The final result may be a total stoppage of your blood flow due to too much plaque. In addition, since the plaque has a roughened surface, a blood clot may form on top of it. And if such a clot occurs in one of your coronary arteries—which are the vessels that feed life-sustaining blood directly to the heart—the result may be sudden death by heart attack.

So this, in a nutshell, is the disturbing scenario that's taking place minute by minute, second by second, in your bloodstream. Your liver, to begin the action, gathers the LDL cholesterol "passengers" and launches them in a VLDL ship. Then, when they reach the various cells in your body, the cargo and passengers of the ship are unloaded.

Some of the LDLs are delivered via receptors to the body's cells for productive work in cell growth. But other LDLs, containing the villain Apo B and cholesterol, are left loose, like unsupervised orphans, in the bloodstream. Some are transported back to the liver and are picked up by liver receptors and disposed of. But some of the cholesterol garbage is never picked up. Eventually the LDLs, carrying Apo B and cholesterol, penetrate arterial walls, where they get stuck and start the growth of plaque.

As more of the LDL "orphans" gravitate toward the artery walls, clogging of the arteries occurs. The final result? Perhaps a fatal heart attack.

Obviously, this is a very complex process. Also, much is still unknown about exactly how the various LDLs, HDLs, and apolipoproteins operate and interact, either to clear out the blood or to clog up the arteries.

But what we do know is this: None of this information that you've been reading is an abstraction. This drama, which so often ends in tragedy, is occuring *in reality* in countless human beings—perhaps even in you and your loved ones—at this very moment.

To understand just how serious the problem is, let's move on now to a consideration of the deadly work that cholesterol has done—and is continuing to do—throughout our population.

PART II

Why Your Cholesterol Must Be in Balance

FOUR

The Great Principle
of Balance

When I was at the University of Oklahoma Medical School during the mid-1950s, we were taught that the normal, "safe" range for cholesterol was 150 to 350 milligrams per deciliter (mg/dl). But how the thinking on this topic has changed during the last thirty years!

Today, if your total cholesterol is above 230, most physicians get concerned. And if your level is 250 or above, you should be placed immediately on a special diet and exercise program, and possibly even on drugs. It's at these higher levels—which used to be considered safe—that cholesterol does its deadliest work.

But your total cholesterol count is not the whole story. It's part of a much broader picture, which is rooted in a principle of balance in your blood. Our information about heart disease and cholesterol—and about the need for balance among the fatty components of the blood—comes directly from solid, well-documented population studies. The most important investigations, called "longitudinal studies," have been conducted with groups of people over a period of years, and sometimes over decades.

Perhaps the most important theme that emerges from these longitudinal studies is this: *If your cholesterol is completely in balance, you probably have almost complete protection against atherosclerosis.* Of course, I can't say there's any absolute guarantee that certain preventive steps can ensure you won't have any problem with coronary artery disease. But I can say that it's possible for most people to arrange their lives to minimize and often eliminate any chance of developing a problem with atherosclerosis.

To this end, then, it's extremely important to think in terms of the individual cholesterol and other fatty components of your blood, in addition to your total cholesterol level. Specifically, you should pay attention to:

1. Your total cholesterol

2. Your LDLs (low-density lipoproteins)

3. Your HDLs (high-density lipoproteins)

4. The ratio of your total cholesterol to your HDL cholesterol

5. Your triglycerides

If any of the components of your cholesterol level are out of balance, you may find yourself confronting a problem that's now being called "dyslipidemia." That means an imbalance of the fats in your body, a condition which can only spell bad news for your blood vessels and ultimately your heart.

Let's turn to a number of the important longitudinal studies which suggest a few guidelines to keep in mind as you try to put your blood values in proper balance.

What the Studies Say About Total Cholesterol

First of all, what should your total cholesterol level be? As we'll see later, there are many factors, such as your age and HDL levels, which have to be taken into account in arriving at your optimum total cholesterol level. But still, it's possible to make a few generalizations in light of various longitudinal studies.

One group of findings has emerged from the Framingham Heart Study, a project begun in Framingham, Massachusetts, in 1948. These suggest that for the average adult, there may be a relatively safe "threshold" level of cholesterol, ranging from 200 to 220 mg/dl. Specifically, the Framingham Study and a number of other investigations indicate that the rates of coronary heart disease remain relatively constant for cholesterol levels up to the 200–220 range. But as cholesterol levels rise above this threshold, the risk for coronary heart disease—

and especially atherosclerosis—accelerates. So, if your cholesterol goes up from 200 to 250, your risk of heart disease doubles. Then, if it goes up from 250 to 300, your risk doubles again.

Another organization studying the long-term effects of a high cholesterol is the National Institutes of Health (NIH). In a recent consensus statement (1984), the following age-adjusted cholesterol risk levels were established:

ACLS*: Total Cholesterol
and All Cause Mortality, 1971–1985

| Age Groups | Cholesterol Groups | | |
	Low	Moderate	High
20–29 years	≤200	201–220	>220
30–39 years	≤220	221–240	>240
40+ years	≤240	241–260	>260

(From NIH Consensus Conference, MG/DL)
*Aerobics Center Longitudinal Study (ACLS, 1971–1985)

Using these cholesterol risk groups, Dr. Steve Blair, Director of Epidemiology at the Institute for Aerobics Research, looked at the relationship between total cholesterol levels and all causes of mortality in 13,509 men. In this Aerobics Center Longitudinal Study (ACLS, 1971–1985), the men were divided into two groups based on whether they were healthy or unhealthy. If any question dealing with a significant medical problem was answered in the affirmative (either past or present), they were placed in the unhealthy group. The healthy group had no known medical problems. Both groups of men were then followed for a total of almost 100,000 person-years. (A person-year is a term to express how long a person has been followed. That is, ten person-years equals either ten people followed for one year, or one person followed for ten years.) The results were most interesting.

If you study the chart on the next page carefully, you will notice that the risk of death in the unhealthy group was equally high in the LOW as it was in the MODERATE risk group. In the HIGH risk group, the age-adjusted death rate was remarkably higher. Why is there no difference between the LOW and MODERATE risk groups? I wonder if it is because of the cholesterol levels established by the NIH for the LOW risk group? My

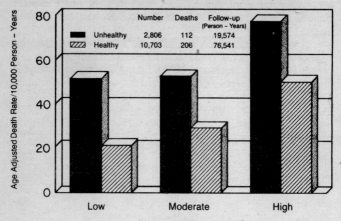

TC AND ALL CAUSE MORTALITY, MEN

	Number	Deaths	Follow-up (Person – Years)
Unhealthy	2,806	112	19,574
Healthy	10,703	206	76,541

feeling is that regardless of age, in men, any level of cholesterol above 213 mg/dl is in the MODERATE risk category. If such a level had been used, I predict that a significant difference in age-adjusted death rate for the unhealthy would have been seen in all three groups.

What about the healthy? As the level of cholesterol increased, a direct linear increase in age-adjusted death rate was seen. This is another large longitudinal study showing a direct correlation between total cholesterol and age-adjusted death rate from all causes. Again, this adds a sense of urgency to the need to lower cholesterol if it is elevated.

Now, let's look at total cholesterol levels and death from cardiovascular disease (heart attacks and strokes). The results can be seen in the chart on page 45.

Studying this chart reveals very little difference in the age-adjusted death rate in all three of the unhealthy groups, but a highly significant difference in the healthy. Again, the lack of a difference in the unhealthy may be due to the cholesterol risk groupings, but notice the marked increase in risk in the healthy. There is almost a five-fold difference between the LOW and HIGH risk groups. In the HIGH risk group, there is very little difference between the healthy and unhealthy. Certainly, this

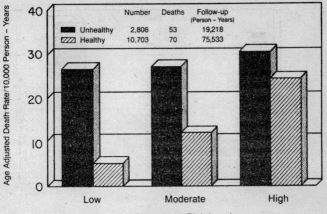

TC AND CVD MORTALITY, MEN

	Number	Deaths	Follow-up (Person – Years)
Unhealthy	2,806	53	19,218
Healthy	10,703	70	75,533

Age Adjusted Death Rate/10,000 Person – Years

Cholesterol Risk Levels

should provide adequate motivation for at least healthy men to want to lower their cholesterol.

But what about women? In the Aerobics Center Longitudinal Study, there were not enough unhealthy women to divide them into healthy and unhealthy groups. Yet, if you use the same cholesterol risk groupings established by the NIH Consensus Conference, there is no question about the relationship between total cholesterol and all cause mortality (see chart on page 46).

In this chart, it is obvious that a healthy woman in the high cholesterol group has an age-adjusted death rate over 3 times higher than a woman in the low cholesterol group.

Why should there be this accelerated risk in both men and women as cholesterol goes up?

According to Dr. Scott M. Grundy, Director of the Center for Human Nutrition at the University of Texas Health Science Center at Dallas and one of the world's foremost authorities on cholesterol, there may be a critical phase in the process of vessel-clogging. This point may be reached when about 60 percent of the surface of your coronary arteries is covered with plaque from the LDL cholesterol and its "partner" Apo B. At that level of blockage in your arteries, you may begin to experience a substantially increased risk of coronary heart disease.

For example, the increased narrowing of the blood vessels

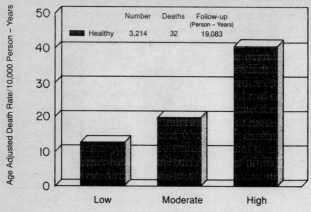

TC AND ALL CAUSE MORTALITY, WOMEN

	Number	Deaths	Follow-up (Person – Years)
Healthy	3,214	32	19,083

Cholesterol Risk Levels

at those high levels of blockage may make it more likely that a blood clot or other obstruction will result in a complete stoppage of blood flow. This would cause a heart attack, death of heart tissue, and perhaps death of the individual.

So it's certainly advisable not to allow your cholesterol to rise above the 200–220 range. Findings by another long-term study, the Multiple Risk Factor Intervention Trial (MRFIT), also suggest that it may indeed be a good idea to get your cholesterol *below* 200.

The MRFIT Study measured cholesterol levels of approximately 360,000 men, from ages 35 to 57. The initial tests were conducted between 1973 and 1975 in eighteen cities in the United States. The participants were followed for six years, and researchers recorded deaths in the group from coronary disease. Among other things, this study showed the risk of heart disease definitely was lower for people with cholesterol levels below 200 mg/dl.

So what's your optimum level of cholesterol?

My recommendation: *The best level for the average adult for total cholesterol should be in the range of 180 to 190 mg/dl.* As a matter of fact, if our entire American population could get its cholesterol into this range or even lower, our rate of coronary heart disease probably would be reduced by 30 to 50 percent!

To put this in different terms, if you reduce the total cholesterol in your blood by a certain percentage, you can expect to reduce your risk of heart disease by a much greater percentage. Specifically, as a rough rule of thumb, each 1 percent reduction in blood cholesterol level is associated with a 2 percent reduction in the risk of heart attack and sudden death. That's the conclusion of a major longitudinal study, the Lipid Research Clinics Coronary Primary Prevention Trial (LRC-CPPT). This study involved 3,806 middle-aged men with high cholesterol levels who were recruited at twelve clinics around the country. The participants were given the drug cholestyramine (Questran) to reduce their cholesterol levels, which were 265 mg/dl or above. But the researchers say the results also support the idea of lowering cholesterol by diet.

What the Studies Say About Balancing Your Total Cholesterol and HDL Cholesterol Levels

As I've already indicated, watching your total cholesterol level is only one message from the major longitudinal studies. It's also important to strike a healthy balance between your total cholesterol and HDL cholesterol, according to the federally funded Framingham Heart Study. To this end, it's essential to keep your LDL cholesterol down and to raise your HDL cholesterol as much as possible.

You'll recall from chapter 3 that HDL cholesterol is associated with a lower risk of heart disease. In fact, as we saw in that chapter, the HDLs may actually be involved as "heroes" in helping to remove excess cholesterol from arterial walls.

Dr. William P. Castelli, director of the Framingham Study, acknowledges first that "cholesterol seems to be the keystone" in causing coronary heart disease. In addition, he believes that it's important to pay close attention to the *ratio* of the total cholesterol to the HDL cholesterol.

In the previously mentioned Aerobics Center Longitudinal Study (page 43), men and women were followed for up to 100,000 person years. A good correlation was shown between the total cholesterol and both all risk mortality and deaths only from cardiovascular disease. In addition, the relation between cholesterol/HDL ratios and all risk mortality in men was studied:

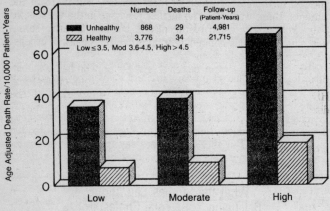

CHOL./HDL RATIO AND ALL CAUSE MORTALITY, MEN

Chol/HDL Risk Levels

In the unhealthy, the death rate was almost twice as great in the HIGH ratio group as it was in the LOW. In the healthy, the death rate, although considerably lower than in any of the unhealthy groups, was still over twice as great in the HIGH ratio group as it was in the LOW.

My recommendations, as we'll see later, are that men should keep the ratio of total cholesterol to HDL cholesterol below 4.6, and women should keep the ratio below 4.0. To illustrate, this means that a woman with a total cholesterol of 200 should have an HDL cholesterol count of 51 or more. If her HDL is 51, her ratio will be 200/51, or about 3.9.

A major study in the Netherlands, known as the Leiden Intervention Trial, has confirmed the importance of this total cholesterol/HDL cholesterol ratio. This investigation involved 39 patients who had at least one coronary artery that was 50 percent obstructed.

The researchers first measured the obstructions by taking pictures of the blood vessels with coronary arteriography. Then, the subjects in the study were put on a vegetarian diet for two years. During this period they consumed fewer than 100 mg. of cholesterol each day. Considering the fact that the average American takes in about 450 mg. per day, you can see that they were on a highly restricted diet.

At the end of the two-year period, 21 of the patients showed further progression of their disease. But in 18 of the patients, there was either no further blockage in the vessels, *or* there was a regression of the plaque buildup. Clearly, something important was happening to improve the health of at least 18 patients—but what was it?

The most important factor among those who had a stabilization or regression of the disease was their total cholesterol/HDL cholesterol ratio. Specifically, the progression of the disease—that is, the worsening of the hardening of the arteries—occurred in patients who had total cholesterol/HDL ratios of more than 6.9. Those who had ratios of *less than* 6.9 showed no further progression of their vessel blockage.

What is the main message of this study? As far as I'm concerned, your total cholesterol/HDL cholesterol ratio should be reduced as much as possible. That means first raising your HDL level through the methods we'll outline later in this book. Also, it means lowering your total cholesterol levels, and especially your LDL cholesterol, through diet or, if necessary, through drugs.

What the Studies Say About Drugs and Your Cholesterol Balance

Drugs are another very important topic addressed by the major longitudinal studies. In particular, the Lipid Research Clinics Coronary Primary Prevention Trial (LRC-CPPT) study has demonstrated that drugs can help put your cholesterol in better balance.

The researchers in this investigation screened more than 480,000 men, ranging from 39 to 59 years of age. Of these, 3,806, who were an average age of 47.8 years, were finally selected for the study. One-half of these men were placed on the drug cholestyramine; the other half took a placebo, a substance having no active healing or curative agent (such as a sugar pill). Neither the patients nor the medical investigators knew which participants were taking the real medication and which were taking the placebo. Finally, members of both groups were also placed on a moderate cholesterol-lowering diet and then were put randomly into one of the two groups.

Because cholestyramine has certain unpleasant side effects

such as constipation, nausea, or bloating, the men who were chosen to take it didn't always comply by taking the full daily dose. Even so, after an average 7.4 years of follow-up on the study, the group that was being treated with the drug developed 19 percent less coronary heart disease than did the untreated group.

In this study, greater lowering of cholesterol by drugs was the decisive factor in the treated group's greater reduction in coronary heart disease. In the drug-treated group, the cholestyramine lowered cholesterol levels by an average of 13.4 percent. In contrast, the nondrug group—which was only on a moderate cholesterol-lowering diet—showed a more modest 4.9 percent decrease in their total cholesterol levels.

Also, note this: There was an 8.5 percent difference in total cholesterol levels between the two groups. Yet, there was a much *larger*—19 percent—reduction in heart disease among those who were being treated with the drug! In other words, if you lower your cholesterol by a certain percentage, the chances are that your risk of getting coronary heart disease will drop by an even greater percentage.

What the Studies Say About Changing Diet and Lifestyle

Although drug therapy may be necessary at times, the longitudinal studies give us an alternative: A change in diet and lifestyle can also balance your cholesterol—sometimes even more dramatically than drugs.

In a study begun in Oslo, Norway, in 1973, researchers followed more than 1,200 men, from ages 40 to 49, for more than five years. They were selected for the study because they had cholesterol levels between 290 and 380 mg/dl, and they were smoking at least one pack of cigarettes per day.

One-half of these men made no changes in diet or lifestyle. The other half were placed in an experimental program designed to help them reduce the cholesterol and saturated fat in their diets and break their cigarette habits. During the course of the study, 25 percent of the men managed to quit smoking; another 45 percent decreased to some extent the number of cigarettes they smoked each day.

The final result? The total cholesterol levels of those in the experimental low-fat, nonsmoking group decreased by 13 percent. Furthermore, after the five-year program had been completed, the subjects who were on the diet-and-lifestyle program were healthier. They showed a 47 percent lower rate of heart attacks and sudden death than those who had made no changes in their lifestyles!

It's likely there were two primary reasons for this: (1) the low-cholesterol diet probably helped lower the "bad" LDLs in their blood, along with the total cholesterol levels; (2) the reduced smoking may have allowed their protective HDLs to increase.

You'll note, by the way, that the 47 percent decrease in coronary heart disease in this Oslo study exceeds by far the 19 percent reduction achieved through drugs in the LRC-CPPT study. Certainly, it was quite important that one-quarter of the Oslo men stopped smoking. But, in addition, the low-cholesterol, low-fat diets had to contribute to the treated group's greater decline in heart disease.

What the Studies Urge You to Do—Right Now!

Finally, the longitudinal studies suggest that heart attacks tend to decrease when people take two important steps:

Step 1. They seek better medical care.

Step 2. They learn as much as they can about how to prevent atherosclerosis—and then they *apply* what they've learned.

These two conclusions match up quite well with developments and trends in the nation at large. By most evaluations, there has been a sustained decrease of at least 28 percent in heart attacks in this country since 1968. Most experts cite at least four major reasons for this:

• *Eating habits—especially with regard to cholesterol—have improved.* By 1980, many Americans had changed their eating habits for reasons of health, with a much lower consumption of fat and high-cholesterol foods. As a result, the average cholesterol level dropped for both men and women. Data from the National Health and Nutrition Examination Surveys, 1960 to 1980, revealed that in men, age-adjusted average blood cholesterol levels decreased from 217 mg/dl to 211 mg/dl. In women, total cholesterol levels went down from 223 mg/dl to 215 mg/dl. Both declines were statistically significant.*

• *High blood pressure (hypertension) has declined.* In the late 1960s, only 10 to 15 percent of hypertension in this country was detected, treated, and effectively controlled. But by 1984, more than 50 percent of high blood pressure patients were receiving adequate treatment.

• *Cigarette smoking is down among American men.* In 1964, more than 50 percent of the American male population smoked cigarettes. Currently, that figure is less than one-third of American men.

• *More people exercise.* In the early 1960s, 24 percent of adult Americans exercised regularly. According to a Gallup poll, by 1984 that number had increased to 59 percent.

What does all this mean to you?

There are at least two conclusions I would draw: First, it seems clear that you should do everything possible to quit smoking and to treat hypertension. Second, you should embark immediately on a program to change your eating habits and lifestyle to conform with practices that will put your cholesterol into better balance.

How to Determine
Your Probable Coronary Risk

As a basic guide to show you if your cholesterol is in proper balance, we've formulated a chart showing your probable coronary risk when the various components of your cholesterol and other blood fats are at certain levels. This chart is based on our best understanding of the many longitudinal studies on cholesterol and heart disease, and also on our ongoing work at the Aerobics Institute in Dallas.

---

*National Center for Health Statistics—National Heart, Lung and Blood Institute Collaborative Lipid Group. "Trends in Serum Cholesterol Levels Among U.S. Adults Aged 20 to 74 Years." *Journal of the American Medical Association,* February 20, 1987, pp. 937–42.

The Cardiovascular Disease Risk Chart for Cholesterol and Lipid Levels

Lipids	Age (yrs)	Excellent Protection 25th percentile (no changes necessary)		Moderate Risk 50th percentile (refer to book for diet and exercise program)		High Risk 75th percentile (consult physician for diet and/or drug therapy)		Very High Risk 90th percentile (seek immediate medical attention)	
		M	F	M	F	M	F*	M	F
Total Cholesterol mg/dl	20-39	162-179	157-176	180-202	177-197	203-225	198-220	>225	>220
	40-59	186-209	186-209	210-233	210-235	234-257	236-259	>257	>259
	60+	189-213	205-227	214-240	228-252	241-262	253-276	>262	>276
LDL Cholesterol mg/dl	20-39	100-117	90-108	118-137	109-127	138-159	128-149	>159	>149
	40-59	119-140	110-128	141-162	129-155	163-183	156-181	>183	>181
	60+	122-143	126-149	144-165	150-175	166-190	176-198	>190	>198
HDL Cholesterol mg/dl	20-39	>51	>63	51-37	63-45	<37	<45*	------	------
	40-59	>52	>69	52-37	69-49	<37	<49	------	------
	60+	>60	>74	60-40	74-50	<40	<50	------	------
Triglycerides mg/dl	20-39	71-93	58-77	94-133	78-106	[134-195	107-146]**	>195	>146
	40-59	89-121	73-98	122-170	99-140	171-231	141-190	>231	>190
	60+	83-110	82-110	111-154	111-146	155-206]	147-206]	>206	>206
Total Cholesterol/ HDL ratio	20-39	2.3-3.6	1.9-2.8	3.7-5.1	2.9-3.6	5.2-6.1	3.7-4.2	>6.1	>4.2
	40-59	2.6-4.2	2.0-3.0	4.3-6.0	3.1-4.0	6.1-7.4	4.1-4.9	>7.4	>4.9
	60+	2.5-4.0	2.0-3.2	4.1-6.0	3.3-4.8	6.1-6.9	4.9-5.5	>6.9	>5.5

M = Male
F = Female

> = "more than"
< = "less than"

*Due to the lack of data, one may question whether HDL cholesterol levels in women in this range truly mean High Risk. However, at this time, this is the best estimate of risk.

**Triglycerides at this level do not warrant drug therapy. Consult your physician/nutritionist for dietary, weight loss, or exercise therapy.

FIVE

The Concern About
Total Cholesterol

As we discussed in the preceding chapter, your total cholesterol count is important for a number of reasons. To name a few, an elevated total cholesterol level may signal that:

• Your low-density lipoproteins, or LDLs, are too high.

• The ratio of your total cholesterol to HDL cholesterol is too high.

• Your apolipoprotein Bs, or "Apo Bs"—those villainous partners of the LDLs which stick to the blood vessel walls—are too prevalent in your bloodstream.

A growing number of researchers feel that the Apo Bs may be the best indicators of all to determine whether a person has or is prone to develop cardiovascular disease. Unfortunately, at the present time we don't have the methods to test the blood of the average patient for the presence of Apo B. These measurements are now being done only as part of special research projects. But the day is fast drawing near when the Apo B level in the blood will become a regular part of every lab test. In fact, this "villainous" component may very well turn out to be the most important part of every cholesterol test!

Apart from these considerations, the total cholesterol level may somehow operate as an *independent* risk factor. In other words, a high total cholesterol—quite separate from LDLs, HDL ratios, or any other components—can indicate the likelihood that you'll develop atherosclerosis.

The Cardiovascular Disease Risk Chart for Cholesterol and Lipid Levels

Lipids	Age (yrs)	Excellent Protection 25th percentile (no changes necessary)		Moderate Risk 50th percentile (refer to book for diet and exercise program)		High Risk 75th percentile (consult physician for diet and/or drug therapy)		Very High Risk 90th percentile (seek immediate medical attention)	
		M	F	M	F	M	F	M	F
Total Cholesterol mg/dl	20–39	162–179	157–176	180–202	177–197	203–225	198–220	>225	>220
	40–59	186–209	186–209	210–233	210–235	234–257	236–259	>257	>259
	60 +	189–213	205–227	214–240	228–252	241–262	253–276	>262	>276
LDL Cholesterol mg/dl	20–39	100–117	90–108	118–137	109–127	138–159	128–149	>159	>149
	40–59	119–140	110–128	141–162	129–155	163–183	156–181	>183	>181
	60 +	122–143	126–149	144–165	150–175	166–190	176–198	>190	>198

M = Male
F = Female

> = "more than"
< = "less than"

To provide a reference point for the following discussion, let's take another look at a relevant part of the risk chart from chapter 4 (see page 53). As you can see, this portion of the chart deals with total cholesterol and LDL cholesterol, the two key risk factors we're concerned with in this chapter.

A Classic Example of Total Cholesterol As a Risk Factor

Total cholesterol was the only signal of the cardiovascular problems that faced 52-year-old James Fixx, the best-selling author on exercise and running. As you may recall, he died in 1984 while jogging on a country road in Vermont. Jim's case, which I discussed in detail in my book *Running Without Fear*, has a number of interesting ramifications. But for our present purposes, the most important points relate to his total cholesterol readings.

According to the autopsy, which was performed immediately after his death, Jim Fixx's total cholesterol was 254—a count which would have placed him well up into the "high risk" category which we've established in this book. Actually, Jim's cholesterol count had almost reached the "critical risk" category, which begins at 258 mg/dl for a person of his age.

The other cholesterol and fatty components in Jim Fixx's blood provided hardly a clue to the deadly work that was being done in his body. For example, his LDL count at the time of his death was 156, a figure which placed him in our "average risk" category. Furthermore, there was no problem at all with his HDLs: they were recorded as 73 mg/dl at the time of his death—a level which put him in our "excellent protection" category. Finally, his total cholesterol/HDL cholesterol ratio was 3.48. This was also an extremely good rating, well below the 4.6 ratio level which we generally regard as the maximum that a healthy man should have.

As you can see, Jim Fixx's blood seemed to be in extremely good shape—*except* for his total cholesterol. Fixx's case and similar ones that we encounter in our clinical examinations flash a definite warning signal. So be wary if your total cholesterol is in the "high risk" category or above for your age, even if all the other components of your cholesterol and blood fats seem to be all right. There just may be something indepen-

dent of all the other factors which can cause your total cholesterol level to operate against you. You should immediately see
a physician who is knowledgeable about this subject and, under
his or her direction, embark on changes in your diet and
lifestyle, such as those described later in this book. Your doctor
may also conclude that drugs are required.

Another very important danger which is often directly
connected with high total cholesterol is a high reading of low-
density lipoprotein, or LDL. In most cases, high total cholesterol and high LDLs go hand-in-hand. And LDLs, as we already
know, are a major culprit in the development of clogging of the
arteries and cardiovascular disease.

One person who confronted great danger because of high
LDLs and a high total cholesterol count was a good friend of
mine in Dallas, Jay Streetman. I began to see Jay in 1972, when
he was 41 years of age, and I was quite impressed with his
level of physical fitness. He did extremely well on his first
treadmill stress test, which measures a person's cardiovascular
fitness by providing an electrocardiogram under exercise conditions. Specifically, he walked for 24 minutes and 30 seconds, a
performance that placed him in the top, or "superior," category
of fitness for his age group according to our standards at the
Aerobics Center.

Jay's total cholesterol level at that time was 263 mg/dl, a
figure which was certainly too high. And I must say, that gave
me some concern. But in those days, as I've indicated previously, we didn't worry too much about a total cholesterol
level in that range. In general, readings in the mid-200s were
considered acceptable.

Unfortunately, we didn't have access to the longitudinal
studies and other recent research which have since indicated
that a cholesterol count of 263 at age 41 would have placed Jay
in the very high risk category although in every other way Jay
was in excellent condition. For several years, his body fat
remained at low, athletic levels, between 10 and 11 percent.
Also, he managed to keep his weight quite consistent—generally
between 133 and 137 pounds. To top it all off, he continued to
improve his walking time on the treadmill. He reached 27
minutes by 1975. Then, ten years later, in 1985, he established
a new personal record of 28 minutes and 31 seconds.

When research revealed that the total cholesterol/HDL
cholesterol ratio could be an important indicator of cardiovascu-

lar disease, we began computing those ratios on Jay. Once again, he seemed the picture of perfect health. Beginning in 1979, his ratios ranged from a high of 4.6 to a low of 3.8. In fact, he had only one HDL ratio which was as high as 4.6. All the others were well below 4.6, a fact which placed him in a relatively low coronary risk category.

As you might expect with such excellent ratios, Jay's HDLs were high: They ranged consistently in the middle-50s during this period of observation, and this level should have given him "excellent protection" in terms of his coronary risk.

Let me digress for a moment on this HDL issue. There has been speculation that if your HDL level and especially your total cholesterol/HDL ratio is in a safe range, it makes little difference how high your total cholesterol is. The rationale behind this view is that the body needs only enough HDLs to clean out the "bad" LDLs and their Apo B partners. According to this understanding, as long as there are sufficient HDLs in relation to LDLs, the person will automatically be protected from the buildup of plaque, which is the key characteristic of atherosclerosis.

But Jay's experience, as well as a number of similar cases, is strong evidence that this view may not be correct. When Jay came in for his regular medical examination in August 1985, his HDLs and ratio were completely normal. Also, he established an all-time personal record on the treadmill at 28 minutes and 31 seconds. But now, for the first time in his medical history, his treadmill stress test, which indicated the condition of his heart and coronary arteries, was clearly abnormal.

Because he was in such good shape otherwise, I thought that this abnormality might be what we call a "false positive." In other words, even though the stress test was abnormal, there was no significant coronary artery disease. Also, Jay's resting electrocardiogram had continued to be perfectly normal. So I felt strongly that there might be something wrong with the way we had conducted the stress test.

Still, I wanted to be sure. So I encouraged him to concentrate on eating a low-fat diet, to continue with his exercise program, and to come back to see me again in four months. Not only did Jay work at his diet, he even intensified his exercise. When he returned to see me in December 1985, his treadmill stress test performance increased once again to another all-time personal record of 29 minutes. Many young professional athletes I've examined don't perform this well—and at the time, Jay was 54 years old! His performance on the treadmill placed him far up into the "superior" category of cardiovascular fitness, even for men approximately half his age.

Unfortunately, Jay's stress electrocardiogram didn't improve. If anything, the results during exercise were even more abnormal.

Now I realized something was seriously wrong. I immediately referred Jay to a cardiologist for a coronary arteriogram. This procedure involves the arterial injection of a radio-opaque dye. In this way, X-ray pictures can be taken of the heart and the coronary arteries which supply blood to the heart. And Jay's test revealed some big trouble.

Sometime prior to his first abnormal stress test in August 1985, Jay had apparently suffered a major silent heart attack. There had been no symptoms—no chest pains, fatigue, or other discomfort indicating that anything was wrong. Yet, at some point during that interval, his right main coronary artery had become completely obstructed. Not only that, the blockage had seriously damaged about one-third of his heart! In addition, several of the other vessels supplying blood to his heart were significantly blocked. Obviously, Jay was in serious danger.

Despite his problems, Jay was fortunate for a number of reasons. First, he had been faithful in coming in for his annual stress test. Two of these tests finally had revealed the fact that he had developed significant obstructive coronary artery disease. As you'll recall, all of his resting EKGs were quite normal, and if we had relied only on them, his coronary problem would never have been diagnosed.

Also, his extensive exercise program had helped him develop an excellent "collateral" circulation. In other words, by running several miles a day for many years, the smaller vessels supplying blood to his heart had grown larger and stronger. Then, when the heart attack occurred, these smaller vessels "stepped in" to save him. The blood which could no longer get to the heart through the blocked coronary artery was diverted through some of the secondary, collateral channels. He had survived a major heart attack without even being aware that he had suffered one! This was a classic case of what doctors call a "silent infarction."

In fact, Jay's blood flow to his heart was so good that he didn't need immediate bypass surgery. He was advised to start in a cardiac rehabilitation program, utilize protective drugs, and continue to restrict his diet. He was told that if he responded well, he could probably avoid surgery—and that's exactly what has happened. Now, almost two years later, Jay continues to be very active physically, is completely without symptoms, and has no further cardiac problems.

Jay, then, is an excellent example of the principle that *you must seek regular evaluations and monitor your total cholesterol* if you want to keep your body in a healthy state of balance. His total cholesterol consistently ranged from the mid-250s to the mid-260s during those early years. As the cardiovascular disease chart shows, these levels usually placed him in the "very high risk" category. In fact, he never dropped below the "high risk" category. Not only that, his LDLs also ranged up consistently into the "high risk" category for his age. Typically, the LDLs were in the neighborhood of 160 to 175 mg/dl.

At the present time, in addition to his diet and exercise program, Jay is on a treatment program that involves the drug Questran, which has lowered his total and LDL cholesterol levels. Also, he's taking what is called a "beta-blocker"— Tenormin—a drug which may protect him from potentially severe heart rhythm irregularities.

As a result, his total cholesterol levels are gradually moving down to a safer range. Also, he's been able to maintain an active and safe exercise program. Most important, his risk of developing more serious cardiovascular disease because of an imbalance in his blood lipids has decreased significantly.

Although Jay's is a success story, his experience should serve as a warning to all of us. The main message is this: You must not become complacent just because you have no symptoms, because you're in superior physical condition, or because a few of your cholesterol risk factors are in the low-risk ranges. Instead, you must look at *all* of the lipid risk categories listed on the Cardiovascular Disease Risk Chart (see p. 53) and be certain that all of them are in proper balance.

How exactly do you treat a condition that involves elevated total cholesterol or elevated LDLs? Jay's case has given us a few important pointers, and we'll consider others in greater detail in part 3 of this book, How to Control Your Cholesterol. For now, let me just summarize the basic approaches to treatment for high total cholesterol or high LDLs:

• Go on a cholesterol-lowering diet, such as those described in chapter 9.

• Reduce your percentage of body fat, in line with the standards outlined in chapter 16. The more obese you are (i.e., the higher your level of body fat), the more likely it is that your total cholesterol, as well as your LDL cholesterol, will be too high.

• If necessary, use cholesterol-lowering drugs, niacin, or other supplements—but only under your doctor's supervision.

We'll discuss each of these approaches to treatment in part 3 of the book. For the moment, however, we're still focusing on why your cholesterol must be completely in balance. So now let's turn to our next important topic—the very important cholesterol ratio.

SIX

Be Aware
of Your Ratio!

Assume you're sitting in on a conversation in a doctor's office about the results of a thorough blood examination. The first question many patients ask in such a situation is, "What's my cholesterol level?"

If the doctor responds that the level is in the low 200s or below—and if the patient knows just a little bit about cholesterol—you'll probably hear a big sigh of relief.

But this sense of well-being may be a bit premature—especially if any of the *components* of the person's cholesterol are out of balance. In fact, 40 percent of patients with coronary artery disease have normal total cholesterol levels, says Dr. Gerald Berenson, Director of the Bogalusa Heart Study and head of Louisiana State University's Specialized Center of Research on Atherosclerosis.

Even with a "safe" level of total cholesterol, there are still several ways that your risk of coronary artery disease may be too high. One major set of problems may involve some of the possible "heroes" in your cholesterol scenario—namely, the high-density lipoproteins, or HDLs.

There are two factors we need to consider in evaluating the role of the HDLs: First, the level of HDLs in your blood is an important factor all by itself. If the HDL level is unusually low, your risk of cardiovascular disease may increase dramatically. On the other hand, if your HDLs are relatively high, you can expect to have some degree of protection against atherosclerosis.

Second, the HDLs are important as they relate to the total cholesterol levels. Specifically, it's important for the *ratio* of your total cholesterol to your HDL cholesterol to be *below* certain levels. The higher your ratio is, the greater your risk of having a cardiovascular problem. In short, as far as your ratio is concerned, the lower, the better!

For example, in men, it's important to keep this ratio below 4.6. So, suppose you are a man and your total cholesterol count is 200 mg/dl—not a bad level according to many longitudinal studies. But if your HDLs are 40 mg/dl, that means your ratio will be 200/40 or 5.0—a figure that's perhaps a little too high to give you adequate protection against cardiovascular disease. To drop your rate, you'll have to take steps to lower your total cholesterol, raise the HDL level, or rely on a combination of both.

Paying attention to your ratio becomes even more important if you already have been diagnosed as having coronary artery disease. As I have already mentioned, in the Leiden Intervention Trial conducted in the Netherlands, a study of 39 patients with stable angina which was reported in the *New England Journal of Medicine,* March 28, 1985, each patient had at least one coronary artery that was more than 50 percent obstructed. All were placed on a strict vegetarian diet, with fewer than 100 mg. of cholesterol per day, and then they were followed for two years.

During that time, their body weight decreased, their cholesterol dropped, and their total cholesterol/HDL ratios all decreased. Twenty-four months later, the researchers once again examined all 39 patients, using computer-assisted coronary angiography.

In 21 of the 39 patients, there was progression of the disease, whereas in 18 of the patients, lesions associated with the disease failed to grow. Furthermore, changes in the coronary lesions didn't correlate with changes in blood pressure, smoking habits, alcohol intake, weight loss, or drug therapy. But there *was* a correlation between coronary artery disease and the ratio.

Specifically, disease progression occurred in those patients who had cholesterol/HDL ratios above 6.9 throughout the twenty-four months. Also, the researchers observed no coronary lesion growth in patients who had a cholesterol/HDL ratio less than 6.9. Likewise, there was no progression of disease in those who initially had values above 6.9, but then were able to significantly lower them by dietary intervention.

The moral to this story is that *if you already have been diagnosed as having coronary artery disease, you must resort to whatever means are necessary to lower your cholesterol/HDL ratio to less than 6.9.* One way this can be accomplished is by increasing your HDL cholesterol level, and an excellent approach, as we'll see in chapter 12, is through exercise. But first, it's important to understand a little more about HDLs and also about the ratio.

As we've seen earlier, the exact way that the HDLs work in your blood is not clear. They may act independently as a kind of "hero" or "garbage-removal agent," which cleans the excess, plaque-forming LDLs and Apo Bs out of the blood. Somehow, according to this view, the HDLs may take the LDLs and Apo Bs back to the liver for final disposal before they can do any damage to the blood vessels.

On the other hand, a second theory says the HDLs may not be particularly active at all. Their presence may simply *signal* the fact that the LDLs and other fatty remnants in the blood are being cleaned out through some other means.

Whatever their particular role, the HDLs and the total cholesterol/ HDL cholesterol ratio are very important indicators of your risk of cardiovascular disease. To help us in this discussion, here is that portion of the Cardiovascular Disease Risk Chart showing the risk ranges for these two lipid factors.

Now let's consider this HDL issue with a practical example:

A patient whom I will call Mike came to our clinic in 1979, when he was 47 years of age. For his age, he seemed in relatively good physical condition. His 213-pound frame consisted of 18.24 percent body fat—a level which we regard as well within normal limits, particularly considering his weight. His total cholesterol level wasn't bad either—192 mg/dl. We checked him out with both a resting and a stress electrocardiogram, and they came out normal.

But then, potential problems began to emerge as we focused on his laboratory results. His HDL level was 30 and his total cholesterol/HDL cholesterol ratio was 6.4—both figures which were in the "high risk" categories.

Even though Mike felt fine and had no signs or symptoms of heart disease, he was still worried because there was a strong history of heart disease in his family. His father had

The Cardiovascular Disease Risk Chart for Cholesterol and Lipid Levels

Lipids	Age (yrs)	Excellent Protection 25th percentile (no changes necessary)		Moderate Risk 50th percentile (refer to book for diet and exercise program)		High Risk 75th percentile (consult physician for diet and/or drug therapy)		Very High Risk 90th percentile (seek immediate medical attention)	
		M	F	M	F	M	F*	M	F
HDL Cholesterol mg/dl	20–39	>51	>63	51–37	63–45	<37	<45*	------	
	40–59	>52	>69	52–37	69–49	<37	<49	------	
	60+	>60	>74	60–40	74–50	<40	<50	------	
Total Cholesterol/ HDL ratio	20–39	2.3–3.6	1.9–2.8	3.7–5.1	2.9–3.6	5.2–6.1	3.7–4.2	>6.1	>4.2
	40–59	2.6–4.2	2.0–3.0	4.3–6.0	3.1–4.0	6.1–7.4	4.1–4.9	>7.4	>4.9
	60+	2.5–4.0	2.0–3.2	4.1–6.0	3.3–4.8	6.1–6.9	4.9–5.5	>6.9	>5.5

M = Male
F = Female

> = "more than"
< = "less than"

*Due to the lack of data, one may question whether HDL cholesterol levels in women in this range truly mean High Risk. However, at this time, this is the best estimate of risk.

suffered his first heart attack at age 53 and had died at age 56, following a second heart attack.

In light of his family background, I agreed with Mike that we should take some precautionary measures. Also, caution seemed appropriate in view of his below-normal HDL level and the elevated ratio. So I put him on a special diet and increased his exercise in an effort to get his cholesterol in better balance. Also, I suggested that the use of certain drugs might help him.

In many ways, Mike was the "perfect" patient, in that he adhered exactly to the program I prescribed for him—with one exception: he preferred not to try any drugs to control his cholesterol. In fact, when he returned one year later, his weight had dropped 15 pounds, and his body fat was down to 15 percent. But his cholesterol situation was getting worse. His total cholesterol went up from 192 to 213, and his HDL cholesterol went down to 28, to give him a ratio of 7.6.

Still, he wasn't displaying any symptoms of cardiovascular disease, and his resting and exercise electrocardiograms continued to be normal. So, despite our advice, he still resisted using drugs at this point. Instead, he restricted his low-fat, low-cholesterol diet even more.

When Mike returned a year later, at age 49, he had managed to maintain his weight, and his total cholesterol had dropped back to a more acceptable 197 mg/dl. Also, his HDL cholesterol level had come up slightly to 32 mg/dl, to give him a better ratio of 6.2—although this ratio was still higher than we wanted. Overall, Mike's exercise program was putting him in even better physical condition. He now tested in the superior category on the treadmill stress test, for his age group, with a personal record time of 24 minutes.

At this point, we were beginning to think that Mike might be one of those people with genetically low HDLs, which don't respond to a lifestyle-changing program. Normally, if a person is on a regular aerobic exercise program, such activity tends to elevate the HDL levels. In fact, exercise is probably the most effective thing available to elevate the HDL cholesterol levels. But despite Mike's exercise regimen and his obvious improvement in conditioning—as evidenced by his outstanding performance on the treadmill stress test—his HDL cholesterol level remained relatively low.

Unfortunately, the advice we had given him about the need for drugs turned out to be correct. Mike suffered a major heart attack just a few months after his third physical exam. At the time, he was only 50 years of age. About a month later, he underwent a coronary arteriogram. The pictures which were taken of his heart and coronary arteries showed that one coronary artery was completely obstructed, and two others were 30 to 40 percent obstructed.

When Mike returned to the clinic a couple of months after his heart attack, we started him on a slowly progressive cardiac rehabilitation program. As a result, his weight dropped even lower, to 192 pounds. In addition, this time he was placed on the lipid-lowering drug Lopid. Soon his total cholesterol level had dropped to 156 mg/dl. But unfortunately, his HDLs went down as well, to 23 mg/dl. This gave him a ratio of 6.78, again a figure which continued to trouble us. So, he became even more aggressive with his diet and lifestyle program.

When Mike was tested eight months later, at age 51, he had responded well. His weight had gone down even further, to 186 pounds, and his body fat was now at 12 percent. Even a well-conditioned athlete would have been pleased with these results. But his total cholesterol level was again up to 198 mg/dl, and with an HDL level of 27, his ratio was 7.3.

Soon after this, I took him off Lopid and placed him on a combination of the cholesterol-lowering drug colestipol hydrochloride (Colestid) and niacin. This change seemed to help. His total cholesterol dropped to 147 mg/dl, and with an HDL level of 25, his ratio was 5.9.

Mike's HDL levels are still much lower than I would like, and his total cholesterol/HDL cholesterol ratio is too high. But at least he's showing some progress in getting his cholesterol in better balance. If he does eventually enjoy a long life, at least two things will have done a great deal to help him accomplish this goal: (1) his willingness to work closely with his physicians to correct a troublesome cholesterol problem; and (2) the availability of certain modern drugs. When the problem is one of genetics as indicated in Mike's case, drugs are nearly always required.

What other lessons can we learn from Mike's situation?

The National Institutes of Health, and also a number of the major longitudinal studies, indicate that a total cholesterol of less than 200 mg/dl should provide significant protection against cardiovascular disease. But Mike's experience demonstrates that it's also absolutely essential to look at all parts of the cholesterol picture—including the very important ratio.

It has been said that "heart attacks do not occur in people who have total cholesterol levels under 150 mg/dl." But let me give you an example which questions the accuracy of that statement. I had followed this man at our clinic for over five years. His cholesterol ranged from 140 to 185 mg/dl, and at the time of a massive heart attack at age 61, his total cholesterol was 147 mg/dl. Only a six-vessel bypass procedure saved his life.

When you look beyond the total cholesterol level, you begin to see this man's real problem. His HDLs had been extremely low, ranging from 20 to 22 mg/dl. As a result, his total cholesterol/HDL cholesterol ratio stayed above 7.0. In this executive's case, as with Mike, the most dangerous, life-threatening factor seemed to be the HDL level and the ratio, *not* the total cholesterol level.

Clearly, then, high-density lipoproteins play a major role in our arteriosclerosis/heart disease scenario. But even as we present these examples, I should add that there's still a great deal that we don't know about HDLs and the various proteins and lipids which are associated with them. Even now, research is under way on several fronts to expand our knowledge in these areas. It's important that you understand something about these efforts so that you can know what to expect in the future.

For example, research in recent years has shown that there may be better indicators of protection against cardiovascular disease in the blood than the level of the HDL cholesterol.

One line of investigation has focused on what's called the "subfractions" of the HDL, including a component labeled HDL-2. This component is rather difficult to measure, and at present evaluations are limited to research laboratories. Still, the HDL-2 has become one of the front-runners for the title of "hero" in preventing clogging of the arteries.

Studies have shown that HDL-2 levels are low in the presence of cardiovascular disease. Also, this subfraction tends to be significantly higher in the blood of women. Interestingly, HDL-2 is the component in HDL which increases significantly in the blood of runners and others involved in aerobic exercise.

The HDL-2 subfraction of the HDL seems to perform a special beneficial role that other subfractions don't perform. For example, another subfraction, HDL-3, may or may not be related to cardiovascular disease. And, interestingly, this HDL-3 subfraction shows no clear relationship to aerobic exercise. But the HDL-3 level tends to increase with the consumption of alcoholic beverages.

So what should we conclude about these subfractions of the HDL?

The jury is still out on this issue. But both Dr. Grundy and I feel that the total HDL cholesterol is probably a better predictor of cardiovascular disease and atherosclerosis than either of the HDL subfractions.

An even more promising risk indicator of cardiovascular disease may be apolipoprotein A-I, or Apo A-I. A number of studies, including one reported in the August 18, 1983, issue of the *New England Journal of Medicine,* have concluded that Apo A-I is "by itself . . . more useful than HDL cholesterol for identifying patients with coronary-artery disease."

How does Apo A-I work? It attaches itself to the HDL, much as the Apo B does with the LDL. But the Apo A-I is definitely a "hero," in contrast to the Apo B, which is one of our major "villains." The Apo B, you'll recall, contributes to the buildup of life-threatening plaque in our blood vessels. This Apo A-I, on the other hand, apparently takes used cholesterol out of the body's cells and blood. Then it wraps up the cholesterol and transports it back to the liver for final disposal. There's still considerable discussion over exactly how the Apo A-I works, and any final word on this topic must await further research.

In the meantime, wherever possible, the Apo A-I should be considered in any complete lab test. Unfortunately, equipment is not generally available to test for Apo A-I at this time. But it's quite likely that soon the average lab will be testing for Apo A-I just as it tests now for HDLs and other cholesterol components in the blood.

The measurement of the blood level of the enzyme HGM-CoA-Reductase is another promising field of research. Since the level of this enzyme is the best indicator of the amount of cholesterol being produced in the body, its measurement may be invaluable in controlling arteriosclerosis.

So stay tuned! In the next few years, the information on the apolipoproteins, the subfractions of HDL, and the enzyme HMG-CoA-Reductase will almost certainly increase dramatically, as will our ability to routinely test for their presence in our blood.

Now, before we get into the details of how to treat the out-of-balance cholesterol and other fats in your blood, there's one more major topic to consider: The question of triglycerides.

SEVEN

What Are Triglycerides— and Why Should You Worry About Them?

Triglycerides are not cholesterol—but they are one of the important fats found in our blood, and they often travel in close contact with various cholesterol packages. In addition, there is a growing body of thought that implicates triglycerides in the destructive process of atherosclerosis.

Here are some of the current connections that are being made with triglycerides, cholesterol, and cardiovascular disease:

• Some studies have shown an inverse correlation between the "good" HDL cholesterol and triglyceride levels in the blood. In other words, if HDL levels tend to be high, the triglyceride levels tend to be low. Conversely, if HDLs are low, the triglycerides tend to be high.

But this relationship isn't by any means inevitable: Sometimes, people with low triglycerides also have low HDLs. Also, certain studies have indicated that lowering triglycerides in a group of patients doesn't necessarily raise their HDL levels. Still, a number of experts believe that for many people—in fact, perhaps for most people—a concerted effort to lower triglycerides may in fact raise the "good" HDL cholesterol levels. But at this time, further studies are needed to prove or disprove this theory.

• When a person has high triglycerides, his or her LDLs tend to be *smaller* than normal. A number of researchers— including myself and Dr. Scott M. Grundy—feel that these small LDLs may pose greater danger than larger LDLs in causing atherosclerosis and plaque buildup in the blood vessels.

• High triglyceride levels tend to be associated with premature coronary heart disease in patients with special types of diseases. These include people with diabetes mellitus, severe hyperlipidemia (high lipid levels), and chronic kidney disease which requires hemodialysis for long periods of time.

• Women aged 38 to 60 with high triglyceride levels have a higher incidence of heart attacks, stroke, and other forms of fatalities than do women who have normal triglyceride values. This was the finding of a twelve-year longitudinal study in Gothenburg, Sweden.

Clearly, then, elevation of the triglycerides may pose a problem for you. But exactly what are they? Triglycerides are lipids or fatty molecules which are formed in the liver from the fats you eat or from the body's own synthesis of internal fat. The VLDL "ship" which we discussed in chapter 3 carries them from the liver and also from the intestines to the body's tissues for use as energy or for storage in fatty tissues. Another molecule, called a "chylomicron," is the main way the triglycerides are transported in the blood.

In general, triglycerides should be less than 100 to 120 mg/dl. For women, who may be at higher risk than men with high triglycerides, the levels should be even lower. To help you see clearly where you stand, here's a reproduction of the triglyceride chart which we presented with the other lipid risk factors in chapter 4.

Before we move more deeply into the subject, a preliminary word of caution is in order about the proper way to be tested for triglycerides. Before you are tested in a medical laboratory, you should engage in an overnight, twelve- to fourteen-hour fast, eating no foods at all and drinking only water. This way, the triglycerides in your blood will consist only of those that are part of the very low-density lipoproteins (VLDLs). This procedure will result in a much better picture of the precise level of triglycerides in your blood.

People whose triglyceride levels range between 250 and 500 mg/dl after such a fast face approximately twice the risk of cardiovascular disease as those with lower levels. When the triglycerides go up even higher, other health problems ensue. For example, triglyceride levels above 1,000 mg/dl will greatly increase a person's risk of getting pancreatitis. This is an

The Cardiovascular Disease Risk Chart for Cholesterol and Lipid Levels

Lipids	Age (yrs)	Excellent Protection 25th percentile (no changes necessary)		Moderate Risk 50th percentile (refer to book for diet and exercise program)		High Risk 75th percentile (consult physician/ nutritionist for dietary/exercise therapy)		Very High Risk 90th percentile (seek immediate medical attention)	
		M	F	M	F	M	F	M	F
Triglycerides	20–39	71–93	58–77	94–133	78–106	[134–195]*	107–146	>195	>146
mg/dl	40–59	89–121	73–98	122–170	99–140	171–231	141–190	>231	>190
	60 +	83–110	82–110	111–154	111–146	[155–206]	147–206	>206	>206

M = Male   > = "more than"
F = Female   < = "less than"

*Triglycerides at this level do not warrant drug therapy. Consult your physician/nutritionist for dietary, weight loss, or exercise therapy.

inflammation of the pancreas, which in its most acute forms may result in hemorrhaging and death.

I recall a 49-year-old patient at our clinic with triglycerides of 296 mg/dl. As you know, a count in the 250 to 500 mg/dl range may signal the possibility of low HDL cholesterol and other blood-fat abnormalities, which may be associated with atherosclerosis. Sure enough, as we tested him further, we discovered that his HDLs were low—only 32 mg/dl. This gave him a total cholesterol/HDL cholesterol ratio of 6.0, a figure much higher than we like to see in the average healthy male.

Yet, his total cholesterol levels weren't bad. In fact, they were hovering around 190 when we saw him. However, if we had been looking only at total cholesterol, we wouldn't have given his condition a second thought. But remember: *It's the overall balance that matters!* You have to look at *all* the lipid risk factors in order to get a complete picture of your atherosclerotic risk.

In this man's case, there was a problem with three lipid risk factors—triglycerides, total HDLs, and the ratio. But he had no symptoms of any sort of disease—that is, no pain or discomfort, and no abnormalities on his resting or stress electrocardiograms.

So I decided to treat him conservatively. I adjusted his diet so that it contained fewer cholesterol-laden foods, and I tried to limit his carbohydrates, which can drive up a person's triglycerides. Unfortunately, this approach didn't do the job. His triglycerides did drop, but his HDLs held steady. In other words, this man was one of those people whose HDL levels are not significantly affected by a lowering of triglycerides.

Without warning, he suffered a heart attack a couple of years later. A coronary arteriogram was done on him, and this indicated total occlusion of one of his coronary arteries. Also, two other vessels had fairly major obstructions.

For treatment I employed several drugs and dietary supplements to control his lipids, including Lopid, or gemfibrozil as it's known generically. At this time, his triglycerides were 450 mg/dl and his HDLs were 23 mg/dl. The gemfibrozil lowered his triglycerides to 146 and his HDLs went up slightly to 27. Finally, the triglycerides dropped to 119 and the HDLs crept up slightly to 28.

But this treatment wasn't good enough. I knew we needed to try something else. The combination of medications we finally settled on was Colestid, known generically as colestipol hydrochloride, and also nicotinic acid. With these two medications, his triglycerides stabilized at a fairly low level of 114—which places him in the "excellent protection" category for a man who is now in his mid-fifties. His HDLs have remained low—in the mid- to upper 20s. And his total cholesterol level is lower, so that the ratio of his total cholesterol/HDL cholesterol is now less than 6.0.

In this case, the treatment hasn't by any means been perfect. With a combination of therapies we have managed to reduce his triglycerides and also to improve his ratio. But his main problem is his heredity: With testing, I learned he has genetically low HDL levels, which seem completely resistant to any type of therapy. As a result, it will be necessary for him to continue to use medication and pay close attention to his diet, probably for the rest of his life. If he does, there is every reason to believe that he may have many years of an active, symptom-free life ahead.

But this case is the exception, not the rule. If you have a modest triglyceride elevation, check first with your physician. Then, consider these three steps, which should be effective in lowering this blood fat:

Step 1. Lose weight. High triglycerides tend to be associated with increases in body weight, particularly body fat.

Step 2. Reduce the carbohydrates in your diet. Excess consumption of carbohydrates such as those found in bread, potatoes, sugar, and fruits tends to elevate the triglycerides.

Step 3. Get started on an aerobic exercise program. Triglycerides respond quite well to good physical conditioning—and especially to endurance-type exercises, such as walking, jogging, cycling, and swimming. In effect, the energy-laden triglycerides in your blood get "burned up" as you participate in these exercises.

If none of these methods works, you may need to consult with your physician further and try some type of drug therapy designed to lower the triglycerides.

Up to this point, we've been dealing primarily with definitions of the various types and subtypes of blood lipids, their normal and abnormal levels, and the importance of their being in proper balance. We've already described ways you can lower your total cholesterol, lower your LDLs, raise your HDLs, lower your total cholesterol/HDL cholesterol ratio, and lower your triglycerides. But those were just introductory remarks. Now, let's move on to the main purpose of this book: how to control your cholesterol, including ways to lower your total cholesterol if it's elevated.

PART III

How to Control Your Cholesterol

EIGHT

Everything You Need to Know About Getting a Cholesterol Test

The first step in evaluating your cholesterol situation is to get a blood test. That's the only way to understand precisely how the various cholesterol and fat components in your blood are affecting you. It's a prerequisite to all your efforts in controlling your risk of cardiovascular disease.

I'm always being asked certain key questions about how to get a test and how to evaluate it. As a result, I've decided that the best way to deal with this topic is in a question-and-answer format, providing you with the best answers available from our current knowledge on the subject.

Q: How often should I get a blood test to determine my cholesterol and other blood lipids?

A: If you've never had a blood test for your blood lipids and are over 35 years of age, you should have one done as soon as possible. Then, if your test shows that all your blood levels are normal, you can wait a while before your next test. As to the time interval, the Center for Disease Control (CDC) recommends that a test be done every five years if your initial readings are normal. But I think it's advisable to have one done more often than that—every two to three years. If there is a history of heart disease in the family, you'll need more frequent tests, starting much earlier than age 35.

If any of the lipid components in your blood are elevated, you should take steps to correct the problem and have another blood test done in three to six months. If any of your lipids are in the higher-risk categories, such as "high risk" or "very high risk," you'll want to begin treatment immediately through diet or drugs, and you should return within six to eight weeks for a reevaluation.

Q: Should I have my children tested?

A: Yes—especially if you have any family history of high cholesterol, high triglycerides, or heart disease. As we've seen earlier in this book, some children develop severe atherosclerosis at an early age because of inherited defects in their cholesterol or lipid metabolism. In general, I believe that it's a good idea for every child to have a complete blood workup, including cholesterol and lipid studies, by the age of puberty. And certainly this should be done by the early to mid-teen years. Then, if the results are normal, there is no reason for undue concern. On the other hand, if your child does have elevated blood lipids, you'll be in a position to deal with it at an early stage, and you probably can correct the situation before serious problems occur.

Q: Should I fast before my blood test?

A: Yes. It's important to stay away from all foods, including liquids other than water, for twelve to fourteen hours before your scheduled blood test.

The reason for fasting before your blood test is primarily to ensure accuracy in determining the triglycerides. The blood cholesterol shouldn't vary appreciably, but the triglycerides normally will be elevated if you fail to fast. By fasting, you'll give your body time to clear out, or "metabolize," the excess triglycerides. This way, the triglycerides which remain will tend to be limited mostly to those linked to VLDLs, or very low-density lipoproteins. These are the ones that are potentially the most damaging.

I recommend to my patients that they eat a normal meal between 6:00 and 7:00 P.M. Then, they report to the laboratory the following morning between 8:00 and 9:00 A.M. This approach ensures a good fast, and it's not that burdensome a routine.

Q: Are all blood labs and blood tests basically the same?

A: No. Currently there is a great deal of discussion in medical circles about the need for common standards in the area of blood testing. Some surveys have shown that cholesterol measurements may vary by as much as 50 mg/dl among different labs. That means you could be told you have a total cholesterol of 200 mg/dl at one lab, 250 at another, and 150 at still another! Obviously, with this sort of variation, it's difficult to plan a proper cholesterol-control program.

At this time, the best that you can do to evaluate a lab is simply to ask if it is accredited or certified by a national agency such as the Lipid Standardization Laboratory of CDC.

Also, you might ask if "quality controls" are used regularly for standardization. This refers to a procedure whereby blood samples of known values are used as a basis to measure patients' samples. This is done to standardize testing procedures and is a common practice in most good laboratories.

Q: But I'm not a physician or medical expert! This sounds like I need a special knowledge to know if I'm getting an accurate cholesterol test! Isn't there anything else I can do?

A: Determine whether the lab you are using employs pathologists (physicians who specialize in examining tissues to identify diseases) or registered medical technologists. If the testing is being done by improperly trained personnel, the possibility for error increases. On the other hand, if the lab is staffed by highly qualified personnel, you can feel more comfortable about the results.

Q: What tests should I ask for?

A: You should ask for at least five studies:

• Total cholesterol

• Low-density lipoprotein (LDL) cholesterol

• High-density lipoprotein (HDL) cholesterol

• Total cholesterol/HDL cholesterol ratio and

• Triglycerides

In our blood lab at the Aerobics Center in Dallas we report on a number of other values in the blood, and we also take a urine specimen. But the five results listed above are the key ones enabling you to determine whether your cholesterol and blood lipids are at normal levels.

Generally speaking, most labs will analyze directly the

total cholesterol, the HDL cholesterol, and the triglycerides. Then, through a mathematical formula, they'll determine the ratio, LDLs and VLDLs. To get the LDLs, for example, the following formula may be used:

$$LDL = \text{total cholesterol} - \text{HDL cholesterol} - \text{triglycerides}/5.$$

To put this in words, the LDL cholesterol is equal to the total cholesterol, minus the HDLs, minus one-fifth of the triglycerides. The value of one-fifth of the triglycerides, by the way, is what we use to determine the level of the VLDL cholesterol.

Here's the way this formula will work with actual numbers. If you want to find your LDL cholesterol, you first determine the total cholesterol value, which we'll assume is 200. Then you subtract the HDLs, which we'll assume are 50. Next, you'll take one-fifth of the triglycerides. Let's say that the triglycerides are 100 mg/dl; so, one-fifth would be 20 (which is also the value of the VLDL). Now, to plug this in to the formula:

$$LDL = 200 - 50 - 100/5 = 130.$$

Q: What does a cholesterol and blood lipid evaluation cost?

A: We did a brief survey just for the purposes of this book and found that the prices for this type of blood test ranged from a low of $18—a real bargain—up to nearly $45. I doubt you'll be able to get a test anywhere for much less than $18. But it's quite conceivable, especially in large cities, that you may have to pay more than $45. In any case, ask what the cost is before you request the test. But remember, certified labs may charge more than noncertified—and less reliable—labs.

Q: Do I need a referral from a doctor to get a cholesterol blood test?

A: If you follow the instructions which follow the index at the back of this book, you should be able to get a test without being referred by a physician. But, as a general rule, most labs do require a physician referral before they'll do the test.

Q: Why is this?

A: In most places, the reason seems not to relate to any state regulations. Rather, a custom has grown up among many labs that it's best to have a doctor, rather than the lab or the patient, interpret the results of laboratory studies.

I certainly agree that if any of the components of your cholesterol or lipids are markedly elevated, you should seek consultation from a physician and then follow his or her advice. But for an initial test or for those who have no major problem with their blood lipids, there is no reason why patients shouldn't be able to refer themselves to testing facilities and then consult with a physician afterward about the results.

Q: Is there anything I should know about the way the test should be administered before I go to the laboratory?

A: You'll be ushered into the lab and asked to sit in a regular chair or a reclining chair while the medical technician prepares to draw your blood. It's important that you be sitting or lying down while your blood is drawn. Why is this? Your blood values, including cholesterol, may be lower when you're in a sitting or lying position—and that will be more likely to result in an accurate test result.

In a study we did at the Cooper Clinic in Dallas, patients experienced a 9 to 10 percent decrease in their cholesterol when they were lying down, rather than standing up. Also, their triglycerides went down by 12 percent in a lying position, and their HDLs were down by 10 to 11 percent.

Most labs will do your blood test when you're in a sitting or semireclining position. For the purposes of comparing the blood tests that are taken over a period of years, it's important that you be in a similar position each time you are tested.

Now for the actual test:

When you're comfortably seated, the technician will place a tourniquet around your upper arm; then he or she will find a prominent vein in the upper part of your forearm and insert a needle with a blood vial attached on the end. In about fifteen seconds a sufficient amount of blood will have been withdrawn to perform all the necessary tests.

This procedure is relatively easy and involves only a slight pinprick type of pain. The technician will apply pressure to the area after the needle is withdrawn to assure proper blood clotting. Usually, the entire procedure takes only two to three minutes, and complications are almost nonexistent, particularly when the above guidelines are followed.

Q: Will my eating patterns in the period immediately before my blood test influence my cholesterol values?

A: Possibly. We know that certain people can bring their cholesterol values down dramatically by reducing their intake of saturated fats and cholesterol-laden foods in the thirty-six to seventy-two hours prior to the test. By the same token, it's reasonable to assume that you could drive your cholesterol levels up by eating a lot of fried foods or eggs during the week preceding the test.

As a rule of thumb, I recommend that you try to eat normal meals the week before the test. That way, you'll have the best chance of getting a true picture of your cholesterol and lipid levels.

Q: *Does it matter what time of year I take the test?*

A: Studies have suggested that there may be seasonal variations in cholesterol levels. Some researchers have found that cholesterol levels tend to be low in summer and high in winter; others have identified other times as being important for high or low points for cholesterol during the course of the year. What should we make of these seemingly contradictory findings?

An article in *Preventive Medicine* in 1981 surveyed a number of these studies and concluded that "the existence of seasonal effects has not been confirmed." On the other hand, for any individual there may be variations in cholesterol levels during the year. These differences may depend in part upon whether the person tends to eat more foods that are high in cholesterol or to exercise more during certain seasons than in others.

If you decide to have more than one test a year, you might watch for seasonal variations with your blood. In this way, you can evaluate whether you should change your diet, reduce your weight, or otherwise change your lifestyle during certain times of the year. Such an approach may help provide you with greater protection against cardiovascular disease risks with regard to cholesterol.

Q: *Are there any cholesterol tests, other than ordinary tests, which I should be aware of?*

A: There are a number of important tests on the horizon which soon may become generally available to the public.

As I've already indicated, tests for apolipoprotein A-I (Apo A-I), the protein associated with the "good" HDL cholesterol, may turn out to be one of the best indicators of cardiovascular disease. Also, HDL-2—that subfraction of HDLs which tends to be lower in the presence of cardiovascular disease—may be a better risk indicator than the total cholesterol level.

At the present time, testing for HDL-2 has some advantages over Apo A-I because it requires lower start-up costs and also lower long-term costs for each lab test. Also, you can do an HDL-2 test faster than an Apo A-I test (the HDL-2 test takes a matter of hours to turn around, while the Apo A-I may take days).

On the other hand, the clinical usefulness of HDL-2 measurements hasn't been well established by research. Also, even though HDL-2 has some advantages over Apo A-I in the lab, both are still more difficult to test for than the total HDL levels. But before long, when the lab problems are worked out, you can expect Apo A-I to occupy an important place in the experts' list of coronary risk factors.

A number of more specialized tests are also becoming available for individuals who have particular cholesterol problems. For example, a group of scientists at the University of Texas Health Science Center at Dallas has developed a blood test to identify those who are genetically inclined to have high cholesterol levels—a condition which can result in heart attacks at a very early age.

About 1 in every 500 Americans inherits a defective gene which allows the person only half of the necessary LDL receptors. The receptors, you'll recall, are those "rescue teams" which pull the deadly LDLs and their partner Apo Bs out of the bloodstream. Without the receptors, the LDLs and Apo Bs tend to enter the artery walls and form plaque, which may clog the vessels and result in a heart attack. Those who have this genetic condition may have heart attacks by age 30 or 40. But if their condition is detected early enough, they can be put on low cholesterol diets or treated with drugs, and perhaps live a normal life.

The test developed by the Dallas group involves isolating white blood cells from patients' blood samples. Then, through a series of complex steps, scientists are able to determine whether patients have a genetic problem. Most important of all, they are able to do this in much less time and at considerably less expense than was possible using other such tests. Unfortunately, this test is not available for routine analyses at this time.

Q: When should I get my first cholesterol and lipoprotein test?

A: As soon as possible!

NINE

Nutrition:
It's Still the
Key to Lowering
Cholesterol

A proper diet should be the first step you consider to control your body's cholesterol. Among other things, a diet designed to control your cholesterol can:

- Reduce your total blood cholesterol level

- Improve the all-important ratio of your total cholesterol/HDL cholesterol

- Lower your risk of heart disease

Of course, it's important to be realistic about what you can expect your diet to do. For most people, a reduction of total cholesterol through diet, without drugs, usually doesn't exceed a maximum, sustained drop of 50 mg/dl. In other words, if your cholesterol level is 250, and you're a person with average bodily responses, you can anticipate that a low cholesterol diet will reduce your cholesterol count to a consistent level of about 200. For some people, however, a change in diet may not work at all. For some reason, their bodies just don't respond to a reduction in cholesterol intake, so the only way they can hope to reduce their cholesterol levels is through the use of drugs.

The encouraging news is that some people can expect to do much better than the average 50 mg/dl decline. And they may see these dramatic changes occur very quickly.

Consider for example, Tim Connolly, an executive at a large eastern corporation. When he came to one of our in-residence seminars at the Aerobics Center in Dallas, his total cholesterol count was 250 mg/dl. He was understandably quite eager to lower that reading, so he embarked on a relatively moderate low-fat diet and exercise regimen.

Specifically, Connolly's daily food intake consisted of 60 percent complex carbohydrates, 15 percent protein, and 25 percent fat. As part of this diet, he consumed less than 300 mg. of cholesterol per day. Also, he walked up to twelve miles daily for a period of ten days.

What was the effect on his cholesterol?

Connolly experienced a dramatic reduction in his total cholesterol and an improvement in his total cholesterol/HDL cholesterol ratio. His total cholesterol count, as I said, stood at 250 mg/dl on June 4, 1985, just before he embarked on the program. Just as bad, his total cholesterol/HDL cholesterol ratio was a risky 7.4. But by June 14, his cholesterol had plunged to 142 mg/dl! And his ratio was down to an enviable 3.9! In some cases, the drop in cholesterol is temporary and will gradually increase, even in the presence of a fat and cholesterol restricted diet.

As I've indicated, not everyone will respond the same way to a given diet and exercise program. But Tim's case was not unusual. Many people find that through diet changes alone, they can dramatically lower their total cholesterol. Consequently, the message for the average reader should be clear: *A relatively moderate but disciplined approach to diet and exercise may well be all that is needed to improve any cholesterol or lipid abnormality in your blood—and in a relatively short period of time.*

So how, exactly, should you structure your diet to lower your cholesterol?

The staff of the Nutrition Department at the Aerobics Center in Dallas and I have designed the following dietary program. Just as bad, his total cholesterol/HDL cholesterol the different components of your cholesterol into better balance. The diets presented in this chapter include two weeks of menus at three levels of fat and cholesterol restriction: there's a basic level, a moderate level, and a strict level. Also, the diets are presented at two calorie amounts—1,500 calories for women and 2,200 for men. Women generally require 1,500 to 1,700 calories per day to maintain their proper weight, while men require 2,000 to 2,500 calories per day.

To use these diets most effectively, there are three dietary "keys" you should understand:

1. The fat and cholesterol restriction level key

2. The food exchange key

3. The basic meal planning key

Here, in more detail, are some explanations of each of these keys.

Key 1: Understand How the Fat and Cholesterol Restriction Levels Work

For the purposes of this book, we are concerned with three types of fats: saturated, monounsaturated, and polyunsaturated.

In general, foods derived from plants, such as vegetables, are rich in polyunsaturates and contain no cholesterol. Foods derived from certain plants, such as olives, tend to be high in monounsaturates. These contain no cholesterol, and may actually work to lower cholesterol, as we'll see in chapter 20. Finally, foods that come from animals are generally the ones which contain saturated fats—and *these* are the main sources of cholesterol in our diets.

But there are a number of exceptions to these generalizations. For example, some plant-derived foods such as palm oil, coconut oil, and cocoa butter (chocolate) are highly saturated. Although these saturated vegetable fats contain no cholesterol, they may be converted to cholesterol and triglycerides after they enter the body.

Furthermore, it's important for the fats in your food to be kept in a healthy proportion to one another, in part because certain fats are essential to your health. For instance, some polyunsaturated fats, which are known as "essential fatty acids," have to come from your diet because your body doesn't manufacture them. If you lack these special polyunsaturated fats, you could encounter problems with your liver, heart, or circulatory system.

Also, as we'll see in chapter 20, there are strong indications in some recent studies that a healthy, cholesterol-lowering diet should include significant proportions of monounsaturated and polyunsaturated fats to balance the intake of saturated fats.

Finally, the most recent research indicates that a particular kind of saturated fat, stearic acid, apparently doesn't increase cholesterol levels.

What are the practical implications of these findings? One of the most interesting is that the fats found in both beef and cocoa butter, which is the fat in chocolate, have relatively high proportions of stearic acid. As a result, the most current thinking suggests that beef and chocolate may not elevate cholesterol levels as much as previously had been supposed.

To sum up this latest research, then, on stearic acid: Coconut oil raises cholesterol levels the most. Butterfat and palm oil are the next most serious offenders. Less serious offenders in raising cholesterol include chocolate and the meat fats, such as beef, pork, and chicken.

To put this another way, Dr. Scott M. Grundy says that "the meat fats and cocoa butter should raise the plasma cholesterol by only about half as much as palm oil and butterfat, and only a third as much as coconut oil."

How to Choose the Diet That's Best for You

In designing the balanced, cholesterol-controlling menus and recipes in this chapter, our Nutrition Department at the Aerobics Center has taken into consideration the precise fat and cholesterol contents of a wide variety of foods. Specifically, these diets contain three levels of progressively stricter menus—"strictness" being defined by the fat and cholesterol content at each level. In general, these levels include:

• The *Basic* diet—for the average person who wants to maintain or achieve normal cholesterol and lipid levels

• The *Moderate* diet—for those who cannot achieve an adequate lowering of their cholesterol after eight weeks on the basic diet

• The *Strict* diet—for those who have found the "moderate" level inadequate after eight weeks and who require an even greater fat and cholesterol reduction in their diets

Nutritional Values of the Cholesterol-Restrictive Diets

The three levels of restriction—*basic, moderate,* and *strict*—have been designed to conform to the following nutritional values of cholesterol, fats, protein, and complex carbohydrates:

Three Fat Levels

Nutrients	Basic*	Moderate	Strict
Cholesterol (mg.)	300	200	100
Fat (% of total calories)	20–30%	15–20%	10–15%
Saturated fat (S)	⅓	⅓	⅓
Monounsaturated fat (M)	⅓	⅓	⅓
Polyunsaturated fat (P)	⅓	⅓	⅓
P/S ratio	1	1	1–2
Protein (% of total calories)	10–20%	10–20%	10–20%
Complex carbohydrates (% of total calories)	50–60%	50–70%	60–70%

Simple carbohydrate (sugar) may account for 10% maximum of daily carbohydrate calories.

*This recommended dietary composition is consistent with the American Heart Association Phase I diet and may be used for the general public.

How to Follow the Diet

How do you decide when to go from one of these levels to the next? It's best to move according to the following steps:

Step 1. Begin by eating at the Basic level for eight weeks. At the end of that time, have your blood cholesterol values evaluated by a medical laboratory. If your total cholesterol has dropped by 10 percent or more, you're doing fine: You should stick with this Basic diet—either until you don't experience any further cholesterol reductions, or until you reach the target cholesterol level you've set for yourself. In fact, it would be wise for most people to maintain this level indefinitely.

Step 2. If you have less than a 10 percent reduction in your total cholesterol after eight weeks on the Basic diet, move to the Moderate diet for another eight weeks. Then recheck your blood cholesterol level.

Step 3. If you fail to achieve a 10 percent reduction with the Moderate diet after eight weeks, shift to the Strict diet. Then check your blood levels once again.

If none of these steps works, the dietary approach may

simply not be the thing for you. Drugs, used under the supervision of your physician, may be the only answer.

Finally, you should understand that fat in our diets comes from two key sources—the fat that we *add* and the fat that is *hidden* in many animal protein foods and bakery products. The added fat tends to come in such foods as margarine, mayonnaise, oils, and salad dressings. The hidden fat, in contrast, is usually found in protein-rich animal foods like fish, poultry, meat, eggs, and dairy products.

The different menus in each of the three levels of our diets have been chosen with these two key sources of fat in mind. In other words, we've restricted the meals according to:

• The amount of fat added daily in the diet. (In our menus, these added fats vary from 2 to 8 teaspoons daily.)

• The amount of animal protein consumed daily, with its hidden fat. (This varies from 4 to 8 ounces each day.)

• The number of eggs eaten per week. (These vary from no eggs on the Strict diet to a maximum of three per week on the Basic diet.)

Key 2: Understand the Food Exchange System

Most people will probably prefer to use our diet menus just as they're presented in order to lower their cholesterol levels as far as possible. But some may want to experiment with different foods. And some people, after they've been on these diets for a while, may want a little more variety. So, we've set up these menus according to a standard "food exchange system," which can best be explained in these terms:

Generally, a well-balanced diet will include three basic nutrients: protein, complex carbohydrates, and fat. Our Basic cholesterol-lowering diet—which I recommend even for those who don't have a cholesterol problem—consists of the following balance of those three nutrients:

• Carbohydrates—50 to 60 percent of the total calories

• Protein—10 to 20 percent of the total calories

• Fat—20 to 30 percent of the total calories

Here are some of the low-fat foods that are included in each of the three main groups:

Protein—fish; poultry; lean meat; eggs; dried peas and beans (such as black-eyed peas, lentils, split peas, navy beans, pinto beans, red beans, kidney beans); skim milk; skim yogurt; skim cheese. (Never use whole-milk products—skim-milk products provide the same amount of protein and a lot less fat to the diet!)

Complex carbohydrates—fresh fruits; unsweetened fruit juices; vegetables; breads and starches (including sliced bread, rolls, tortillas, bagels, oats, cereal, pasta, rice, corn, popcorn, and potatoes).

Fat—added fats: margarine, oil, salad dressing, mayonnaise, and similar products.

—Hidden fats: These are found in fish, poultry, lean meat, eggs, and a variety of processed foods which usually include fat listings in the "ingredients" list.

With these basic food categories in mind, the following menus have been set up so that they can be used according to a simple "food category" system. Here's how the system works: after each food listing in the menus you will find the key food category noted in parentheses. For example, (Milk) refers to milk products, and (Meat) refers to various types of protein-rich foods, such as fish, poultry, lean meat, or beans. Also, you'll find a number, such as 1 or 2, to indicate the portion size of a particular food.

With this information in hand, you can freely substitute one type of meat for another, or one type of fruit for another—provided you use the same portion sizes. If you vary the portion sizes, you'll also vary your calories—and may find that you're consuming too much or too little food. If you keep the food types and portion sizes constant, you can vary your menus and at the same time keep your calories and nutrients at the proper levels.

Here, in more detail, are all the key food categories you will use. The second column shows the portion size for one item in each food category. The third column indicates the number of calories in each portion.

Key Food Categories

Food Category	Size of One Portion	Calories	Fat
(Milk)—skim milk/yogurt*	1 cup	80–90	0
(Meat)*—lean meat, fish, poultry, egg	1 ounce	60	3
(Fruit)—fresh or frozen fruit or juice	½ cup fruit/juice **or** 1 small fruit	40	0
(Vegetable)—fresh or frozen	½ cup cooked **or** 1 dinner salad	25	0
(Bread/Starch)	½ cup cooked **or** 1 slice bread	70	0
(Fat)	1 teaspoon	45	5

*1 ounce of low-fat cheese (60 to 80 calories per ounce) may count as "1 ounce lean meat."

Here are two handy charts to use as you create your own cholesterol-restrictive menus. I've included one chart for one day's menus for women at the 1,500-calorie level and another chart for one day's menus for men at the 2,200-calorie range. When the term "portions" is used, refer to the above explanation of portion sizes for more precise information. As with the other menus, these are divided into Basic, Moderate, and Strict levels for your fat and cholesterol intake.

Daily Food Exchange Charts

1,500 Calories (Female)			
Food Category	Basic	Moderate	Strict
(Milk)	2 cups	2 cups	2 cups
(Meat)*	6 ounces	5 ounces	4 ounces
(Fruit)	4 portions	6 portions	7 portions
(Vegetable)	4 portions	4 portions	4 portions
(Bread/Starch)	8 portions	9 portions	9 portions
(Fat)	3 teaspoons	2 teaspoons	2 teaspoons
*Includes eggs per week	3	2	0

Food Category	2,200 Calories (Male)		
	Basic	Moderate	Strict
(Milk)	2 cups	2 cups	2 cups
(Meat)*	8 ounces	6 ounces	4 ounces
(Fruit)	7 portions	8 portions	8 portions
(Vegetable)	6 portions	6 portions	6 portions
(Bread/Starch)	12 portions	14 portions	16 portions
(Fat)	8 teaspoons	6 teaspoons	4 teaspoons
*Includes eggs per week	2	2	0

Key 3: Understand the Basic Meal Planning Behind the Diets

The time has arrived to focus on a few rules of thumb that apply to these cholesterol-lowering diets. First, let's accentuate the positive. Here are a dozen food types that you can include in your daily menus, within the indicated limits.

1. Seafood—approximately 16 ounces each week (for healthy Omega-3 fish oils).

2. Poultry—at least 5 servings each week (for monounsaturated fat).

3. Lean meat—at most, 6 to 12 ounces each week (to limit saturated fat).

4. Skim milk—14+ servings each week (at least 2 each day for healthy bones from calcium).

5. Low-fat cheese (80 calories or less per ounce)—7 ounces maximum each week (count 1 ounce low-fat cheese = 1 ounce lean meat).

6. Oats, beans, apples—at least 7 servings each week (for beneficial fiber, which lowers cholesterol).

7. Vegetable oils—½ polyunsaturated oils and soft margarines (corn, safflower, sunflower, soybean, etc.) and ½ mono-unsaturated oils (olive) (for the beneficial cholesterol-lowering effects of both fats). *Tip:* In cooking, mix olive and saf-flower oil, half and half. Avoid butter because it is full of **cholesterol and saturated fat.**

8. Fruits and juices—consume fresh fruit more often than fruit juice (for more fiber).

9. Bread and grain products—choose whole grains and a mixture of grains (for their varied nutrients and fiber). These include whole wheat, oats, wheat bran, cereals, brown rice, whole wheat pasta, and pumpernickel or rye bread.

10. "Diet" fats—use diet margarine, diet mayonnaise, and diet salad dressing to cut fat and calories in half (generally, 1 tablespoon of regular margarine = 2 tablespoons of diet margarine, etc.).

11. Salad dressings—French and Ranch are lowest in fat and calories (50 calories per tablespoon); choose low-calorie dressings that are 20 or fewer calories per tablespoon.

12. "Sweeteners"—raisins, bananas, fruit, cinnamon, and vanilla extract may be added to foods as healthy "sweeteners." "Lite" syrups, "diet" jellies, and apple butter also are lower-calorie options.

Now, let's turn to some negatives. As a general rule, if your cholesterol or triglycerides are elevated, you should avoid or minimize your intake of the foods listed under the following food categories:

Milk and Milk Products

Whole-milk products such as chocolate, condensed, dried, or evaporated milk; buttermilk (made from whole milk); flavored milk drink mixes; instant breakfast drinks; flavored yogurts; eggnog; ice cream; custard; pudding.

Meat and Meat Substitutes

Poultry: duck; goose; poultry skin.
Fish: fish roe (caviar); limit shrimp.
Meats: In general, eliminate those that are fried, or prepared with gravies, sauces, or breading, or in casseroles. Also, eliminate high-fat meats such as:

• Beef—brisket, corned beef, ground hamburger, club or rib steaks, rib roasts, spareribs

• Pork—bacon, deviled ham, loin, spareribs, sausage, cold cuts, hot dogs, luncheon meats

Cheese: eliminate all except skim-milk or cholesterol-free cheese.

Convenience foods: canned or frozen meats; cream cheese; cheese spreads; dips; chips; packaged dinners; pork and beans; pizza; fast foods; cold cuts; fried foods.

Carbohydrates

Croissants; doughnuts; fried foods; commercial granola cereals (with coconut); pancakes; waffles; pastries; potato chips; bakery products (such as sweet rolls, biscuits, cornbread).

Vegetables

Creamed or fried vegetables; vegetables with gravies or sauces.

Fats

Bacon and bacon drippings; butter; egg and cheese sauces; chicken fat and skin; chocolate; cocoa butter; coconut and palm oil; commercial popcorn (made with coconut oil); creamy salad dressings (blue cheese, sour cream, etc.); cream, including liquid, sour, whipping (sweet); dips and chips; hydrogenated oils (as first-listed ingredient on label); lard; nondairy creamers (read labels—avoid those containing coconut); whipped topping; salt pork; shortening; food labeled with nonspecific "vegetable oil."

The Low-Cholesterol Menus

The following menus, which have been formulated by the Nutrition Department at the Aerobics Center in Dallas, have been analyzed thoroughly by computer to assure a proper nutritional balance. As you compare the foods in these menus, you may want to refer to the recipe section which follows it for guidelines about specific food preparation. Also, remember that you can substitute some of those recipes for the items included in the main menus—as long as you follow the basic food principles that we've already outlined.

Remember: You should begin with the Basic plan and then check your cholesterol values after eight weeks. If you've achieved at least a 10 percent reduction in your total cholesterol, you're on the right track. If the *Basic* level fails to help you adequately after eight weeks, you can move on to the *Moderate* or *Strict* levels, in accordance with the three-step approach outlined under "Key 1," on p. 90.

As you move from one fat-cholesterol level to another, you'll notice that certain foods may be added or omitted, or the amounts may be varied. In other words, in one day's menus, you may find that a banana and an oat bran muffin are added, while an ounce of chicken may be subtracted, when you move from the *Basic* to the *Moderate* levels. These changes are necessary to keep the calorie levels the same while changing the balance of nutrients (less fat, more carbohydrate).

So, don't be misled and think we've made a mistake if you sometimes seem to be eating a bigger breakfast with the more restrictive levels than with the Basic menus. The important thing is to look at what happens to your meals over the course of an *entire day.*

Finally, here are some guidelines to keep in mind as you prepare these menus:

• Drink 1 cup of water with or after each meal. Make sure that you have a daily intake of at least 4 glasses of water and 4 glasses of other fluids (or 2 quarts of fluids each day).

• The Strict diet menus may be low in calcium and fish because the protein portions have to be limited to 4 ounces a day in order to restrict the "hidden" fat. Take a calcium supplement according to your physician's prescribed level (usually 800 to 1,200 mg. per day) and eat fish more frequently (approximately 16 ounces per week).

• Assume that all the vegetables are steamed, unless otherwise specified.

• Assume that all the fruits and vegetables are fresh—though you can substitute unsweetened fresh-frozen fruit or frozen vegetables if you like.

• Include in your fruit salads some apples and citrus fruits (oranges, grapefruit). This will ensure that you get enough pectin (apple fiber) and vitamin C (from the citrus fruits).

• Count ½ cup of tomato sauce as "1 Vegetable" and 1 cup of tomato sauce as "1 Bread". The reason for this is that it's necessary to take into account the higher carbohydrate content of the larger sauce portion.

• If you use "diet" fats (such as low-calorie dressings and margarine), you can double the portions of "regular fat" servings and still maintain the same number of calories.

PROTEIN

MILK & MILK PRODUCTS

One serving contains **80 calories**
(8 grams protein, 12 grams carbohydrate)

Eat

Milk (non-fat, skim, ½%, 1%)	1 cup
evaporated	½ cup
powdered	¼ cup
Low-fat 2% milk	¾ cup
Buttermilk (made from non-fat milk)*	1 cup
Yogurt	
from skim milk, plain, unflavored	1 cup
from low-fat milk, plain, unflavored	½ cup
Low-calorie hot cocoa or milkshake (i.e., Alba, Swiss Miss, Carnation, etc.)	1 cup

Avoid

Whole milk products:
    chocolate
    condensed
    dried
    evaporated
Buttermilk (made from whole milk)*
Flavored milk drink mixes*

Instant breakfast drinks*
Flavored yogurts
Eggnog
Ice cream
Custard
Pudding

*-high in salt (sodium)

MEAT/SUBSTITUTES

One serving (1 ounce) contains **70 calories**
(8 grams protein, 3-5 grams fat)

Eat 4-8 oz. meat or substitutes daily.

Eat

Choose 10+ meals per week:
Poultry (without skin)
    chicken, turkey, cornish hen, squab ....1 oz.
Fish—any kind (fresh or frozen) ....1 oz.
    water-packed tuna or salmon, crab or lobster* ....¼ cup
    clams, oysters, scallops, shrimp ....1 oz. or 5
    sardines, drained* 3
Veal—any lean cut ....1 oz.
Peanut butter*, not hydrogenated (read labels) ....1 Tbsp.
Dried beans, peas (count as 1 meat + 1 bread) ....½ cup
Chicken or turkey cold cuts*
    turkey ham, turkey bologna ....1 oz.

Limit to 4 meals per week:
Lean beef cuts
    tenderloin (sirloin, filet, T-bone, porterhouse),
    round, cube, flank ....1 oz.
    roasts, stews—sirloin tip, round, rump, chuck, arm....1 oz.
    other—ground round or chuck (15% fat ground beef),
    chipped beef, venison ....1 oz.
Lean lamb cuts—leg, chops, loin, shoulder ....1 oz.
Lean pork & ham*
    center cut steaks, loin chops, smoked ham* ....1 oz.

Limit to 3-5 ounces per week:
Cholesterol-free cheese*
    Cheezola, Countdown, Kraft "Golden Image", etc......1 oz.
Low-fat cheese*
    low-fat cottage cheese, mozzarella, farmer's,
    parmesan, ricotta, neufchatel ....1 oz. or ¼ cup

Limit to 1-3 egg yolks per week:
Whole egg 1
Egg substitutes* (cholesterol-free) ....¼ cup
Egg whites ....as desired

Limit to 2 meals per month:
Shrimp ....1 oz. or 5
Organ meats—liver, heart, brains, kidney ....1 oz.

*-high in salt (sodium)

MEAT TIPS

Avoid

Poultry—duck, goose, poultry skin
Fish—fish row (caviar); limit shrimp
Meats—fried, with gravies, sauces, breading, casseroles
    —high fat meats:
        beef—brisket, corned beef, ground hamburger, club
           or rib steaks, rib roasts, spare ribs
        pork—bacon*, deviled ham*, loin, spare ribs, sausage*,
           cold cuts*
        pork—hot dogs*, luncheon meats*
Cheese*—all except skim milk or cholesterol-free cheese (see
    protein list p. 100)
Convenience foods—canned* or frozen meats, cream cheese,
    cheese spreads*, dips*, packaged dinners*, pork and
    beans*, pizza*, fast foods*, cold cuts*.

*-high in salt (sodium)

TIPS TO REDUCE FATS

COOKING SUBSTITUTES

Recipe calls for:	Substitute:
1 whole egg	¼ c. egg substitute or 2 egg whites
1 c. shortening or butter	¾ c. liquid oil
1 T. shortening or butter	1 T. liquid oil
1 square chocolate	3 T. dry cocoa powder + ½ T. liquid oil
1 c. whole milk	1 c. skim milk + 2 tsp. liquid oil or 1 c. evaporated skim milk
1 c. sour cream	1 c. nonfat yogurt
1 oz. cream cheese	1 oz. cottage cheese

COOKING TIPS TO REDUCE FAT

• Use non-stick sprays and non-stick pans.

• Chill soups and stews and lift off congealed fat or use a strainer to pour off fat.

• Make gravies with fat-free broth, skim milk, and cornstarch.

• Cook onions, green pepper and other vegetables in a little broth instead of sautéing them in fat; add garlic powder and onion powder to enhance flavor.

• Season vegetables with herbs and spices and chicken or beef broth rather than bacon, butter, ham hocks or salt pork.

• Cheese sauce—use skim milk and low-fat cheese rather than whole milk, regular cheese and butter.

• Serve foods without added sauces.

• Instead of using milk in a recipe, use nonfat dry milk, or evaporated skim milk instead of evaporated milk or light cream.

• Eliminate dabs of butter on casseroles. Reduce fat to ½ of the amount stated.

• Instead of sour cream or vegetable dips, use plain yogurt blended with cottage cheese and seasonings; or mix plain low-fat yogurt and a ranch dressing packet. Also, use on baked potatoes and sandwiches.

• Reduce sugar in recipes ¼ to ⅓ without much effect on the final product.

• Use naturally sweet flavors instead of excess sugar—vanilla, cinnamon, almond and cherry extracts; raisins, banana, concentrated apple juice.

• Substitute fresh fruits for sweet desserts.

Note: frequently, you'll find that more food is used in a recipe than remains in the final yields for serving. The reason for this is that weight is often lost during cooking.

Here are the menus—first, the two weeks of 1,500-calorie diets for women; then the two weeks of 2,200-calorie diets for men. You should repeat your chosen diet for a total of eight weeks so that your blood lipids will have sufficient time to respond to the adjustments in your food intake.

The Controlling Cholesterol Diet

Recipes for The Controlling Cholesterol Diet, indicated in the menu plans by an asterisk(*), are found on pages 176–228.

1,500-CALORIE MENUS

Week 1—Monday

	BREAKFAST	LUNCH

BASIC	½ grapefruit (1 Fruit)
	2 whole wheat toast (2 Bread)
	    with 1 teaspoon margarine
	    (1 Fat)
	1 cup skim milk (1 Milk)
		Tuna Sandwich
		  2 whole wheat bread slices (2
		    Bread)
		  ¾ cup tuna (4.5 ounces),
		    water-packed with 1 tea-
		    spoon mayonnaise (3 Meat,
		    1 Fat)
		    and lettuce and tomato
		    slices (0)
		  ½ cup coleslaw (1 Vegetable)
		    with 1 tablespoon lemon
		    juice (0)
		    and 1 tablespoon vinegar (0)
		1 medium apple (2 Fruit)
		1 cup skim milk (1 Milk)

MODERATE	½ grapefruit (1 Fruit)
	2 whole wheat toast (2 Bread)
	    with 2 teaspoons diet mar-
	    garine (½ Fat)
	1 cup skim milk (1 Milk)
		Tuna Sandwich
		  2 whole wheat bread slices
		    (2 Bread)
		  ½ cup tuna (3 ounces), water-
		    packed with 2 teaspoons
		    diet mayonnaise (2 Meat, ½
		    Fat)
		    and lettuce and tomato
		    slices (0)
		  ½ cup coleslaw (1 Vegetable)
		    with 1 tablespoon lemon
		    juice (0)
		    and 1 tablespoon vinegar (0)
		1 medium apple (2 Fruit)
		1 cup skim milk (1 Milk)

STRICT	½ grapefruit (1 Fruit)
	2 whole wheat toast (2 Bread)
	    with 2 teaspoons diet mar-
	    garine (½ Fat)
	1 cup skim milk (1 Milk)
		Tuna Sandwich
		  2 whole wheat bread slices (2
		    Bread)
		  ¼ cup tuna (1.5 ounces), water-
		    packed with 2 teaspoons
		    diet mayonnaise (1 Meat, ½ Fat)
		    and lettuce and tomato
		    slices (0)
		  ½ cup coleslaw (1 Vegetable)
		    with 1 tablespoon lemon
		    juice (0)
		    and 1 tablespoon vinegar (0)
		1 medium apple (2 Fruit)
		1 cup skim milk (1 Milk)

SUPPER

3 ounces Baked Chicken (skin-
    less)* (3 Meat), see p.
    177
1 medium baked potato (2 Bread)
    with 1 tablespoon lemon
    juice (0)
½ cup carrots (1 Vegetable)
½ cup green beans (1 Vegetable)
1 tomato and lettuce salad
    (1 Vegetable) with 1 table-
    spoon Ranch or French
    Dressing (1 Fat)
2 whole wheat rolls (2 Bread)
½ cup pineapple, fresh or un-
    sweetened (1 Fruit)

---

3 ounces Baked Chicken (skin-
    less)* (3 Meat), see p.
    177
1 medium baked potato (2 Bread)
    with 1 tablespoon lemon
    juice (0)
½ cup carrots (1 Vegetable)
½ cup green beans (1 Vegetable)
1 tomato and lettuce salad
    (1 Vegetable) with 1 table-
    spoon Ranch or French
    Dressing (1 Fat)
2 whole wheat rolls (2 Bread)
*1 cup pineapple, fresh or unsweet-
    ened (2 Fruit)*

---

3 ounces Baked Chicken (skin-
    less)* (3 Meat), see p.
    177
1 medium baked potato (2 Bread)
    with 1 tablespoon lemon
    juice (0)
½ cup carrots (1 Vegetable)
½ cup green beans (1 Vegetable)
1 tomato and lettuce salad
    (1 Vegetable) with 1 table-
    spoon Ranch or French
    dressing (1 Fat)
2 whole wheat rolls (2 Bread)
*1 cup pineapple, fresh or unsweet-
    ened (2 Fruit)*

SNACKS

*3 cups popcorn (1½ tablespoons
    dry kernels) plain and air-
    popped (1 Bread)*
4 ounces orange juice (1 Fruit)

---

*3 cups popcorn (1½ tablespoons
    dry kernels), plain and air-
    popped (1 Bread)*
8 ounces orange juice (2 Fruit)

Week 1—Tuesday

	BREAKFAST	LUNCH

BASIC	¼ cantaloupe (1 Fruit)
	1 whole wheat English muffin (2 Bread) with 1 teaspoon margarine (1 Fat)
	(or 1 tablespoon apple butter)
	1 cup skim milk (1 Milk)
		Turkey Sandwich
		  2 whole-wheat bread slices (2 Bread)
		  3 ounces turkey (3 Meat)
		  1 teaspoon mayonnaise (1 Fat)
		  and lettuce and tomato slices (0)
		1 cup raw vegetables (1 Vegetable)
		1 small pear (1 Fruit)
		1 cup skim milk (1 Milk)

MODERATE	½ cantaloupe (2 Fruit)
	1 whole wheat English muffin (2 Bread) with 1 teaspoon margarine (1 Fat)
	(or 1 tablespoon apple butter)
	1 cup skim milk (1 Milk)
		Turkey Sandwich
		  2 whole wheat bread slices (2 Bread)
		  2 ounces turkey (2 Meat)
		  2 teaspoons mustard (0)
		  (omit mayonnaise)
		  and lettuce and tomato slices (0)
		1 cup raw vegetables (1 Vegetable)
		25 salt-free pretzel sticks (1 Bread)
		1 medium pear (2 Fruit)
		1 cup skim milk (1 Milk)

STRICT	½ cantaloupe (2 Fruit)
	1 whole wheat English muffin (2 Bread) with 1 teaspoon margarine (1 Fat)
	(or 1 tablespoon apple butter)
	1 cup skim milk (1 Milk)
		Turkey Sandwich
		  2 whole wheat bread slices (2 Bread)
		  1 ounce turkey (1 Meat)
		  2 teaspoons mustard (0)
		  (omit mayonnaise)
		  and lettuce and tomato slices (0)
		1 cup raw vegetables (1 Vegetable)
		25 salt-free pretzel sticks (1 Bread)
		1 medium pear (2 Fruit)
		1 cup skim milk (1 Milk)

SUPPER   SNACKS

3 ounces Baked Seafood Sea-
    soned with Mixed Vegeta-
    bles* (3 Meat, 2 Vegetable),
    see p. 185
½ cup Carrot Raisin Salad* (1
    Vegetable, 1 Fruit, 1 Fat),
    see p. 209
1 corn-on-the-cob or 1 cup corn
    (2 Bread)
½ cup green peas (1 Bread)
1 whole wheat roll (1 Bread)
½ cup seedless grapes (1 Fruit)

3 ounces Baked Seafood Sea-
    soned with Mixed Vegeta-
    bles* (3 Meat, 2 Vegetable),
    see p. 185
½ cup Carrot Raisin Salad* (1
    Vegetable, 1 Fruit, 1 Fat),
    see p. 209
1 corn-on-the-cob or 1 cup corn
    (2 Bread)
½ cup green peas (1 Bread)
1 whole wheat roll (1 Bread)
½ cup seedless grapes (1 Fruit)

3 ounces Baked Seafood Sea-
    soned with Mixed Vegeta-
    bles* (3 Meat, 2 Vegetable),
    see p. 185
½ cup Carrot Raisin Salad* (1
    Vegetable, 1 Fruit, 1 Fat),
    see p. 209
1 corn-on-the-cob or 1 cup corn
    (2 Bread)
½ cup green peas (1 Bread)
1 whole wheat roll (1 Bread)
1 cup seedless grapes (2 Fruit)

Week 1—Wednesday

	BREAKFAST	LUNCH
BASIC	½ banana (1 Fruit) 1 cup oat bran cereal (2 Bread) 1 cup skim milk (1 Milk)	Pasta Salad #1* (2 Bread, 2 Vegetable, 3 Meat, 3 Fat), see p. 211 1 cup Seasonal Fruit Salad (2 Fruit), see p. 218 1 cup skim milk (1 Milk)
MODERATE	*1 banana (2 Fruit)* 1 cup oat bran cereal (2 Bread) 1 cup skim milk (1 Milk)	Pasta Salad #2* (2 Bread, 2 Vegetable, 2 Meat, 2 Fat), see pp. 211–212 *1½ cups Seasonal Fruit Salad (3 Fruit)*, see p. 218 1 cup skim milk (1 Milk)
STRICT	*1 banana (2 Fruit)* 1 cup oat bran cereal (2 Bread) *with 2 tablespoons raisins (1 Fruit)* 1 cup skim milk (1 Milk)	Pasta Salad #3* (2 Bread, 2 Vegetable, 1 Meat, 2 Fat), see p. 212 *1½ cups Seasonal Fruit Salad (3 Fruit)*, see p. 218 1 cup skim milk (1 Milk)

SUPPER	SNACKS

2 soft tortillas topped with hot
   sauce (2 Bread)
2 Mexican Fajitas #1* (with 3
   ounces meat) (2 Bread, 3
   Meat, 1 Vegetable), see p.
   197
1 raw carrot (1 Vegetable)
¾ cup strawberries (1 Fruit)

---

*3 soft tortillas (3 Bread) topped
   with hot sauce (0)*
2 Mexican Fajitas #1* (with 3
   ounces meat) (2 Bread, 3
   Meat, 1 Vegetable), see p.
   197
1 raw carrot (1 Vegetable)
¾ cup strawberries (1 Fruit)

---

*3 soft tortillas (3 Bread) topped
   with hot sauce (0)*
2 Mexican Fajitas #1* (with 3
   ounces meat) (2 Bread, 3
   Meat, 1 Vegetable), see p.
   197
1 raw carrot (1 Vegetable)
¾ cup strawberries (1 Fruit)

Week 1—Thursday

	BREAKFAST	LUNCH
BASIC	2 Homemade Cheese Danish Rolls* (2 Bread, 1 Meat, 1 Fruit), see p. 225 1 cup skim milk (1 Milk)	2½ cups Cajun Beans with Brown Rice #1* (4 Bread, 2 Meat, 1 Vegetable), see p. 200 1 tomato and lettuce salad (1 Vegetable) with 1 tablespoon French dressing (1 Fat) 1 medium orange (1 Fruit) 1 cup skim milk (1 Milk)
MODERATE	8 ounces orange juice (2 Fruit) 2 Homemade Cheese Danish Rolls* (2 Bread, 1 Meat, 1 Fruit), see p. 225 1 cup skim milk (1 Milk)	2½ cups Cajun Beans with Brown Rice #1* (4 Bread, 2 Meat, 1 Vegetable), see p. 200 1 tomato and lettuce salad (1 Vegetable) with 1 tablespoon French dressing (1 Fat) 1 medium orange (1 Fruit) 1 cup skim milk (1 Milk)
STRICT	8 ounces orange juice (2 Fruit) 2 Homemade Cheese Danish Rolls* (2 Bread, 1 Meat, 1 Fruit), see p. 225 1 cup skim milk (1 Milk)	2½ cups Cajun Beans with Brown Rice #1* (4 Bread, 2 Meat, 1 Vegetable), see p. 200 1 tomato and lettuce salad (1 Vegetable) with 1 tablespoon French dressing (1 Fat) 1 medium orange (1 Fruit) 1 cup skim milk (1 Milk)

SUPPER

SNACKS·

1 cup pasta (2 Bread)
½ cup Easy Meat Sauce #1 (2
    ounces meat, ½ cup to-
    mato sauce)* (2 Meat, 1
    Vegetable), see pp. 194–195
3 tablespoons Parmesan cheese
    (1 Meat)
½ cup stir-fried zucchini in 2
    teaspoons olive oil (1 Veg-
    etable, 2 Fat)
1 medium apple, fresh or baked
    (2 Fruit)

1½ cups pasta (3 Bread)
½ cup Easy Meat Sauce #1 (2
    ounces meat, ½ cup to-
    mato sauce)* (2 Meat, 1
    Vegetable), see pp. 194–195
(omit cheese)
½ cup stir-fried zucchini *in 1
    teaspoon olive oil* (1 Vege-
    table, 1 Fat)
1 medium apple, fresh or baked
    (2 Fruit)

1½ cups pasta (3 Bread)
*½ cup Easy Meat Sauce #2 (1
    ounce meat, ½ cup to-
    mato sauce)** (1 Meat, 1
    Vegetable), see p. 195
(omit cheese)
½ cup stir-fried zucchini *in 1
    teaspoon olive oil* (1 Vege-
    table, 1 Fat)
1 medium apple, fresh or baked
    (2 Fruit)

1 small peach (1 Fruit)

Week 1—Friday

	BREAKFAST	LUNCH

BASIC	½ banana (1 Fruit)
	1 pumpernickel bagel (2 Bread)
	1 poached egg (1 Meat)
	1 cup skim milk (1 Milk)
		2 cups vegetable soup (2 Bread)
		1 Stuffed Tomato
		  1 tomato (1 Vegetable)
		  ½ cup tuna (3 ounces), water-packed, with 1 tablespoon diet mayonnaise (2 Meat, 1 Fat)
		4 melba toast (1 Bread)
		1 medium apple (2 Fruit)
		1 cup skim milk (1 Milk)

MODERATE	*4 ounces orange juice (1 Fruit)*
	1 banana (2 Fruit)
	1 pumpernickel bagel (2 Bread)
	(omit egg)
	1 cup skim milk (1 Milk)
		2 cups vegetable soup (2 Bread)
		1 Stuffed Tomato
		  1 tomato (1 Vegetable)
		  ½ cup tuna (3 ounces), water-packed, *or ⅔ cup 1% cottage cheese (2 Meat)*
		  (omit mayonnaise)
		4 melba toast (1 Bread)
		1 medium apple (2 Fruit)
		1 cup skim milk (1 Milk)

STRICT	*8 ounces orange juice (2 Fruit)*
	1 banana (2 Fruit)
	1 pumpernickel bagel (2 Bread)
	(omit egg)
	1 cup skim milk (1 Milk)
		2 cups vegetable soup (2 Bread)
		1 Stuffed Tomato
		  1 tomato (1 Vegetable)
		  ¼ cup tuna (1.5 ounces), water-packed, *or ⅓ cup 1% cottage cheese (1 Meat)*
		  (omit mayonnaise)
		4 melba toast (1 Bread)
		1 medium apple (2 Fruit)
		1 cup skim milk (1 Milk)

SUPPER	SNACKS
3 ounces Grilled or Poached Salmon* (3 Meat), see pp. 188–189 ½ cup brown rice (1 Bread) ½ cup spinach with 1 teaspoon margarine (1 Vegetable, 1 Fat) ½ cup yellow squash or carrots with 1 teaspoon margarine (1 Vegetable, 1 Fat) 1 whole wheat roll (1 Bread) 1 3-inch slice Angel Food Cake* (1 Bread), see pp. 226–227 topped with ½ cup fruit, fresh or unsweetened (1 Fruit)	1 cup raw vegetables (1 Vegetable)
3 ounces Grilled or Poached Salmon* (3 Meat), see pp. 188–189 ½ cup brown rice (1 Bread) ½ cup spinach with 1 teaspoon margarine (1 Vegetable, 1 Fat) ½ cup yellow squash or carrots with 1 teaspoon margarine (1 Vegetable, 1 Fat) 2 whole wheat rolls (2 Bread) 1 3-inch slice Angel Food Cake* (1 Bread), see pp. 226–227 topped with ½ cup fruit, fresh or unsweetened (1 Fruit)	1 cup raw vegetables (1 Vegetable)
3 ounces Grilled or Poached Salmon* (3 Meat), see pp. 188–189 ½ cup brown rice (1 Bread) ½ cup spinach with 1 teaspoon margarine (1 Vegetable, 1 Fat) ½ cup yellow squash or carrots with 1 teaspoon margarine (1 Vegetable, 1 Fat) 2 whole wheat rolls (2 Bread) 1 3-inch slice Angel Food Cake* (1 Bread), see pp. 226–227 topped with ½ cup fruit, fresh or unsweetened (1 Fruit)	1 cup raw vegetables (1 Vegetable)

Week 1—Saturday

	BREAKFAST	LUNCH
BASIC	1 cup oatmeal (2 Bread) with 2 tablespoons raisins (1 Fruit) 1 cup skim milk (1 Milk)	1 cup minestrone soup (1 Bread) 1 tomato and lettuce salad (1 Vegetable) with 1 tablespoon Ranch dressing (1 Fat) 1 medium baked potato (2 Bread) with 1 tablespoon lemon juice (0) or picante sauce (0) 1 large orange (2 Fruit) 1 cup skim milk (1 Milk)
MODERATE	*1 banana (2 Fruit)* *1½ cups oatmeal (3 Bread)* with 2 tablespoons raisins (1 Fruit) 1 cup skim milk (1 Milk)	1 cup minestrone soup (1 Bread) 1 tomato and lettuce salad (1 Vegetable) *with 1 tablespoon herb vinegar (0)* *or lemon juice (0)* *(omit Ranch dressing)* 1 medium baked potato (2 Bread) with 1 tablespoon lemon juice (0) or picante sauce (0) 1 large orange (2 Fruit) 1 cup skim milk (1 Milk)
STRICT	*4 ounces orange juice (1 Fruit)* *1 banana (2 Fruit)* *1½ cups oatmeal (3 Bread)* with 2 tablespoons raisins (1 Fruit) 1 cup skim milk (1 Milk)	1 cup minestrone soup (1 Bread) 1 tomato and lettuce salad (1 Vegetable) *with 1 tablespoon herb vinegar (0)* *or lemon juice (0)* *(omit Ranch dressing)* 1 medium baked potato (2 Bread) with 1 tablespoon lemon juice (0) or picante sauce (0) 1 large orange (2 Fruit) 1 cup skim milk (1 Milk)

SUPPER   SNACKS

6 ounces Broiled Seafood* (6
    Meat), see p. 186, with
    lemon wedges (0)
½ cup pasta (1 Bread) with ½
    cup Marinara Sauce* (1
    Vegetable), see pp. 221–222
½ cup stir-fried mixed vegeta-
    bles in 1 teaspoon oil (1
    Vegetable, 1 Fat)
1 tomato and lettuce salad (1
    Vegetable) with lemon
    wedges (0)
    or herb vinegar (0)
2 French or Italian bread slices
    (each slice, 3 inches long)
    (2 Bread) with 1 teaspoon
    margarine (1 Fat)
½ cup berries (1 Fruit)

5 ounces Broiled Seafood (5
    Meat), see p. 186, with
    lemon wedges (0)
½ cup pasta (1 Bread) with ½
    cup Marinara Sauce* (1
    Vegetable), see pp. 221–222
½ cup stir-fried mixed vegeta-
    bles in 1 teaspoon oil (1
    Vegetable, 1 Fat)
1 tomato and lettuce salad (1
    Vegetable) with lemon
    wedges (0)
    or herb vinegar (0)
2 French or Italian bread slices
    (each slice, 3 inches long)
    (2 Bread) with 1 teaspoon
    margarine (1 Fat)
½ cup berries (1 Fruit)

4 ounces Broiled Seafood (4
    Meat), see p. 186, with
    lemon wedges (0)
½ cup pasta (1 Bread) with ½
    cup Marinara Sauce* (1
    Vegetable), see pp. 221–222
½ cup stir-fried mixed vegeta-
    bles in 1 teaspoon oil (1
    Vegetable, 1 Fat)
1 tomato and lettuce salad (1
    Vegetable) with lemon
    wedges (0) or herb
    vinegar (0)

Week 1—Saturday (cont'd)

BREAKFAST	LUNCH

SUPPER   SNACKS

2 French or Italian bread slices
    (each slice, 3 inches long)
    (2 Bread) with 1 teaspoon
    margarine (1 Fat)
½ cup berries (1 Fruit)

Week 1—Sunday

	BREAKFAST	LUNCH
BASIC	4 ounces orange juice (1 Fruit) 2 Oat Bran Muffins* (2 Bread), see p. 224 1 cup skim milk (1 Milk)	6 ounces Hawaiian Chicken #1* (6 Meat, 1 Fruit, 1 Fat), see pp. 181–182 1 cup wild rice with 1 teaspoon margarine (2 Bread, 1 Fat) ½ cup broccoli with 1 teaspoon margarine (1 Vegetable, 1 Fat) 2 whole wheat dinner rolls (2 Bread) ½ cup peach slices (1 Fruit)
MODERATE	4 ounces orange juice (1 Fruit) *1 banana (2 Fruit)* *3 Oat Bran Muffins* (3 Bread)*, see p. 224 1 cup skim milk (1 Milk)	*5 ounces Hawaiian Chicken #2* (5 Meat, 1 Fruit, 1 Fat)*, see p. 182 1 cup wild rice (2 Bread) *(omit margarine)* ½ cup broccoli with 1 teaspoon margarine (1 Vegetable, 1 Fat) 2 whole wheat dinner rolls (2 Bread) ½ cup peach slices (1 Fruit)
STRICT	*8 ounces orange juice (2 Fruit)* *1 banana (2 Fruit)* *3 Oat Bran Muffins* (3 Bread)*, see p. 224 1 cup skim milk (1 Milk)	*4 ounces Hawaiian Chicken #3* (4 Meat, 1 Fruit, 1 Fat)*, see pp. 182–183 1 cup wild rice (2 Bread) *(omit margarine)* ½ cup broccoli with 1 teaspoon margarine (1 Vegetable, 1 Fat) 2 whole wheat dinner rolls (2 Bread) ½ cup peach slices (1 Fruit)

SUPPER	SNACKS
1 whole wheat pita pocket filled with 1 cup steamed mixed vegetables (2 Bread, 2 Vegetable)` 1 raw carrot (1 Vegetable) ½ cup seedless grapes (1 Fruit) 1 cup skim milk (1 Milk)	
1 whole wheat pita pocket filled with 1 cup steamed mixed vegetables (2 Bread, 2 Vegetable) 1 raw carrot (1 Vegetable) ½ cup seedless grapes (1 Fruit) 1 cup skim milk (1 Milk)	
1 whole wheat pita pocket filled with 1 cup steamed mixed vegetables (2 Bread, 2 Vegetable) 1 raw carrot (1 Vegetable) ½ cup seedless grapes (1 Fruit) 1 cup skim milk (1 Milk)	

Week 2—Monday

	BREAKFAST	LUNCH
BASIC	¼ cantaloupe (1 Fruit) 1 pumpernickel or whole wheat bagel (2 Bread) 1 cup skim milk (or 4 tablespoons skim ricotta cheese on bagel) (1 Milk)	2 cups Gumbo* (2 Meat, 2 Bread), see p. 204 6 shrimp (1 Meat) with 1 tablespoon cocktail sauce (0) or fresh lemon juice (0) 1 large tomato and lettuce salad (2 Vegetable) with 2 tablespoons herb vinegar (0) or lemon juice (0) 4 melba toast (1 Bread) 1 large apple (2 Fruit) 1 cup skim milk (1 Milk)
MODERATE	½ cantaloupe (2 Fruit) 2 pumpernickel or whole wheat bagels (4 Bread) 1 cup skim milk (or 4 tablespoons skim ricotta cheese on bagels) (1 Milk)	1 cup Gumbo* (1 Meat, 1 Bread), see p. 204 6 shrimp (1 Meat) with 1 tablespoon cocktail sauce (0) or fresh lemon juice (0) 1 large tomato and lettuce salad (2 Vegetable) with 2 tablespoons herb vinegar (0) or lemon juice (0) 4 melba toast (1 Bread) 1 large apple (2 Fruit) 1 cup skim milk (1 Milk)
STRICT	4 ounces orange juice (1 Fruit) ½ cantaloupe (2 Fruit) 2 pumpernickel or whole wheat bagels (4 Bread) 1 cup skim milk (or 4 tablespoons skim ricotta cheese on bagels) (1 Milk)	1 cup Gumbo* (1 Meat, 1 Bread), see p. 204 6 shrimp (1 Meat) with 1 tablespoon cocktail sauce (0) or fresh lemon juice (0) 1 large tomato and lettuce salad (2 Vegetable) with 2 tablespoons herb vinegar (0) or lemon juice (0) 4 melba toast (1 Bread) 1 large apple (2 Fruit) 1 cup skim milk (1 Milk)

SUPPER   SNACKS

3 ounces Barbecued Chicken
(skinless)* (3 Meat, 1 Fat),
see pp. 180 and 220
½ cup Potato Salad* (1 Bread, 1
Fat), see p. 210
1 corn-on-the-cob or 1 cup corn
(2 Bread)
½ cup coleslaw with 1 tablespoon diet mayonnaise (1
Vegetable, 1 Fat)
½ banana, frozen (1 Fruit)

---

3 ounces Barbecued Chicken
(skinless)* (3 Meat, 1 Fat),
see pp. 180 and 220
½ cup Potato Salad* (1 Bread, 1
Fat), see p. 210
1 corn-on-the-cob or 1 cup corn
(2 Bread)
*1 cup coleslaw (2 Vegetable) with
2 tablespoons lemon juice (0)
and 2 tablespoons vinegar (0)*
1 banana, frozen (2 Fruit)

---

*2 ounces Barbecued Chicken (skin-
less)* (2 Meat, 1 Fat), see
pp. 180 and 220
½ cup Potato Salad* (1 Bread, 1
Fat), see p. 210
1 corn-on-the-cob or 1 cup corn
(2 Bread)
*1 cup coleslaw (2 Vegetable) with
2 tablespoons lemon juice (0)
and 2 tablespoons vinegar (0)*
1 banana, frozen (2 Fruit)

Week 2—Tuesday

	BREAKFAST	LUNCH

BASIC	½ grapefruit (1 Fruit)
	2 Oat Bran Muffins* (2 Bread), see p. 224
	1 cup skim milk (1 Milk)
		1 cup lentil soup (1 Meat, 1 Bread, 1 Vegetable)
		Turkey Sandwich
		  2 whole wheat bread slices (2 Bread)
		  2 ounces turkey (2 Meat)
		  1 teaspoon mayonnaise (1 Fat)
		  and lettuce and tomato slices (0)
		1 large pear (2 Fruit)
		1 cup skim milk (1 Milk)

MODERATE	½ grapefruit (1 Fruit)
	2 Oat Bran Muffins* (2 Bread), see p. 224
	1 cup skim milk (1 Milk)
		1 cup lentil soup (1 Meat, 1 Bread, 1 Vegetable)
		Turkey Sandwich
		  2 whole wheat bread slices (2 Bread)
		  2 ounces turkey (2 Meat)
		  2 teaspoons mustard (0)
		  (omit mayonnaise)
		  and lettuce and tomato slices (0)
		1 large pear (2 Fruit)
		1 cup skim milk (1 Milk)

STRICT	½ grapefruit (1 Fruit)
	2 Oat Bran Muffins* (2 Bread), see p. 224
	1 cup skim milk (1 Milk)
		1 cup lentil soup (1 Meat, 1 Bread, 1 Vegetable)
		Turkey Sandwich
		  2 whole wheat bread slices (2 Bread)
		  1 ounce turkey (1 Meat)
		  2 teaspoons mustard (0)
		  (omit mayonnaise)
		  and lettuce and tomato slices (0)
		1 large pear (2 Fruit)
		1 cup skim milk (1 Milk)

SUPPER	SNACKS
Shishkabob #1* (3 Meat, 1 Vegetable), see p. 192 1 cup brown or wild rice (2 Bread) 1 whole wheat roll (1 Bread) 1 large tomato and lettuce salad (2 Vegetable) with 2 tablespoons Ranch or buttermilk dressing (2 Fat) ½ cup pineapple, fresh or unsweetened (1 Fruit)	
Shishkabob #2* (2 Meat, 1 Vegetable), see pp. 192–193 1 cup brown or wild rice (2 Bread) *2 whole wheat rolls (2 Bread)* 1 large tomato and lettuce salad (2 Vegetable) with 2 tablespoons Ranch or buttermilk dressing (2 Fat) ½ cup fresh or unsweetened pineapple (1 Fruit)	*1 snack box (1.5 ounces) raisins (2 Fruit)*
Shishkabob #2* (2 Meat, 1 Vegetable), see pp. 192–193 1 cup brown or wild rice (2 Bread) *2 whole wheat rolls (2 Bread)* 1 large tomato and lettuce salad (2 Vegetable) with 2 tablespoons Ranch or buttermilk dressing (2 Fat) *1 cup pineapple, fresh or unsweetened (2 Fruit)*	*1 snack box (1.5 ounces) raisins (2 Fruit)*

Week 2—Wednesday

	BREAKFAST	LUNCH

BASIC	4 ounces orange juice (1 Fruit)
	Egg and Muffin Sandwich
	   1 whole wheat English muffin
	     (2 Bread)
	   1 poached egg (1 Meat)
	   1 ounce turkey ham (1 Meat)
	1 cup skim milk (1 Milk)
		1 cup Bean Chili #1* (2 Meat, 2
		   Bread, 1 Fat, 1 Vegeta-
		   ble), see pp. 198–199
		1 whole wheat roll (1 Bread)
		   with 1 teaspoon margarine
		   (1 Fat)

MODERATE	4 ounces orange juice (1 Fruit)
	Egg and Muffin Sandwich
	   1 whole wheat English muffin
	     (2 Bread)
	   1 poached egg (1 Meat)
	   (omit ham)
	1 cup skim milk (1 Milk)
		1 cup Bean Chili #1* (2 Meat, 2
		   Bread, 1 Fat, 1 Vegeta-
		   ble), see pp. 198–199
		1 whole wheat roll (1 Bread)
		   (omit margarine)

STRICT	*8 ounces orange juice (2 Fruit)*
	1 whole wheat English muffin (2
	   Bread)
	   (omit egg)
	   (omit ham)
	1 cup skim milk (1 Milk)
		1 cup Bean Chili #1* (2 Meat, 2
		   Bread, 1 Fat, 1 Vegeta-
		   ble), see pp. 198–199
		1 whole wheat roll (1 Bread)
		   (omit margarine)

SUPPER	SNACKS
1 cup Shrimp Creole #1* (2 Meat, 1 Bread, 1 Vegetable), see pp. 189–190 1 cup brown rice (2 Bread) ½ cup yellow squash (1 Vegetable) 1 cup Citrus Spinach Salad* (1 Vegetable, 1 Fruit), see p. 214, with 1 tablespoon Ranch or French dressing (1 Fat)	Milkshake 1 cup skim milk (1 Milk) ½ cup frozen strawberries (1 Fruit) ½ banana (1 Fruit)
1 cup Shrimp Creole #1* (2 Meat, 1 Bread, 1 Vegetable), see pp. 189–190 1 cup brown rice (2 Bread) ½ cup yellow squash (1 Vegetable) *1 whole wheat roll (1 Bread)* 1 cup Citrus Spinach Salad* (1 Vegetable, 1 Fruit), see p. 214, with 1 tablespoon Ranch or French dressing (1 Fat)	Milkshake 1 cup skim milk (1 Milk) *1 cup frozen strawberries (2 Fruit)* *1 banana (2 Fruit)*
1 cup Shrimp Creole #1* (2 Meat, 1 Bread, 1 Vegetable), see pp. 189–190 1 cup brown rice (2 Bread) ½ cup yellow squash (1 Vegetable) *1 whole wheat roll (1 Bread)* 1 cup Citrus Spinach Salad* (1 Vegetable, 1 Fruit), see p. 214, with 1 tablespoon Ranch or French dressing (1 Fat)	Milkshake 1 cup skim milk (1 Milk) *1 cup frozen strawberries (2 Fruit)* *1 banana (2 Fruit)*

Week 2—Thursday

	BREAKFAST	LUNCH

BASIC	2 small Oatmeal or Whole Wheat Pancakes* (2 Bread), see pp. 225 or 226, with ½ cup blueberries (1 Fruit) and 1 tablespoon diet margarine (or 1 tablespoon light syrup) (1 Fat)
	1 cup skim milk (or 4 tablespoons skim ricotta cheese) (1 Milk)
		Tuna Sandwich
		  2 whole wheat bread slices (2 Bread)
		  ¾ cup tuna (4.5 ounces), water-packed (3 Meat) with 3 tablespoons diet mayonnaise (1 Fat)
		  and lettuce and 4 pickle slices (0)
		½ tomato, sliced (1 Vegetable)
		½ cup artichoke hearts marinated in oil-free Italian Salad Dressing (1 Vegetable), see pp. 218–219
		1 medium apple (2 Fruit)
		1 cup skim milk (1 Milk)

MODERATE	*4 ounces orange juice (1 Fruit)*
	3 small Oatmeal or Whole Wheat Pancakes (3 Bread), see pp. 225 or 226, with ½ cup blueberries (1 Fruit)*
	and 1 tablespoon diet margarine (or 1 tablespoon light syrup) (1 Fat)
	1 cup skim milk (or 4 tablespoons skim ricotta cheese) (1 Milk)
		Tuna Sandwich
		  2 whole wheat bread slices (2 Bread)
		  ½ cup tuna (3 ounces), water-packed (2 Meat) with 3 teaspoons diet mayonnaise (1 Fat)
		  and lettuce and 4 pickle slices (0)
		½ tomato, sliced (1 Vegetable)
		½ cup artichoke hearts marinated in oil-free Italian Salad Dressing (1 Vegetable), see pp. 218–219
		1 medium apple (2 Fruit)
		1 cup skim milk (1 Milk)

SUPPER   SNACKS

Nachos
    2 soft corn tortillas baked and
      broken into chips (2 Bread)
    topped with 1 ounce mozza-
      rella cheese, grated and
      melted (1 Meat)
    and ¼ cup green chili or
      jalapeno peppers (0)
Beef Chalupas
    2 soft corn or flour tortillas (2
      Bread)
    topped with 3 ounces lean
      ground beef, browned and
      drained (3 Meat); with 2
      teaspoons chili powder (0);
    ½ tomato, diced (1 Vegetable);
      onion and lettuce slices (0);
      and hot sauce (optional) (0)
1 cup raw vegetables (broccoli,
    carrots, cauliflower) (1
    Vegetable) with 1 tablespoon
    Ranch or Yogurt dressing
    (1 Fat)
½ cup seedless grapes (1 Fruit)

Nachos
    2 soft corn tortillas baked and
      broken into chips (2 Bread)
    topped with 1 ounce mozza-
      rella cheese, grated and
      melted (1 Meat)
    and ¼ cup green chili or
      jalapeno peppers (0)
Beef Chalupas
    2 soft corn or flour tortillas (2
      Bread)
    *topped with 2 ounces lean
      ground beef, browned and
      drained (2 Meat)*; with 2
      teaspoons chili powder (0);
    ½ tomato, diced (1 Vegetable);
      onion and lettuce slices (0);
      and hot sauce (optional) (0)
1 cup raw vegetables (broccoli,
    carrots, cauliflower) (1
    Vegetable)
    (omit dressing)
1 cup seedless grapes (2 Fruit)

Week 2—Thursday (cont'd)

	BREAKFAST	LUNCH
STRICT	8 ounces orange juice (2 Fruit) 3 small Oatmeal or Whole Wheat Pancakes* (3 Bread), see pp. 225 or 226, with ½ cup blueberries (1 Fruit) and 1 tablespoon diet margarine (or 1 tablespoon light syrup) (1 Fat) 1 cup skim milk (or 4 tablespoons skim ricotta cheese) (1 Milk)	Tuna Sandwich 2 whole wheat bread slices (2 Bread) ½ cup tuna (3 ounces), water-packed (2 Meat) with 3 teaspoons diet mayonnaise (1 Fat) and lettuce and 4 pickle slices (0) ½ tomato, sliced (1 Vegetable) ½ cup artichoke hearts marinated in oil-free Italian Salad Dressing (1 Vegetable), see pp. 218–219 1 medium apple (2 Fruit) 1 cup skim milk (1 Milk)

SUPPER	SNACKS

Nachos
    2 soft corn tortillas baked and
      broken into chips (2 Bread)
    topped with 1 ounce mozza-
      rella cheese, grated and
      melted (1 Meat)
    and ¼ cup green chili or
      jalapeno peppers (0)
Beef Chalupas
    2 soft corn or flour tortillas (2
      Bread)
    topped with 1 ounce lean ground
      beef, browned and drained
      (1 Meat); with 2 teaspoons
      chili powder (0);
    ½ tomato, diced (1 Vegetable);
    onion and lettuce slices (0);
    and hot sauce (optional) (0)
1 cup raw vegetables (broccoli,
    carrots, cauliflower) (1
    Vegetable)
    (omit dressing)
1 cup seedless grapes (2 Fruit)

Week 2—Friday

	BREAKFAST	LUNCH

BASIC	Peanut Butter Sandwich
	  2 whole wheat bread slices (2 Bread)
	  1 tablespoon peanut butter (1 Meat)
	  and ½ banana, sliced (1 Fruit)
	1 cup skim milk (1 Milk)
		Turkey Sandwich
		  2 whole wheat bread slices (2 Bread)
		  2 ounces turkey (2 Meat)
		  1 teaspoon mustard (0)
		  1 teaspoon mayonnaise (1 Fat)
		  and lettuce and tomato slices (0)
		1 large peach or apple (2 Fruit)
		1 cup skim milk (1 Milk)

MODERATE	*4 ounces orange juice (1 Fruit)*
	Peanut Butter Sandwich
	  2 whole wheat bread slices (2 Bread)
	  1 tablespoon peanut butter (1 Meat)
	  and ½ banana, sliced (1 Fruit)
	1 cup skim milk (1 Milk)
		Turkey Sandwich
		  2 whole wheat bread slices (2 Bread)
		  1 ounce turkey (1 Meat)
		  1 teaspoon mustard (0)
		  omit mayonnaise
		  and lettuce and tomato slices (0)
		1 large peach or apple (2 Fruit)
		25 salt-free pretzel sticks (1 Bread)
		1 cup skim milk (1 Milk)

STRICT	*8 ounces orange juice (2 Fruit)*
	Peanut Butter Sandwich
	  2 whole wheat bread slices (2 Bread)
	  1 tablespoon peanut butter (1 Meat)
	  and ½ banana, sliced (1 Fruit)
	1 cup skim milk (1 Milk)
		Turkey Sandwich
		  2 whole wheat bread slices (2 Bread)
		  1 ounce turkey (1 Meat)
		  1 teaspoon mustard (0)
		  omit mayonnaise
		  and lettuce and tomato slices (0)
		1 large peach or apple (2 Fruit)
		25 salt-free pretzel sticks (1 Bread)
		1 cup skim milk (1 Milk)

SUPPER   SNACKS

1 cup won ton soup (2 Bread)
1 cup steamed rice (2 Bread)
2 cups oriental chicken and stir-
    fried vegetables
  3 ounces chicken (skinless) (3
    Meat)
  2 cups mixed vegetables (4
    Vegetable)
  in 2 teaspoons oil (2 Fat)
*½ cup Seasonal Fruit Salad (1
    Fruit), see p. 218*

---

1 cup won ton soup (2 Bread)
1 cup steamed rice (2 Bread)
2 cups oriental chicken and stir-
    fried vegetables
  3 ounces chicken (skinless) (3
    Meat)
  2 cups mixed vegetables (4
    Vegetable)
  in 2 teaspoons oil (2 Fat)
*1 cup Seasonal Fruit Salad (2
    Fruit), see p. 218*

---

1 cup won ton soup (2 Bread)
1 cup steamed rice (2 Bread)
2 cups oriental chicken and stir-
    fried vegetables
  *2 ounces chicken (skinless) (2
    Meat)*
  2 cups mixed vegetables (4
    Vegetable)
  in 2 teaspoons oil (2 Fat)
*1 cup Seasonal Fruit Salad (2
    Fruit), see p. 218*

Week 2—Saturday

	BREAKFAST	LUNCH
BASIC	1 cup oatmeal (2 Bread) with 2 tablespoons raisins (1 Fruit) and 1 teaspoon margarine (or 1 tablespoon light syrup or 2 tablespoons honey or syrup) (1 Fat) 1 cup skim milk (1 Milk)	Vegetarian mini-pizzas 2 whole wheat English muffin halves (2 Bread) ¼ cup tomato sauce with ¼ cup sliced onions, green peppers, mushrooms (1 Vegetable) 1 ounce mozzarella cheese, grated and melted (1 Meat) 1 large orange or small grapefruit (2 Fruit) 1 cup skim milk (1 Milk)
MODERATE	*1 banana (2 Fruit)* 1 cup oatmeal (2 Bread) with 2 tablespoons raisins (1 Fruit) *(omit margarine, honey, or syrup)* 1 cup skim milk (1 Milk)	Vegetarian mini-pizzas *3 whole wheat English muffin halves (3 Bread)* ¼ cup tomato sauce with ¼ cup sliced onions, green peppers, mushrooms (1 Vegetable) 1 ounce mozzarella cheese, grated and melted (1 Meat) 1 large orange or small grapefruit (2 Fruit) 1 cup skim milk (1 Milk)
STRICT	*1 banana (2 Fruit)* 1 cup oatmeal (2 Bread) with 2 tablespoons raisins (1 Fruit) *(omit margarine, honey, or syrup)* 1 cup skim milk (1 Milk)	Vegetarian mini-pizzas *3 whole wheat English muffin halves (3 Bread)* ¼ cup tomato sauce with ¼ cup sliced onions, green peppers, mushrooms (1 Vegetable)

SUPPER	SNACKS
1 cup vegetable soup (1 Bread) 5 ounces Baked or Broiled Seafood* (5 Meat), see pp. 185 or 186 with lemon wedges (0) ½ cup red potatoes with skins (1 Bread) with 1 teaspoon margarine (1 Fat) 1 cup mixed vegetables (zucchini, carrots, broccoli, cauliflower) (2 Vegetable) with 1 teaspoon margarine (1 Fat) 1 tomato and lettuce salad (1 Vegetable) with 1 tablespoon herb vinegar (0) or lemon juice (0) 2 French bread slices (each slice, 3 inches long) (2 Bread) ½ cup raspberries (1 Fruit)	
1 cup vegetable soup (1 Bread) *4 ounces Baked or Broiled Seafood* (4 Meat), see pp. 185 or 186, with lemon wedges (0) ½ cup red potatoes with skins (1 Bread) with 1 teaspoon margarine (1 Fat) 1 cup mixed vegetables (zucchini, carrots, broccoli, cauliflower) (2 Vegetable) with 1 teaspoon margarine (1 Fat) 1 tomato and lettuce salad (1 Vegetable) with 1 tablespoon herb vinegar (0) or lemon juice (0) 2 French bread slices (each slice, 3 inches long) (2 Bread) ½ cup raspberries (1 Fruit)	
1 cup vegetable soup (1 Bread) *3 ounces Baked or Broiled Seafood* (3 Meat), see pp. 185 or 186, with lemon wedges (0) ½ cup red potatoes with skins (1 Bread) with 1 teaspoon	

Week 2—Saturday (cont'd)

BREAKFAST	LUNCH
	1 ounce mozzarella cheese, grated and melted (1 Meat)
	1 large orange or small grape-fruit (2 Fruit)
	1 cup skim milk (1 Milk)

SUPPER	SNACKS

margarine (1 Fat)

1 cup mixed vegetables (zucchini, carrots, broccoli, cauliflower) (2 Vegetable) with 1 teaspoon margarine (1 Fat)

1 tomato and lettuce salad (1 Vegetable) with 1 tablespoon herb vinegar (0) or lemon juice (0)

2 French bread slices (each slice, 3 inches long) (2 Bread)

1 cup raspberries (2 Fruit)

Week 2—Sunday

	BREAKFAST	LUNCH

BASIC	French Toast
	  2 whole wheat bread slices (2 Bread)
	  1 egg and 2 tablespoons skim milk, blended (1 Meat)
	Toppings
	  2 teaspoons honey or jelly (or 1 tablespoon light syrup) (1 Fat)
	  1 small apple, sliced and baked (1 Fruit)
	1 cup skim milk (1 Milk)
		Taco Salad
		  2 soft tortillas, baked and broken in chips (2 Bread)
		  2 cups lettuce salad (0)
		  ½ tomato, diced (1 Vegetable)
		  ½ cup pinto or kidney beans seasoned with 2 teaspoons chili powder (0) (1 Meat, 1 Bread)
		  1 ounce mozzarella cheese, shredded (1 Meat)
		  3 tablespoons hot sauce (0)
		  1 tablespoon Ranch dressing (1 Fat)
		1 cup seedless grapes (2 Fruit)

MODERATE	*4 ounces orange juice (1 Fruit)*
	French Toast
	  3 whole wheat bread slices (3 Bread)
	  1 egg and 2 tablespoons skim milk, blended (1 Meat)
	Toppings
	  2 teaspoons honey or jelly (or 1 tablespoon light syrup) (1 Fat)
	  1 small apple, sliced and baked (1 Fruit)
	1 cup skim milk (1 Milk)
		Taco Salad
		  2 soft tortillas, baked and broken in chips (2 Bread)
		  2 cups lettuce salad (0)
		  ½ tomato, diced (1 Vegetable)
		  ½ cup pinto or kidney beans seasoned with 2 teaspoons chili powder (0) (1 Meat, 1 Bread)
		  1 ounce mozzarella cheese, shredded (1 Meat)
		  3 tablespoons hot sauce (0)
		  (omit Ranch dressing)
		1 cup seedless grapes (2 Fruit)

STRICT	*8 ounces orange juice (2 Fruit)*
	French Toast
	  3 whole wheat bread slices (3 Bread) with ¼ cup egg substitute or 2 egg whites with 2 tablespoons skim milk, blended (1 Meat)
	Toppings
	  2 teaspoons honey or jelly (or 1 tablespoon light syrup) (1 Fat)
	  1 small apple, sliced and baked (1 Fruit)
	1 cup skim milk (1 Milk)
		Taco Salad
		  2 soft tortillas, baked and broken in chips (2 Bread)
		  2 cups lettuce salad (0)
		  ½ tomato, diced (1 Vegetable)
		  ½ cup pinto or kidney beans seasoned with 2 teaspoons chili powder (0) (1 Meat, 1 Bread)
		  1 ounce mozzarella cheese, shredded (1 Meat)
		  3 tablespoons hot sauce (0)
		  (omit Ranch dressing)
		1 cup seedless grapes (2 Fruit)

SUPPER   SNACKS

1 serving (4 × 4½-inch square) Spinach Lasagna #1* (2 Bread,
3 Meat, 2 Vegetable), see
pp. 215–216
½ of French bread roll (6 inches
long) (1 Bread) with 1
teaspoon margarine (1 Fat)
and ½ teaspoon garlic powder
seasoning (0)
½ cup carrots (1 Vegetable)
¼ cantaloupe (1 Fruit)
1 cup skim milk (1 Milk)

*1 serving (4 × 4½-inch square) Spin-
ach Lasagna #2* (2 Bread,
2 Meat, 2 Vegetable), see p.
216*
½ of French bread roll (6 inches
long) (1 Bread) with 1
teaspoon margarine (1 Fat)
and ½ teaspoon garlic powder
seasoning (0)
½ cup carrots (1 Vegetable)
½ cantaloupe (2 Fruit)
1 cup skim milk (1 Milk)

*1 serving (4 × 4½-inch square) Spin-
ach Lasagna #2* (2 Bread,
2 Meat, 2 Vegetable), see p.
216*
½ of French bread roll (6 inches
long) (1 Bread) with 1
teaspoon margarine (1 Fat)
and ½ teaspoon garlic powder
seasoning (0)
½ cup carrots (1 Vegetable)
½ cantaloupe (2 Fruit)
1 cup skim milk (1 Milk)

2,200-CALORIE MENUS

Week 1—Monday

	BREAKFAST	LUNCH

BASIC	½ grapefruit (1 Fruit)
	2 whole wheat toast (2 Bread) with 2 teaspoons margarine (2 Fat)
	1 cup skim milk (1 Milk)
		2 Tuna Sandwiches
		  4 whole wheat bread slices (4 Bread)
		  1 cup tuna (6 ounces), water-packed (4 Meat) with 2 tablespoons diet mayonnaise (2 Fat)
		  and lettuce and tomato slices (0)
		1 cup coleslaw with 1 teaspoon mayonnaise (2 Vegetable, 1 Fat)
		1 medium apple (2 Fruit)
		1 cup skim milk (1 Milk)

MODERATE	½ grapefruit (1 Fruit)
	2 whole wheat toast (2 Bread) with 2 teaspoons margarine (2 Fat)
	1 cup bran cereal (2 Bread)
	1 cup skim milk (1 Milk)
		2 Tuna Sandwiches
		  4 whole wheat bread slices (4 Bread)
		  ¾ cup tuna (4.5 ounces), water-packed (3 Meat) with 2 tablespoons diet mayonnaise (2 Fat)
		  and lettuce and tomato slices (0)
		1 cup coleslaw (2 Vegetable) *with 1 tablespoon lemon juice and 1 tablespoon vinegar (0)*
		1 medium apple (2 Fruit)
		1 cup skim milk (1 Milk)

STRICT	½ grapefruit (1 Fruit)
	2 whole wheat toast (2 Bread) *with 1 teaspoon margarine (1 Fat)*
	1 cup bran cereal (2 Bread)
	1 cup skim milk (1 Milk)
		2 Tuna Sandwiches
		  4 whole wheat bread slices (4 Bread)
		  ½ cup tuna (3 ounces), water-packed (2 Meat) with 1 tablespoon diet mayonnaise (1 Fat)
		  and lettuce and tomato slices (0)
		1 cup coleslaw (2 Vegetables) *with 1 tablespoon lemon juice and 1 tablespoon vinegar (0)*
		1 medium apple (2 Fruit)
		1 cup skim milk (1 Milk)

SUPPER	SNACKS
4 ounces Baked Chicken (skinless)* (4 Meat), see p. 177	3 cups popcorn (1½ tablespoons dry kernels), plain and air-popped (1 Bread)
1 medium baked potato (2 Bread) with 2 teaspoons margarine (2 Fat)	8 ounces orange juice (2 Fruit)
¾ cup carrots (1½ Vegetable)	
¾ cup green beans (1½ Vegetable)	
1 tomato and lettuce salad (1 Vegetable) with 1 tablespoon Ranch or French dressing (1 Fat)	
3 whole wheat rolls (3 Bread)	
1 cup pineapple, fresh or unsweetened (2 Fruit)	
3 ounces Baked Chicken (skinless) (3 Meat), see p. 177*	3 cups popcorn (1½ tablespoons dry kernels), plain and air-popped (1 Bread)
1 medium baked potato (2 Bread) *with 1 teaspoon margarine (1 Fat)*	*12 ounces orange juice (3 Fruit)*
¾ cup carrots (1½ Vegetable)	
¾ cup green beans (1½ Vegetable)	
1 tomato and lettuce salad (1 Vegetable) with 1 tablespoon Ranch or French dressing (1 Fat)	
3 whole wheat rolls (3 Bread)	
1 cup pineapple, fresh or unsweetened (2 Fruit)	
2 ounces Baked Chicken (skinless) (2 Meat), see p. 177*	*9 cups popcorn (4½ tablespoons dry kernels), plain and air-popped (1 Bread)*
1 medium baked potato (2 Bread) *with 1 teaspoon margarine (1 Fat)*	*12 ounces orange juice (3 Fruit)*
¾ cup carrots (1½ Vegetable)	
¾ cup green beans (1½ Vegetable)	
1 tomato and lettuce salad (1 Vegetable) with 1 tablespoon Ranch or French dressing (1 Fat)	
3 whole wheat rolls (3 Bread)	
1 cup pineapple, fresh or unsweetened (2 Fruit)	

Week 1—Tuesday

	BREAKFAST	LUNCH

BASIC	½ cantaloupe (2 Fruit)
	2 whole wheat English muffins (4 Bread) with 2 teaspoons margarine (or 2 tablespoons apple butter) (2 Fat)
	1 cup skim milk (1 Milk)
		2 Turkey Sandwiches
		  4 whole wheat bread slices (4 Bread)
		  4 ounces turkey (4 Meat)
		  2 teaspoons mayonnaise (2 Fat)
		  and lettuce and tomato slices (0)
		2 cups raw vegetables (2 Vegetable)
		1 medium pear (2 Fruit)
		1 cup skim milk (1 Milk)

MODERATE	½ cantaloupe (2 Fruit)
	2 whole wheat English muffins (4 Bread) with 2 teaspoons margarine (or 2 tablespoons apple butter) (2 Fat)
	1 cup skim milk (1 Milk)
		2 Turkey Sandwiches
		  4 whole wheat bread slices (4 Bread)
		  3 ounces turkey (3 Meat)
		  2 teaspoons mayonnaise (2 Fat)
		  and lettuce and tomato slices (0)
		2 cups raw vegetables (2 Vegetable)
		1 medium pear (2 Fruit)
		1 cup skim milk (1 Milk)

STRICT	½ cantaloupe (2 Fruit)
	2 whole wheat English muffins (4 Bread) with 1 teaspoon margarine (or 1 tablespoon apple butter) (1 Fat)
	1 cup skim milk (1 Milk)
		2 cups vegetable soup (2 Bread)
		1 Turkey Sandwich
		  2 whole wheat bread slices (2 Bread)
		  1 ounce turkey (1 Meat)
		  1 teaspoon mayonnaise (1 Fat)
		  and lettuce and tomato slices (0)
		2 cups raw vegetables (2 Vegetable)
		1 medium pear (2 Fruit)
		1 cup skim milk (1 Milk)

SUPPER   SNACKS

4 ounces Baked Seafood Sea-
     soned With Mixed Vege-
     tables* (4 Meat,
     2 Vegetable), see p. 185
1 cup Carrot Raisin Salad* (2
     Vegetable, 2 Fruit, 2 Fat),
     see p. 209
1 corn-on-the-cob or 1 cup corn
     (2 Bread) with 1 teaspoon
     margarine (1 Fat)
½ cup green peas (1 Bread)
1 whole wheat roll (1 Bread)
     with 1 teaspoon margarine
     (1 Fat)
½ cup seedless grapes (1 Fruit)

---

*3 ounces Baked Seafood Seasoned
     With Mixed Vegetables* (3
     Meat, 2 Vegetable), see p.
     185*
1 cup Carrot Raisin Salad* (2
     Vegetable, 2 Fruit, 2 Fat),
     see p. 209
1 corn-on-the-cob or 1 cup corn
     (2 Bread)
     (omit margarine)
1 cup green peas (2 Bread)
2 whole wheat rolls (2 Bread)
     (omit margarine)
1 cup seedless grapes (2 Fruit)

---

3 ounces Baked Seafood Seasoned   *1 bagel (2 Bread)*
     With Mixed Vegetables (3*
     Meat, 2 Vegetable), see p.
     185
1 cup Carrot Raisin Salad* (2
     Vegetable, 2 Fruit, 2 Fat),
     see p. 209
1 corn-on-the-cob or 1 cup corn
     (2 Bread)
     (omit margarine)
1 cup green peas (2 Bread)
2 whole wheat rolls (2 Bread)
     (omit margarine)
1 cup seedless grapes (2 Fruit)

Week 1—Wednesday

	BREAKFAST	LUNCH

BASIC	1 banana (2 Fruit)
	2 cups oat bran cereal (4 Bread)
	   with 2 tablespoons raisins
	   (1 Fruit)
	1 cup skim milk (1 Milk)
		Pasta Salad #4* (2 Bread, 2
		   Vegetable, 3 Meat, 4 Fat),
		   see pp. 212–213
		1½ cups Seasonal Fruit Salad (3
		   Fruit), see p. 218
		1 cup skim milk (1 Milk)

MODERATE	1 banana (2 Fruit)
	2 cups oat bran cereal (4 Bread)
	   with 2 tablespoons raisins
	   (1 Fruit)
	1 cup skim milk (1 Milk)
		Pasta Salad #5* (3 Bread, 2
		   Vegetable, 2 Meat, 4 Fat),
		   see p. 213
		1½ cups Seasonal Fruit Salad (3
		   Fruit), see p. 218
		1 cup skim milk (1 Milk)

STRICT	1 banana (2 Fruit)
	2 cups oat bran cereal (4 Bread)
	   with 2 tablespoons raisins
	   (1 Fruit)
	1 cup skim milk (1 Milk)
		Pasta Salad #6* (3 Bread, 2
		   Vegetable, 4 Fat), see pp.
		   213–214
		1½ cups Seasonal Fruit Salad (3
		   Fruit), see p. 218
		2 whole wheat rolls (2 Bread)
		1 cup skim milk (1 Milk)

SUPPER   SNACKS

2 soft tortillas topped with hot
    sauce (2 Bread)
3 Mexican Fajitas #2* (4 ounces
    meat) (3 Bread, 4 Meat, 1
    Vegetable), see p. 197
½ cup Pinto Beans #1* (1 Bread,
    1 Meat, 1 Vegetable, 2
    Fat), see p. 203
1 raw carrot (1 Vegetable)
½ cup raw bell pepper (1 Vege-
    table) with 2 tablespoons
    Ranch dressing as dip (2
    Fat)
¾ cup strawberries (1 Fruit)

*3 soft tortillas topped with hot
    sauce (3 Bread)*
3 Mexican Fajitas #3 (3 ounces
    meat) (3 Bread, 3 Meat, 1
    Vegetable), see p. 198*
½ cup Pinto Beans #1* (1 Bread,
    1 Meat, 1 Vegetable, 2
    Fat), see p. 203
1 raw carrot (1 Vegetable)
½ cup raw bell pepper
    (1 Vegetable)
(omit dip)
1½ cups strawberries (2 Fruit)

*3 soft tortillas topped with hot
    sauce (3 Bread)*
3 Mexican Fajitas #3 (3 ounces
    meat) (3 Bread, 3 Meat, 1
    Vegetable), see p. 198*
½ cup Pinto Beans #2* (1 Bread,
    1 Meat, 1 Vegetable), see
    p. 203
1 raw carrot (1 Vegetable)
½ cup raw bell pepper
    (1 Vegetable)
(omit dip)
1½ cups strawberries (2 Fruit)

Week 1—Thursday

	BREAKFAST	LUNCH
BASIC	8 ounces orange juice (2 Fruit) 2 Homemade Cheese Danish Rolls* (2 Bread, 1 Meat, 1 Fruit), see p. 225 1 cup skim milk (1 Milk)	2½ cups Cajun Beans #2* (2 Bread, 2 Meat, 1 Vegetable, 2 Fat), see pp. 200–201 1 cup brown rice (2 Bread) 1 tomato and lettuce salad (1 Vegetable) with 1 tablespoon Italian Salad Dressing (2 Fat), see pp. 218–219 1 Cornbread Muffin* (1 Bread, 1 Fat), see pp. 223–224, with 1 teaspoon margarine (1 Fat) 1 large orange (2 Fruit) 1 cup skim milk (1 Milk)
MODERATE	*12 ounces orange juice (3 Fruit)* 2 Homemade Cheese Danish Rolls* (2 Bread, 1 Meat, 1 Fruit), see p. 225 1 cup skim milk (1 Milk)	2½ cups Cajun Beans #2* (2 Bread, 2 Meat, 1 Vegetable, 2 Fat), see pp. 200–201 1 cup brown rice (2 Bread) 1 tomato and lettuce salad (1 Vegetable) *with 1 tablespoon herb vinegar (0)* *2 Cornbread Muffins* (2 Bread, 2 Fat), see pp. 223–224 (omit margarine)* 1 large orange (2 Fruit) 1 cup skim milk (1 Milk)
STRICT	*12 ounces orange juice (3 Fruit)* 2 Homemade Cheese Danish Rolls* (2 Bread, 1 Meat, 1 Fruit), see p. 225 1 cup skim milk (1 Milk)	*3 cups Cajun Beans #1* (2 Bread, 2 Meat, 1 Vegetable), see p. 200* *1½ cup brown rice (3 Bread)* 1 tomato and lettuce salad (1 Vegetable) *with 1 tablespoon herb vinegar (0)* *2 Cornbread Muffins* (2 Bread, 2 Fat), see pp.223–224 (omit margarine)* 1 large orange (2 Fruit) 1 cup skim milk (1 Milk)

SUPPER	SNACKS

1½ cups pasta (3 Bread)
1 cup Easy Meat Sauce #1 (4
    ounces meat, 1 cup to-
    mato sauce)* (4 Meat, 1
    Bread), see pp. 194–195
3 tablespoons Parmesan cheese
    (1 Meat)
2 cups stir-fried vegetables (zuc-
    chini, carrots, cauliflower,
    broccoli) in 2 teaspoons olive
    oil (4 Vegetable, 2 Fat)
1 Italian bread slice (3 inches
    long) (1 Bread)
1 medium apple, fresh or baked
    (2 Fruit)

2 cups pasta (4 Bread)
1 cup Easy Meat Sauce #3 (3
    ounces meat, 1 cup tomato
    sauce) (3 Meat, 1 Bread),*
    see p. 195
(omit cheese)
2 cups stir-fried vegetables (zuc-
    chini, carrots, cauliflower,
    broccoli) in 2 teaspoons olive
    oil (4 Vegetable, 2 Fat)
1 Italian bread slice (3 inches
    long) (1 Bread)
1 medium apple, fresh or baked
    (2 Fruit)

2 cups pasta (4 Bread)
1 cup Easy Meat Sauce #4 (1
    ounce meat, 1 cup tomato
    sauce) (1 Meat, 1 Bread),*
    see pp. 195–196
(omit cheese)
2 cups stir-fried vegetables (zuc-
    chini, carrots, cauliflower,
    broccoli) in 2 teaspoons olive
    oil (4 Vegetable, 2 Fat)
2 Italian bread slices (each slice,
    3 inches long) (2 Bread)
1 medium apple, fresh or baked
    (2 Fruit)

Week 1—Friday

	BREAKFAST	LUNCH

BASIC	8 ounces orange juice (2 Fruit)
	1 banana (2 Fruit)
	1 pumpernickel bagel (2 Bread)
	    with 1 teaspoon margarine
	    (1 Fat)
	1 cup skim milk (1 Milk)
		2 cups vegetable soup (2 Bread)
		1 Stuffed Tomato
		    1 tomato (1 Vegetable)
		    ¾ cup tuna (4.5 ounces),
		      water-packed (3 Meat)
		      with 3 teaspoons mayon-
		      naise (3 Fat)
		8 melba toast (2 Bread)
		1 medium apple (2 Fruit)
		1 cup skim milk (1 Milk)

MODERATE	8 ounces orange juice (2 Fruit)
	1 banana (2 Fruit)
	2 pumpernickel bagels (4 Bread)
	    (omit margarine)
	1 cup skim milk (1 Milk)
		2 cups vegetable soup (2 Bread)
		1 Stuffed Tomato
		    1 tomato (1 Vegetable)
		    ½ cup tuna (3 ounces), water-
		      packed (2 Meat) with 2
		      teaspoons mayonnaise (2 Fat)
		8 melba toast (2 Bread)
		1 medium apple (2 Fruit)
		1 cup skim milk (1 Milk)

STRICT	8 ounces orange juice (2 Fruit)
	1 banana (2 Fruit)
	2 pumpernickel bagels (4 Bread)
	    (omit margarine)
	1 cup skim milk (1 Milk)
		2 cups vegetable soup (2 Bread)
		1 Stuffed Tomato
		    1 tomato (1 Vegetable)
		    ½ cup tuna (3 ounces), water-
		      packed (2 Meat) with 2
		      teaspoons mayonnaise (2 Fat)
		8 melba toast (2 Bread)
		1 medium apple (2 Fruit)
		1 cup skim milk (1 Milk)

SUPPER	SNACKS
5 ounces Grilled or Poached Salmon* (5 Meat), see pp. 188 or 188–189 ½ cup rice with 1 teaspoon margarine (1 Bread, 1 Fat) 1 cup spinach with 1 teaspoon margarine (2 Vegetable, 1 Fat) 1 cup yellow squash or carrots with 1 teaspoon margarine (2 Vegetable, 1 Fat) 2 whole wheat rolls (2 Bread) with 1 teaspoon margarine (1 Fat) 1 3-inch slice Angel Food Cake* (1 Bread), see pp. 226–227 topped with ½ cup fruit, fresh or unsweetened (1 Fruit)	4 graham cracker squares (2 Bread) 1 cup raw vegetables (1 Vegetable)
4 ounces Grilled or Poached Salmon (4 Meat), see pp. 188 or 188–189* ½ cup rice with 1 teaspoon margarine (1 Bread, 1 Fat) 1 cup spinach with 1 teaspoon margarine (2 Vegetable, 1 Fat) 1 cup yellow squash or carrots with 1 teaspoon margarine (2 Vegetable, 1 Fat) 2 whole wheat rolls (2 Bread) with 1 teaspoon margarine (1 Fat) 1 3-inch slice Angel Food Cake* (1 Bread), see pp. 226–227 *topped with 1 cup fruit, fresh or unsweetened (2 Fruit)*	4 graham cracker squares (2 Bread) 1 cup raw vegetables (1 Vegetable)
2 ounces Grilled or Poached Salmon (2 Meat), see pp. 188 or 188–189* ½ cup rice (1 Bread) *(omit margarine)* 1 cup spinach with 1 teaspoon margarine (2 Vegetable, 1 Fat) 1 cup yellow squash or carrots with 1 teaspoon margarine (2 Vegetable, 1 Fat)	*8 graham cracker squares (4 Bread)* 1 cup raw vegetables (1 Vegetable)

Week 1—Friday (cont'd)

BREAKFAST	LUNCH

SUPPER   SNACKS

2 whole wheat rolls (2 Bread)
    (omit margarine)
1 3-inch slice Angel Food Cake*
    (1 Bread), see pp. 226–227
    topped with 1 cup fruit, fresh or
    unsweetened (2 Fruit)

Week 1—Saturday

	BREAKFAST	LUNCH
BASIC	4 ounces orange juice (1 Fruit) 1 banana (2 Fruit) 1½ cups oatmeal (3 Bread) with 2 tablespoons raisins (1 Fruit) 1 whole wheat toast (1 Bread) with 1 teaspoon margarine (1 Fat) 1 cup skim milk (1 Milk)	1 cup minestrone soup (1 Bread) 1 large tomato and lettuce salad (2 Vegetable) with 2 tablespoons Ranch dressing (2 Fat) 1 medium baked potato (2 Bread) with 2 teaspoons margarine (or 2 tablespoons Ranch dressing) (2 Fat) or picante sauce (0) 8 whole wheat crackers or melba toast (2 Bread) 1 large orange (2 Fruit) 1 cup skim milk (1 Milk)
MODERATE	*8 ounces orange juice (2 Fruit)* 1 banana (2 Fruit) 1½ cups oatmeal (3 Bread) with 2 tablespoons raisins (1 Fruit) *2 whole wheat toast (2 Bread)* with 1 teaspoon margarine (1 Fat) 1 cup skim milk (1 Milk)	1 cup minestrone soup (1 Bread) 1 large tomato and lettuce salad (2 Vegetable) with 2 tablespoons Ranch dressing (2 Fat) 1 medium baked potato (2 Bread) with 2 teaspoons margarine (or 2 tablespoons Ranch dressing) (2 Fat) or picante sauce (0) 8 whole wheat crackers or melba toast (2 Bread) *1 large fresh orange (2 Fruit)* 1 cup skim milk (1 Milk)
STRICT	*8 ounces orange juice (2 Fruit)* 1 banana (2 Fruit) 1½ cups oatmeal (3 Bread) with 2 tablespoons raisins (1 Fruit) *2 whole wheat toast (2 Bread)* with 1 teaspoon margarine (1 Fat) 1 cup skim milk (1 Milk)	1 cup minestrone soup (1 Bread) 1 large tomato and lettuce salad (2 Vegetable) with 2 tablespoons Ranch dressing (2 Fat) 1 medium baked potato (2 Bread) *with lemon juice (0)* *or picante sauce (0)* 8 whole wheat crackers or melba toast (2 Bread) 1 large orange (2 Fruit) 1 cup skim milk (1 Milk)

SUPPER	SNACKS

8 ounces Broiled Seafood* (8
    Meat), see p. 186, with
    lemon wedges (0)
1 cup pasta (2 Bread) with ¾
    cup Marinara Sauce* (2
    Vegetable), see pp. 221–222
½ cup stir-fried mixed vegeta-
    bles in 1 teaspoon oil (1
    Vegetable, 1 Fat)
1 tomato and lettuce salad (1
    Vegetable) with 2 table-
    spoons Ranch dressing (2
    Fat)
1 French or Italian bread slice
    (3 inches long)
    (1 Bread)
½ cup berries (1 Fruit)

6 ounces Broiled Seafood (6
    Meat), see p. 186, with
    lemon wedges (0)*
1 cup pasta (2 Bread) with ¾
    cup Marinara Sauce* (2
    Vegetable), see pp. 221–222
½ cup stir-fried mixed vegeta-
    bles in 1 teaspoon oil (1
    Vegetable, 1 Fat)
1 tomato and lettuce salad (1
    Vegetable) *with 1 table-
    spoon herb vinegar (0)
    or lemon (0)*
2 *French or Italian bread slices
    (each slice 3 inches long)
    (2 Bread)*
½ cup berries (1 Fruit)

4 ounces Broiled Seafood (4
    Meat), see p. 186, with
    lemon wedges (0)*
1 cup pasta (2 Bread) with ¾
    cup Marinara Sauce* (2
    Vegetable), see pp. 221–222
½ cup stir-fried mixed vegeta-
    bles in 1 teaspoon oil (1
    Vegetable, 1 Fat)
1 tomato and lettuce salad (1
    Vegetable) *with 1 table-
    spoon herb vinegar (0)
    or lemon (0)*

*1 cup homemade trail mix of
    cereals: Shredded Wheat,
    Bran Chex, Wheat Chex,
    Corn Chex, pretzels (2
    Bread)*

Week 1—Saturday (cont'd)

BREAKFAST	LUNCH

SUPPER	SNACKS

2 French or Italian bread slices
  (each slice 3 inches long)
  (2 Bread)
½ cup berries (1 Fruit)

Week 1—Sunday

	BREAKFAST	LUNCH
BASIC	8 ounces orange juice (2 Fruit) 1 banana (2 Fruit) 3 Oat Bran Muffins* (3 Bread), see p. 224 1 cup skim milk (1 Milk)	6 ounces Hawaiian Chicken #1* (6 Meat, 1 Fruit, 1 Fat), see pp. 181–182 1 cup wild rice with 2 teaspoons margarine (2 Bread, 2 Fat) 1 cup broccoli with 1 teaspoon margarine (2 Vegetable, 1 Fat) 1 tomato and lettuce salad (1 Vegetable) with 1 tablespoon French or Ranch dressing (1 Fat) 2 whole wheat rolls (2 Bread) with 2 teaspoons margarine (2 Fat) ½ cup peach slices (1 Fruit)
MODERATE	8 ounces orange juice (2 Fruit) 1 banana (2 Fruit) 3 Oat Bran Muffins* (3 Bread), see p. 224 1 cup skim milk (1 Milk)	6 ounces Hawaiian Chicken #1* (6 Meat, 1 Fruit, 1 Fat), see pp. 181–182 1 cup wild rice with 2 teaspoons margarine (2 Bread, 2 Fat) 1 cup broccoli with 1 teaspoon margarine (2 Vegetable, 1 Fat) 1 tomato and lettuce salad (1 Vegetable) with 1 tablespoon French or Ranch dressing (1 Fat) 2 whole wheat rolls (2 Bread) *with 1 teaspoon margarine (1 Fat)* ½ cup peach slices (1 Fruit)
STRICT	8 ounces orange juice (2 Fruit) 1 banana (2 Fruit) 3 Oat Bran Muffins* (3 Bread), see p. 224 1 cup skim milk (1 Milk)	*4 ounces Hawaiian Chicken #3* (4 Meat, 1 Fruit, 1 Fat), see pp. 182–183* 1 cup wild rice with 2 teaspoons margarine (2 Bread, 2 Fat) 1 cup broccoli with 1 teaspoon margarine (2 Vegetable, 1 Fat) 1 tomato and lettuce salad (1 Vegetable) with 1 tablespoon French or Ranch dressing (1 Fat) 2 whole wheat rolls (2 Bread) *with 1 teaspoon margarine (1 Fat)* ½ cup peach slices (1 Fruit)

SUPPER	SNACKS
2 whole wheat pita pockets (4 Bread)	25 unsalted pretzel sticks (1 Bread)
one filled with 1 cup steamed mixed vegetables (2 Vegetable)	
one filled with 2 ounces turkey (2 Meat) with 1 teaspoon mayonnaise (1 Fat)	
and lettuce and tomato slices (0)	
1 raw carrot (1 Vegetable)	
½ cup seedless grapes (1 Fruit)	
1 cup skim milk (1 Milk)	
2 whole wheat pita pockets (4 Bread)	*6 graham cracker squares (3 Bread)*
each filled with 1 cup steamed mixed vegetables (2 Vegetable)	*(omit pretzels)*
(omit mayonnaise, lettuce and tomato)	
(omit turkey)	
1 raw carrot (1 Vegetable)	
1 cup seedless grapes (2 Fruit)	
1 cup skim milk (1 Milk)	
2 whole wheat pita pockets (4 Bread)	*10 graham cracker squares (5 Bread)*
each filled with 1 cup steamed mixed vegetables (2 Vegetable)	*(omit pretzels)*
(omit mayonnaise, lettuce and tomato)	
(omit turkey)	
1 raw carrot (1 Vegetable)	
1 cup seedless grapes (2 Fruit)	
1 cup skim milk (1 Milk)	

Week 2—Monday

	BREAKFAST	LUNCH
BASIC	4 ounces orange juice (1 Fruit) ½ cantaloupe (2 Fruit) 2 pumpernickel or whole wheat bagels (4 Bread) 1 cup skim milk (or 4 tablespoons skim ricotta cheese on bagels) (1 Milk)	2 cups Gumbo* (2 Meat, 2 Bread), see p. 204 6 shrimp (1 Meat) with 1 tablespoon cocktail sauce (0) or fresh lemon (0) 1 large tomato and lettuce salad (2 Vegetable) with 2 tablespoons herb vinegar (0) or lemon juice (0) 8 melba toast (2 Bread) 1 large apple (2 Fruit)
MODERATE	*8 ounces orange juice (2 Fruit)* ½ cantaloupe (2 Fruit) 2 pumpernickel or whole wheat bagels (4 Bread) 1 cup skim milk (or 4 tablespoons skim ricotta cheese on bagels) (1 Milk)	2 cups Gumbo* (2 Meat, 2 Bread), see p. 204 6 shrimp (1 Meat) with 1 tablespoon cocktail sauce (0) or fresh lemon (0) 1 large tomato and lettuce salad (2 Vegetable) with 2 tablespoons herb vinegar (0) or lemon juice (0) 8 melba toast (2 Bread) 1 large apple (2 Fruit)
STRICT	*8 ounces orange juice (2 Fruit)* ½ cantaloupe (2 Fruit) 2 pumpernickel or whole wheat bagels (4 Bread) 1 cup skim milk (or 4 tablespoons skim ricotta cheese on bagels) (1 Milk)	2 cups Gumbo* (2 Meat, 2 Bread), see p. 204 *(omit shrimp and sauce)* 1 large tomato and lettuce salad (2 Vegetable) with 2 tablespoons herb vinegar (0) or lemon juice (0) 8 melba toast (2 Bread) 1 large apple (2 Fruit)

SUPPER	SNACKS
5 ounces Barbecued Chicken (skinless)* (5 Meat, 1 Fat), see pp. 180 and 220 ½ cup Potato Salad* (1 Bread, 1 Fat) see p. 210 1 corn-on-the-cob or 1 cup corn (2 Bread) 1½ cups coleslaw with 3 tablespoons diet mayonnaise (3 Vegetable, 3 Fat) 1 whole wheat roll (1 Bread) ½ tomato, sliced (1 Vegetable) 1 banana, frozen (2 Fruit)	1 cup skim milk (1 Milk)
3 ounces Barbecued Chicken (skinless) (3 Meat, 1 Fat), see pp. 180 and 220 ½ cup Potato Salad* (1 Bread, 1 Fat) see p. 210 1 corn-on-the-cob or 1 cup corn (2 Bread) 1½ cups coleslaw with 4 teaspoons diet mayonnaise (3 Vegetable, 2 Fat) 1 whole wheat roll (1 Bread) ½ tomato, sliced (1 Vegetable) 1 banana, frozen (2 Fruit)*	1 cup skim milk (1 Milk) *1 cinnamon raisin English muffin, toasted (2 Bread)*
2 ounces Barbecued Chicken (skinless) (2 Meat, 1 Fat), see pp. 180 and 220 ½ cup Potato Salad* (1 Bread, 1 Fat) see p. 210 1 corn-on-the-cob or 1 cup corn (2 Bread) 1½ cups coleslaw (3 Vegetable) with 3 tablespoons lemon juice (0) and 3 tablespoons vinegar (0) 1 whole wheat roll (1 Bread) ½ tomato, sliced (1 Vegetable) 1 banana, frozen (2 Fruit)*	1 cup skim milk (1 Milk) *2 cinnamon raisin English muffins, toasted (4 Bread)*

Week 2—Tuesday

	BREAKFAST	LUNCH

BASIC	½ grapefruit (1 Fruit)
	3 Oat Bran Muffins* (3 Bread), see p. 224
	1 cup skim milk (1 Milk)
		1 cup lentil soup (1 Meat, 1 Bread, 1 Vegetable)
		Turkey Sandwich
		  2 whole wheat bread slices (2 Bread)
		  3 ounces turkey (3 Meat)
		  2 teaspoons mayonnaise (2 Fat)
		  and lettuce and tomato slices (0)
		1 large pear (2 Fruit)
		1 cup skim milk (1 Milk)

MODERATE	*1 grapefruit (2 Fruit)*
	3 Oat Bran Muffins* (3 Bread), see p. 224
	1 cup skim milk (1 Milk)
		1 cup lentil soup (1 Meat, 1 Bread, 1 Vegetable)
		Turkey Sandwich
		  2 whole wheat bread slices (2 Bread)
		  2 ounces turkey (2 Meat)
		  2 teaspoons mayonnaise (2 Fat)
		  and lettuce and tomato slices (0)
		1 large pear (2 Fruit)
		1 cup skim milk (1 Milk)

STRICT	*1 grapefruit (2 Fruit)*
	3 Oat Bran Muffins* (3 Bread), see p. 224
	1 cup skim milk (1 Milk)
		1 cup lentil soup (1 Meat, 1 Bread, 1 Vegetable)
		Turkey Sandwich
		  2 whole wheat bread slices (2 Bread)
		  1 ounce turkey (1 Meat)
		  (omit mayonnaise)
		  and lettuce and tomato slices (0)
		1 large pear (2 Fruit)
		1 cup skim milk (1 Milk)

SUPPER

Shishkabob #3* (4 Meat, 2 Vegetable, 4 Fat), see p. 193
1 cup brown or wild rice (2 Bread) seasoned with ½ cup mushrooms and onions (1 Vegetable)
2 whole wheat rolls (2 Bread)
1 large tomato and lettuce salad (2 Vegetable) with 2 tablespoons Ranch or buttermilk dressing (2 Fat)
1 cup pineapple, fresh or unsweetened (2 Fruit)

SNACKS

1 snack box (1.5 ounces) raisins (2 Fruit)
1 cup cereal mix of Shredded Wheat, Wheat Chex, Bran Chex, Rice Chex, Corn Chex (2 Bread)

Shishkabob #4* (3 Meat, 2 Vegetable, 2 Fat), see p. 193
1 cup brown or wild rice (2 Bread) seasoned with ½ cup mushrooms and onions (1 Vegetable)
2 whole wheat rolls (2 Bread)
1 large tomato and lettuce salad (2 Vegetable) with 2 tablespoons Ranch or buttermilk dressing (2 Fat)
1 cup fresh or unsweetened pineapple (2 Fruit)

1 snack box (1.5 ounces) raisins (2 Fruit)
1 bagel (2 Bread)
1 cup cereal mix of Shredded Wheat, Wheat Chex, Bran Chex, Rice Chex, Corn Chex (2 Bread)

Shishkabob #5* (2 Meat, 2 Vegetable, 2 Fat), see p. 194
1 cup brown or wild rice (2 Bread) seasoned with ½ cup mushrooms and onions (1 Vegetable)
2 whole wheat rolls (2 Bread)
1 large tomato and lettuce salad (2 Vegetable) with 2 tablespoons Ranch or buttermilk dressing (2 Fat)
1 cup pineapple, fresh or unsweetened (2 Fruit)

1 snack box (1.5 ounces) raisins (2 Fruit)
1 bagel (2 Bread)
2 cup cereal mix of Shredded Wheat, Wheat Chex, Bran Chex, Rice Chex, Corn Chex (4 Bread)

Week 2—Wednesday

	BREAKFAST	LUNCH
BASIC	4 ounces orange juice (1 Fruit) Egg and Muffin Sandwich 1 whole wheat English muffin (2 Bread) 1 poached egg (1 Meat) 1 ounce turkey ham (1 Meat) 1 cup skim milk (1 Milk)	2 cups Bean Chili #1* (4 Meat, 4 Bread, 2 Fat, 2 Vegeta- ble), see pp. 198–199 1 whole wheat roll (1 Bread) with 1 teaspoon margarine (1 Fat) 1 cup Seasonal Fruit Salad (2 Fruit), see p. 218
MODERATE	*8 ounces orange juice (2 Fruit)* Egg and Muffin Sandwich 1 whole wheat English muffin (2 Bread) 1 poached egg (1 Meat) *(omit ham)* 1 cup skim milk (1 Milk)	*2 cups Bean Chili #2* (3 Meat, 4 Bread, 2 Fat, 2 Vegeta- ble),* see p. 199 1 whole wheat roll (1 Bread) with 1 teaspoon margarine (1 Fat) 1 cup Seasonal Fruit Salad (2 Fruit), see p. 218
STRICT	*8 ounces orange juice (2 Fruit)* 1 whole wheat English muffin (2 Bread) *(omit egg)* *(omit ham)* 1 cup skim milk (1 Milk)	*2 cups Bean Chili #3* (3 Meat, 4 Bread, 1 Fat, 2 Vegeta- ble),* see pp. 199–200 *3 whole wheat rolls (3 Bread)* with 1 teaspoon margarine (1 Fat) 1 cup Seasonal Fruit Salad (2 Fruit), see p. 218

SUPPER

1 cup Shrimp Creole #2* (2
   Meat, 1 Bread, 1 Vegetable, 2 Fat), see p. 190
1 cup brown rice (2 Bread)
1 cup yellow squash (2 Vegetable) with 1 teaspoon margarine (1 Fat)
2 whole wheat rolls (2 Bread)
   with 1 teaspoon margarine
   (1 Fat)
1 cup Citrus Spinach Salad* (1
   Vegetable, 1 Fruit), see
   p. 214 with 1 tablespoon
   Ranch or French dressing
   (1 Fat)

SNACKS

Milkshake
   1 cup skim milk (1 Milk)
   ½ cup frozen strawberries (1
      Fruit)
   1 banana (2 Fruit)

---

1 cup Shrimp Creole #3 (2
   Meat, 1 Bread, 1 Vegetable, 1 Fat), see p. 190*
1 cup brown rice (2 Bread)
1 cup yellow squash (2 Vegetable) with 1 teaspoon margarine (1 Fat)
2 whole wheat rolls (2 Bread)
   (omit margarine)
1 cup Citrus Spinach Salad* (1
   Vegetable, 1 Fruit), see
   p. 214 with 1 tablespoon
   Ranch or French dressing
   (1 Fat)

Milkshake
   1 cup skim milk (1 Milk)
   ½ cup frozen strawberries (1
      Fruit)
   1 banana (2 Fruit)
   *4 graham cracker squares (2
      Bread)*

---

1 cup Shrimp Creole #4 (1
   Meat, 1 Bread, 1 Vegetable, 1 Fat), see pp. 190–191*
1 cup brown rice (2 Bread)
1 cup yellow squash (2 Vegetable)
   (omit margarine)
2 whole wheat rolls (2 Bread)
   (omit margarine)
1 cup Citrus Spinach Salad* (1
   Vegetable, 1 Fruit), see
   p. 214 with 1 tablespoon
   Ranch or French dressing
   (1 Fat)

Milkshake
   1 cup skim milk (1 Milk)
   ½ cup frozen strawberries (1
      Fruit)
   1 banana (2 Fruit)
   *4 graham cracker squares (2
      Bread)*

Week 2—Thursday

	BREAKFAST	LUNCH
BASIC	8 ounces orange juice (2 Fruit) 4 small Oatmeal or Whole Wheat Pancakes* (4 Bread), see pp. 225 or 226, with ½ cup blueberries (1 Fruit) and 2 tablespoons diet margarine (or 2 tablespoons light syrup) (2 Fat) 1 cup skim milk (or 4 tablespoons skim ricotta cheese) (1 Milk)	Tuna Sandwich 2 whole wheat bread slices (2 Bread) ¾ cup tuna (4.5 ounces), water-packed (3 Meat) with 2 tablespoons diet mayonnaise (2 Fat) and lettuce and pickle slices (0) ½ tomato, sliced (1 Vegetable) ½ cup artichoke hearts marinated in 1 tablespoon Italian Salad Dressing* (1 Vegetable, 2 Fat), see pp. 218–219 1 medium apple (2 Fruit) 1 cup skim milk (1 Milk)
MODERATE	8 ounces orange juice (2 Fruit) 4 small Oatmeal or Whole Wheat Pancakes* (4 Bread), see pp. 225 or 226, with ½ cup blueberries (1 Fruit) and 2 tablespoons diet margarine (or 2 tablespoons light syrup) (2 Fat) 1 cup skim milk (or 4 tablespoons skim ricotta cheese) (1 Milk)	Tuna Sandwich 2 whole wheat bread slices (2 Bread) *½ cup tuna (3 ounces), water-packed (2 Meat) with 1 tablespoon diet mayonnaise (1 Fat)* and lettuce and pickle slices (0) ½ tomato, sliced (1 Vegetable) ½ cup artichoke hearts marinated in 1 tablespoon Italian Salad Dressing* (1 Vegetable, 2 Fat), see pp. 218–219 1 medium apple (2 Fruit) 1 cup skim milk (1 Milk)

SUPPER	SNACKS

Nachos
    2 soft corn tortillas baked and
      broken into chips (2 Bread)
    topped with 1 ounce mozza-
      rella cheese, grated and
      melted (1 Meat)
    and ¼ cup green chili or
      jalapeno peppers (0)
Beef Chalupas
    4 soft corn or flour tortillas (4
      Bread)
    topped with 3 ounces lean
      ground beef, browned and
      drained (3 Meat); with ½ cup
      tomato sauce (1 Vegetable)
      and 1 teaspoon chili
      powder (0)
    1 tomato, diced (2 Vegetable)
      and onion and lettuce
      slices (0)
      and 1 ounce mozzarella
      cheese, grated (1 Meat)
1 cup raw vegetables (broccoli,
    carrots, cauliflower) (1
    Vegetable) with 2 table-
    spoons Ranch or Yogurt
    dressing (2 Fat)
1 cup seedless grapes (2 Fruit)

Nachos   *1 small peach (1 Fruit)*
    2 soft corn tortillas baked and
      broken into chips (2 Bread)
    topped with 1 ounce mozza-
      rella cheese, grated and
      melted (1 Meat)
    and ¼ cup green chili or
      jalapeno peppers (0)
Bean Chalupas
    4 soft corn or flour tortillas (4
      Bread)
    topped with 1 cup Pinto Beans
      #2* (2 Meat, 2 Bread),
      see p. 203
    1 tomato, diced (2 Vegetable)
      onion and lettuce slices (0)
      and 1 ounce mozzarella
      cheese, grated (1 Meat)

Week 2—Thursday (cont'd)

	BREAKFAST	LUNCH

STRICT

BREAKFAST

8 ounces orange juice (2 Fruit)
4 small Oatmeal or Whole Wheat
   Pancakes* (4 Bread), see
   pp. 225 or 226, with ½ cup
   blueberries (1 Fruit)
   and 2 tablespoons diet
   margarine
   (or 2 tablespoons light syrup)
   (2 Fat)
1 cup skim milk
   (or 4 tablespoons skim ricotta
   cheese) (1 Milk)

LUNCH

Tuna Sandwich
   2 whole wheat bread slices (2
   Bread)
   *¼ cup tuna (1.5 ounces), water-
   packed (1 Meat) with 1
   tablespoon diet mayonnaise
   (1 Fat)*
   and lettuce and pickle slices
   (0)
½ tomato, sliced (1 Vegetable)
½ cup artichoke hearts mari-
   nated in *2 tablespoons commercial low-calorie Italian
   salad dressing (1 Vegetable, 1 Fat)*
1 medium apple (2 Fruit)
1 cup skim milk (1 Milk)

SUPPER	SNACKS

1 cup raw vegetables (broccoli, carrots, cauliflower) (1 Vegetable) *with 1 tablespoon Ranch or Yogurt dressing (1 Fat)*
1 cup seedless grapes (2 Fruit)

Nachos
   3 soft corn tortillas baked and broken into chips (3 Bread)
   topped with 1 ounce mozzarella cheese, grated and melted (1 Meat)
   and ¼ cup green chili or jalapeno peppers (0)

Bean Chalupas
   4 soft corn or flour tortillas (4 Bread)
   topped with 1 cup Pinto Beans #2* (2 Meat, 2 Bread), see p. 203
   1 tomato, diced (2 Vegetable), and onion and lettuce slices (0)
   (omit cheese)
1 cup raw vegetables (broccoli, carrots, cauliflower) (1 Vegetable)
   (omit dressing)
1 cup seedless grapes (2 Fruit)

1 small peach (1 Fruit)
1 Oat Bran Muffin* (1 Bread), see p. 224

Week 2—Friday

	BREAKFAST	LUNCH

BASIC	8 ounces orange juice (2 Fruit)
	Peanut Butter Sandwich
	    2 whole wheat bread slices (2 Bread)
	    1 tablespoon peanut butter (1 Meat)
	    and 1 banana, sliced (2 Fruit)
	1 cup skim milk (1 Milk)
		Turkey Sandwich
		    2 whole wheat bread slices (2 Bread)
		    2 ounces turkey (2 meat)
		    1 teaspoon mustard (0)
		    and lettuce and tomato slices (0)
		1 cup shredded cabbage-carrot-radish coleslaw with 3 teaspoons mayonnaise (2 Vegetable, 3 Fat)
		    and 1 tablespoon each of lemon juice and vinegar (0)
		1 large peach or apple (2 Fruit)
		1 cup skim milk (1 Milk)

MODERATE	8 ounces orange juice (2 Fruit)
	Peanut Butter Sandwich
	    2 whole wheat bread slices (2 Bread)
	    1 tablespoon peanut butter (1 Meat)
	    and 1 banana, sliced (2 Fruit)
	(omit milk)
		Turkey Sandwich
		    2 whole wheat bread slices (2 Bread)
		    2 ounces turkey (2 meat)
		    1 teaspoon mustard (0)
		    and lettuce and tomato slices (0)
		1 cup shredded cabbage-carrot-radish coleslaw with 3 teaspoons mayonnaise (2 Vegetable, 3 Fat)
		    and 1 tablespoon each of lemon juice and vinegar (0)
		1 large peach or apple (2 Fruit)
		1 cup skim milk (1 Milk)

STRICT	8 ounces orange juice (2 Fruit)
	Peanut Butter Sandwich
	    2 whole wheat bread slices (2 Bread)
	    1 tablespoon peanut butter (1 Meat)
	    and 1 banana, sliced (2 Fruit)
	(omit milk)
		Turkey Sandwich
		    2 whole wheat bread slices (2 Bread)
		    1 ounce turkey (1 meat)
		    1 teaspoon mustard (0)
		    and lettuce and tomato slices (0)
		1 cup shredded cabbage-carrot-radish coleslaw *with 3 teaspoons diet mayonnaise (2 Vegetable, 1 Fat)*
		    and 1 tablespoon each of lemon juice and vinegar (0)
		1 large peach or apple (2 Fruit)
		1 cup skim milk (1 Milk)

SUPPER

1 cup won ton soup (2 Bread)
1½ cups steamed rice (3 Bread)
2 cups oriental chicken and stir-
fried vegetables
  3 ounces chicken (skinless) (3
  Meat)
  2 cups mixed vegetables (4
  Vegetables) in 3 teaspoons
  oil (3 Fat)
2 fortune cookies (1 Bread)
½ cup Seasonal Fruit Salad (1
Fruit), see p. 218

1 cup won ton soup (2 Bread)
1½ cups steamed rice (3 Bread)
2 cups oriental chicken and stir-
fried vegetables
  3 ounces chicken (skinless) (3
  Meat)
  2 cups mixed vegetables (4
  Vegetables) in 3 teaspoons
  oil (3 Fat)
2 fortune cookies (1 Bread)
*1 cup Seasonal Fruit Salad (2
Fruit), see p. 218*

1 cup won ton soup (2 Bread)
1½ cups steamed rice (3 Bread)
2 cups oriental chicken and stir-
fried vegetables
  *2 ounces chicken (skinless) (2
  Meat)*
  2 cups mixed vegetables (4
  Vegetable) in 3 teaspoons
  oil (3 Fat)
2 fortune cookies (1 Bread)
*1 cup Seasonal Fruit Salad (2
Fruit), see p. 218*

SNACKS

Tuna Melt
1 whole wheat pita pocket (2
Bread)
¼ cup tuna (1 ounce), water-
packed (1 Meat) with 2
teaspoons mayonnaise (2 Fat)
3 tablespoons (1 ounce) mozzarella cheese, grated (1 Meat)

(omit tuna melt)
2 cups bran cereal (4 Bread)
1 cup skim milk (1 Milk)

(omit tuna melt)
2 cups bran cereal (4 Bread)
1 cup skim milk (1 Milk)
*4 graham cracker squares (2
Bread)*

Week 2—Saturday

	BREAKFAST	LUNCH
BASIC	1 banana (2 Fruit) 2 cups oatmeal (4 Bread) with 2 tablespoons raisins (1 Fruit) and 2 teaspoons margarine (or 2 tablespoons light syrup or 4 teaspoons honey or regular syrup) (2 Fat) 1 whole wheat toast (1 Bread) with 1 teaspoon margarine (1 Fat) 1 cup skim milk (1 Milk)	Vegetarian Mini-pizzas 4 whole wheat pita pocket halves or 4 tortillas (4 Bread) ½ cup tomato sauce with 1 cup sliced onion, green peppers, mushrooms (3 Vegetable) 2 ounces mozzarella cheese, grated and melted (2 Meat) 1 large orange or small grapefruit (2 Fruit) 1 cup skim milk (1 Milk)
MODERATE	1 banana (2 Fruit) 2 cups oatmeal (4 Bread) with 2 tablespoons raisins (1 Fruit) 2 teaspoons margarine (or 2 tablespoons light syrup or 4 teaspoons honey or regular syrup) (2 Fat) *2 whole wheat toast (2 Bread)* with 1 teaspoon margarine (1 Fat) 1 cup skim milk (1 Milk)	Vegetarian Mini-pizzas 4 whole wheat pita pocket halves or 4 tortillas (4 Bread) ½ cup tomato sauce with 1 cup sliced onion, green peppers, mushrooms (3 Vegetable) 1 ounce mozzarella cheese, grated and melted (1 Meat) 1 large orange or small grapefruit (2 Fruit) 1 cup skim milk (1 Milk)
STRICT	1 banana (2 Fruit) 2 cups oatmeal (4 Bread) with 2 tablespoons raisins (1 Fruit) *(omit margarine, syrup, or honey)* *2 whole wheat toast (2 Bread)*	Vegetarian Mini-pizzas 4 whole wheat pita pocket halves or 4 tortillas (4 Bread) ½ cup tomato sauce with 1

SUPPER	SNACKS
1 cup vegetable soup (1 Bread) 6 ounces Baked or Broiled Seafood* (6 Meat), see pp. 185 or 186 with lemon wedges (0) ½ cup red potatoes with skins (1 Bread) with 1 teaspoon margarine (1 Fat) 1 cup mixed vegetables (zucchini, carrots, broccoli, cauliflower) (2 Vegetable) with 2 teaspoons margarine (2 Fat) 1 tomato and lettuce salad (1 Vegetable) with 1 tablespoon Italian Salad Dressing (1 Fat), see pp. 218–219 1 French bread slice (3 inches long) (1 Bread) with 1 teaspoon margarine (1 Fat) 1 cup raspberries (2 Fruit)	
1 cup vegetable soup (1 Bread) *5 ounces Baked or Broiled Seafood* (5 Meat), see pp. 185 or 186 with lemon wedges (0) ½ cup red potatoes with skins (1 Bread) with 1 teaspoon margarine (1 Fat) 1 cup mixed vegetables (zucchini, carrots, broccoli, cauliflower) (2 Vegetable) with 2 teaspoons margarine (2 Fat) 1 tomato and lettuce salad (1 Vegetable) *with 1 tablespoon herb vinegar or lemon juice (0)* *2 French bread slices (each slice 3 inches long) (2 Bread) (omit margarine)* 1 cup raspberries (2 Fruit)	*1 small apple (1 Fruit)*
1 cup vegetable soup (1 Bread) *3 ounces Baked or Broiled Seafood* (3 Meat), see pp. 185 or 186 with lemon wedges (0)	*1 small apple (1 Fruit)*

Week 2—Saturday (cont'd)

BREAKFAST	LUNCH
with 1 teaspoon margarine (1 Fat) 1 cup skim milk (1 Milk)	cup sliced onion, green peppers, mushrooms (3 Vegetable) 1 ounce mozzarella cheese, grated and melted (1 Meat) 1 large orange or small grapefruit (2 Fruit) 1 cup skim milk (1 Milk)

SUPPER	SNACKS
½ cup red potatoes with skins (1 Bread) with 1 teaspoon margarine (1 Fat) 1 cup mixed vegetables (zucchini, carrots, broccoli, cauliflower) (2 Vegetable) with 2 teaspoons margarine (2 Fat) 1 tomato and lettuce salad (1 Vegetable) *with 1 tablespoon herb vinegar or lemon juice (0)* *2 French bread slices (each slice 3 inches long) (2 Bread) (omit margarine)* 1 cup raspberries (2 Fruit) *3-inch slice Angel Food Cake* (2 Bread), see pp. 226–227*	

Week 2—Sunday

	BREAKFAST	LUNCH

BASIC	4 ounces orange juice (1 Fruit)
	French Toast
	   3 whole wheat bread slices (3 Bread)
	   1 egg and 2 tablespoons skim milk, blended (1 Meat)
	Toppings
	   2 teaspoons honey, jelly (or 1 tablespoon light syrup) (1 Fat)
	   1 small apple, sliced and baked (1 Fruit)
	1 cup skim milk (1 Milk)
		Taco Salad
		   2 soft tortillas, baked and broken in chips (2 Bread)
		   2 cups lettuce salad (0)
		   ½ tomato, diced (1 Vegetable)
		   1 cup pinto or kidney beans (2 Meat, 2 Bread), seasoned with 2 teaspoons chili powder (0)
		   2 teaspoons olive oil (2 Fat)
		   2 ounces chicken, baked and sliced (2 Meat)
		   3 tablespoons hot sauce (0)
		   1 tablespoon Ranch dressing (1 Fat)
		   1 cup seedless grapes (2 Fruit)
		   8 ounces tomato juice (2 Vegetable)

MODERATE	8 ounces orange juice (2 Fruit)
	French Toast
	   3 whole wheat bread slices (3 Bread)
	   1 egg and 2 tablespoons skim milk, blended (1 Meat)
	Toppings
	   2 teaspoons honey, jelly (or 1 tablespoon light syrup) (1 Fat)
	   1 small apple, sliced and baked (1 Fruit)
	1 cup skim milk (1 Milk)
		Taco Salad
		   2 soft tortillas, baked and broken in chips (2 Bread)
		   2 cups lettuce salad (0)
		   ½ tomato, diced (1 Vegetable)
		   1 cup pinto or kidney beans (2 Meat, 2 Bread), seasoned with 2 teaspoons chili powder (0)
		   2 teaspoons olive oil (2 Fat)
		   (omit chicken)
		   3 tablespoons hot sauce (0)
		   (omit Ranch dressing)
		   1 cup seedless grapes (2 Fruit)
		   8 ounces tomato juice (2 Vegetable)

STRICT	8 ounces orange juice (2 Fruit)
	French Toast
	   3 whole wheat bread slices (3 Bread) *with ¼ cup egg substitute*
	   or 2 egg whites with 2 tablespoons skim milk, blended (1 Meat)
	Toppings
	   2 teaspoons honey, jelly (or 1 tablespoon light syrup) (1 Fat)
	   1 small apple, sliced and baked (1 Fruit)
	1 cup skim milk (1 Milk)
		Taco Salad
		   2 soft tortillas, baked and broken in chips (2 Bread)
		   2 cups lettuce salad (0)
		   ½ tomato, diced (1 Vegetable)
		   1 cup pinto or kidney beans (2 Meat, 2 Bread), seasoned with 2 teaspoons chili powder (0)
		   2 teaspoons olive oil (2 Fat)
		   (omit chicken)
		   3 tablespoons hot sauce (0)
		   (omit Ranch dressing)
		   1 cup seedless grapes (2 Fruit)
		   8 ounces tomato juice (2 Vegetable)

SUPPER   SNACKS

1 serving Spinach Lasagna #3*
   (4 Bread, 3 Meat, 1 Vegetable, 2 Fat), see p. 216
3-inch French bread roll (1 Bread)
   with 2 teaspoons margarine (2 Fat) and
   1 teaspoon garlic powder
   seasoning (0)
½ cup carrots (1 Vegetable)
½ cup brussels sprouts (1
   Vegetable)
½ cantaloupe (2 Fruit)

---

1 serving Spinach Lasagna #3*   *3 cups popcorn (1½ tablespoons*
   (4 Bread, 3 Meat, 1 Veg-   *dry kernels), plain and*
   etable, 2 Fat), see p. 216   *air-popped (1 Bread)*
6-inch French bread roll (2 Bread)
   with 2 teaspoons diet mar-
   garine (1 Fat) and
   1 teaspoon garlic powder
   seasoning (0)
½ cup carrots (1 Vegetable)
½ cup brussels sprouts (1
   Vegetable)
½ cantaloupe (2 Fruit)

---

1 serving Spinach Lasagna #4   *9 cups popcorn (4½ tablespoons*
   (4 Bread, 1 Meat, 1 Vege-   *dry kernels), plain and*
   table), see p. 217   *air-popped (3 Bread)*
6-inch French bread roll (2 Bread)
   with 2 teaspoons diet mar-
   garine (1 Fat) and
   1 teaspoon garlic powder
   seasoning (0)
½ cup carrots (1 Vegetable)
½ cup brussels sprouts (1
   Vegetable)
½ cantaloupe (2 Fruit)

Recipes to Control
Your Cholesterol

To help you in your low-cholesterol food preparations, here are some recipes which have been developed by our Nutrition Department at the Aerobics Center. These include "quick" chicken and fish entrees, a number of other main dishes that may take a little longer to prepare, and some easy side dishes. You'll find recipes for vegetables, baked goods, sauces, dressings—and even desserts!

These recipes have been designed so that you can use them with the menus and food exchange system I've explained on pp. 105–175. You'll find that each entry includes values for calories, fat, cholesterol, and food exchanges (such as "3 Meat," "½ Fat," and so on).

The recipes, including the variations on a number of the dishes, have been grouped by category in the following order for your easy reference:

- Chicken

- Seafood

- Meat

- Bean Dishes and Soups*

- Vegetable Specialties

- Salad Dressings and Sauces

- Muffins, Rolls, Pancakes, and Desserts

Bon appétit!

---

*Wherever soups are referred to in the menus, you can either use the soups described in the recipe section or canned soups from your local grocery store.

Baked Chicken

Yields: 4 servings
1 serving (3 ounces): calories = 180
                      fat = 9 gm
                      cholesterol = 60 mg
                      exchanges = 3 Meat

4 small chicken breasts without skin or bone (1-pound package) or 4 small chicken breasts with skin and bone (2-pound package)
1 cup commercial oil-free Italian Salad dressing

Skin and wash chicken pieces. Pat dry. Place chicken pieces in shallow pan. Pour dressing over pieces. Cover with foil. Marinate chicken overnight in dressing, turning pieces once.

Preheat oven to 350°F. Pour off marinade. Bake in foil-covered pan for 1 to 1½ hours until done, or juices run clear when punctured with a fork. Remember, boneless chicken will cook faster. To brown, place under broiler for 5 minutes on each side.

Variations:

Lime Ginger Chicken

Marinate in Lime Ginger Sauce, see pp. 220–221

Teriyaki Chicken

Marinate in Teriyaki Sauce, see p. 223

Red Wine and Mushroom Chicken

Bake plain chicken and serve with Red Wine and Mushroom Sauce, see p. 222

———— Baked Chicken with Brown Rice and Nut Dressing ————

Yields: 6 servings
1 serving:

calories	= 410
fat	= 20 gm
cholesterol	= 79 mg
exchanges	= 4 Meat +
	1 Bread +
	1 Vegetable +
	2 Fat

6 chicken breasts (skinned) (2-pound package)
1 cup brown rice, uncooked
2½ cups fat-free chicken broth
1 tablespoon oil-based margarine or 1 tablespoon olive oil
1 cup chopped onion
1 cup chopped celery
1 clove garlic, minced
1 teaspoon salt-free spice/herb blend
dash of pepper
1 cup chopped walnuts

Preheat oven to 325°F. Bake chicken breasts in pan covered with foil, about 1½ hours, or broil at 450° F or less, 7 to 9 inches from broiler 20 to 30 minutes per side, or grill. Combine rice and chicken broth in saucepan. Bring to a boil. Stir once. Reduce heat, cover, and simmer 45 minutes (or follow package directions for rice). Melt margarine in saucepan. Sauté onion, celery, and garlic until tender. (*Fat-free Alternate—spray pan with nonstick cooking spray, or steam onion, celery, and garlic in 2 tablespoons of water.*) Stir cooked onion, celery, and garlic into cooked rice. Add spice/herb blend, pepper, and walnuts. Serve with chicken.

Variation:
Omit the nuts and oil.

Yields: 6 servings
1 serving:

calories	= 260
fat	= 9 gm
cholesterol	= 79 mg
exchanges	= 3 Meat +
	1 Bread +
	1 Vegetable

Suggestion:
If menu calls for 2-ounce portions, buy smaller chicken breasts. If menu calls for 4-ounce portions, buy larger chicken breasts.

======================= Lemon Baked Chicken =======================

Yields: 4 servings
1 serving (4 ounces):
calories	= 265
fat	= 12 gm
cholesterol	= 100 mg
exchanges	= 4 Meat + ½ Fat

Yields: 5 servings
1 serving (3 ounces):
calories	= 210
fat	= 10 gm
cholesterol	= 80 mg
exchanges	= 3 Meat + ½ Fat

1 chicken (2½ to 3 pounds), cut into serving pieces
1 tablespoon fresh lemon juice
1 tablespoon olive oil
1 garlic clove, crushed
salt-free spice/herb blend
dash of pepper
chopped parsley

Preheat oven to 350°F. In a bowl, combine lemon juice, oil, garlic, herb blend and pepper. Arrange chicken in a shallow casserole or baking pan, and pour over it the lemon and oil mixture. Cover and bake until tender, about 40 minutes, basting occasionally. Uncover casserole and bake 10 minutes longer to allow chicken to brown. Sprinkle with chopped parsley and serve.

Variation:
Replace oil with 1 tablespoon oil-free Italian Salad Dressing, see pp. 218–219.

Yields: 4 servings

1 serving (4 ounces):	calories	= 240
	fat	= 8 gm
	cholesterol	= 100 mg
	exchanges	= 4 meat

Yields: 5 servings

1 serving (3 ounces):	calories	= 190
	fat	= 7 gm
	cholesterol	= 80 mg
	exchanges	= 3 Meat

_____ Barbecued Chicken _____

Yields: 4 servings

1 serving (3 ounces):	calories	= 180
	fat	= 9 gm
	cholesterol	= 60 mg
	exchanges	= 3 Meat

With barbecue sauce:

	calories	= 225
	fat	= 15 gm
	cholesterol	= 60 mg
	exchanges	= 3 Meat + 1 Fat

4 small chicken breasts without skin or bone (1-pound package) **or** 4 small chicken breasts with skin and bone (2-pound package)
1 cup Barbecue Sauce, see p. 220

Preheat oven to 350°F. Skin and wash chicken pieces. Pat dry. Pour Barbecue Sauce over chicken in a shallow baking pan. Cover with foil and bake for 60 minutes. Uncover and bake 10 minutes more to allow chicken to brown.

Suggestion:
If menu calls for 2-ounce portions, buy smaller chicken breasts. If menu calls for 4-ounce or 5-ounce portions, buy larger chicken breasts.

===================== Broiled Chicken =====================

Yields: 4 servings
1 serving (3 ounces): calories   = 180
                      fat   = 9 gm
                      cholesterol   = 60 mg
                      exchanges   = 3 Meat

4 small chicken breasts without skin or bone (1-pound package)
   or 4 small chicken breasts with skin and bone (2-pound
   package)
1 teaspoon paprika

Preheat oven at BROIL. Skin and wash chicken pieces. Pat dry.
Place chicken on broiler pan. Broil 4 to 6 inches from broiler
until brown on each side. Keep turning pieces until cooked, but
not overly browned. Sprinkle paprika on chicken.

Suggestion:
If menu calls for 2-ounce portions, buy smaller chicken breasts.
If menu calls for 4-ounce or 5-ounce portions, buy larger chicken
breasts.

===================== Hawaiian Chicken =====================

Standard Recipe—Hawaiian Chicken #1

Yields: 4 servings
1 serving (1 breast): calories   = 415
                      fat   = 12 gm
                      cholesterol   = 155 mg
                      exchanges   = 6 Meat +
                                      1 Fruit +
                                      1 Fat

Note: 6 ounces chicken = 6 Meat
        ½ cup pineapple with juice = 1 Fruit
        1 teaspoon oil = 1 Fat

4 chicken breasts (approximately a 3¼-pound package)
1 16-ounce can crushed pineapple, with juice
½ cup soy sauce ("lite" if available to reduce salt)
4 teaspoons olive oil
¼ teaspoon ginger

Skin, wash, and drain chicken breasts. Place in a shallow pan. Mix pineapple, juice, soy sauce, oil, and ginger. Cover chicken with marinade and cover. Refrigerate at least 8 hours, turning pieces over once. .

Preheat oven to 350°F. Pour off marinade, reserving liquid. Bake chicken for 20 minutes, basting every 5 to 10 minutes. Turn chicken pieces over and continue baking 20 to 30 minutes more, basting every 5 to 10 minutes, until chicken is done, or juices run clear when punctured with a fork. Serve chicken with 1 tablespoon marinade sauce.

Variations:

Hawaiian Chicken #2

Use 4 smaller chicken breasts (approximately a 2¾-pound package). Follow same directions as Standard Recipe.

Yields: 4 servings
1 serving (1 breast):　calories　　= 375
　　　　　　　　　　　fat　　　　= 11 gm
　　　　　　　　　　　cholesterol = 133 mg
　　　　　　　　　　　exchanges　= 5 Meat +
　　　　　　　　　　　　　　　　　1 Fruit +
　　　　　　　　　　　　　　　　　1 Fat

Hawaiian Chicken #3

Use 4 smaller chicken breasts (approximately a 2¼-pound package). Follow same directions as Standard Recipe.

Yields: 4 servings
1 serving (1 breast): calories   = 325
                       fat   = 10 gm
                       cholesterol = 110 mg
                       exchanges   = 4 Meat +
                                      1 Fruit +
                                      1 Fat

=============== Microwaved Chicken ===============

Yields: 4 servings
1 serving (3 ounces): calories   = 180
                       fat   = 9 gm
                       cholesterol = 60 mg
                       exchanges   = 3 Meat

4 small chicken breasts without skin or bone (1-pound package)
  or 4 small chicken breasts with skin and bone (2-pound
  package)
2 tablespoons lemon juice

Skin and wash chicken pieces. Pat dry. Arrange chicken pieces
in a microwave pan, with thick pieces to the outside, thin
pieces toward the center. Sprinkle with lemon juice. Cover
and bake on HIGH for 7 minutes per pound. Check for done-
ness (when liquids run clear as chicken is pierced with a
fork).

Variation:
Instead of lemon juice, sprinkle chicken with herb-blend
seasonings.

Suggestion:
If menu calls for 2-ounce portions, buy smaller chicken breasts.
If menu calls for 4-ounce portions, buy larger chicken breasts.

———————————— Stir-Fried Chicken ————————————

Yields: 4 servings
1 serving (3 ounces cooked chicken, 1 cup vegetables):

calories	= 275
fat	= 14 gm
cholesterol	= 60 mg
exchanges	= 3 Meat +
	2 Vegetable +
	1 Fat

4 small chicken breasts without skin or bone (1-pound package) **or** 4 small chicken breasts with skin and bone (2-pound package)
1 tablespoon olive oil
2 tablespoons soy sauce
use any combination of vegetables:
2 medium carrots, julienne sliced
2 cups broccoli florets
1 stalk celery, chopped
or
2 medium zucchini, sliced
2 cups cauliflowerets
or
2 cups snow pea pods
2 cups sliced fresh mushrooms

Skin and wash chicken pieces. Pat dry. Cut up chicken into bite-size pieces. Add olive oil to electric wok. Heat wok on MEDIUM-HIGH setting. Stir-fry chicken for about 5 minutes. Toss every few minutes to assure that all pieces brown evenly and don't stick to wok. Add cut-up vegetables. Stir-fry vegetables another 3 minutes. Add 2 tablespoons soy sauce during last 2 minutes of cooking.

Suggestion:
If menu calls for 2-ounce portions, buy smaller chicken breasts. If menu calls for 4-ounce portions, buy larger chicken breasts.

————————————— Baked Seafood —————————————

Yields: 2 servings
1 serving (3 ounces): calories   = 150 to 180
                       fat   = 3 to 9 gm
                       cholesterol = 60 mg
                       exchanges   = 3 Meat

8 ounces white fish fillet (cod, scrod, sole, red snapper, trout,
    grouper)
½ cup commercial oil-free Italian Salad Dressing
1 fresh lemon

Preheat oven to 350°F for 10 minutes. Place fish in shallow
pan. Pour dressing over fish and let stand 5 minutes. Pour off
marinade. Bake for 10 to 20 minutes or until fish flakes easily
with a fork. Season after baking with fresh lemon juice.

Variations:

Baked Seafood Seasoned with Mixed Vegetables

Place 1 cup of chopped mixed vegetables (mushrooms, onion,
tomato, green pepper, parsley) on top of fish to flavor it. Bake.

1 serving (3 ounces): calories   = 200 to 230
                       fat   = 3 to 9 gm
                       cholesterol = 60 mg
                       exchanges   = 3 Meat +
                                      2 Vegetable

Lemon Baked Seafood

Omit marinade. After baking, squeeze lemon juice over fish.

Yields: 2 servings
1 serving (3 ounces): calories   = 150 to 180
                       fat   = 3 to 9 gm
                       cholesterol = 60 mg
                       exchanges   = 3 Meat

Suggestion:
If menu calls for 2-ounce portions, buy smaller fillets. If menu calls for 4-ounce portions, buy larger fillets.

―――――――――― Broiled Seafood ――――――――――

Yields: 4 servings
1 serving (3 ounces): calories   = 150 to 180
                       fat   = 3 to 9 gm
                       cholesterol = 60 mg
                       exchanges   = 3 Meat

1 pound white fish fillets (red snapper, orange roughy, tuna, swordfish, sole, cod)
1 teaspoon paprika
½ lemon, cut in wedges

Preheat oven at BROIL. Place fish on broiler pan. Broil 4 to 6 inches from element about 5 minutes* on one side only or until fish flakes easily with a fork. Sprinkle paprika on top and serve with lemon wedges.

Suggestion:
If menu calls for 4-ounce, 5-ounce, 6-ounce, or 8-ounce portions, buy larger fillets.

―――――――――― Microwaved Seafood ――――――――――

Yields: 4 servings
1 serving (3 ounces): calories   = 180
                       fat   = 9 gm
                       cholesterol = 60 mg
                       exchanges   = 3 Meat

*For each inch of thickness, cook 10 minutes. As fish cooks, it turns from translucent white (or pink) to opaque white.

1 pound white fish fillets (red snapper, orange roughy, tuna, swordfish, sole, cod)
1 tablespoon herb blend seasoning
1 tablespoon fresh lemon juice
½ lemon cut in wedges

Arrange fish in a microwave pan, with thick pieces to the outside, thin pieces toward the center. Sprinkle with commercial herb blend seasoning or seasoning of choice and lemon juice. Cover and bake on HIGH for 5 minutes per pound or until fish flakes easily with a fork. Serve with lemon wedges.

Suggestion:
If menu calls for 2-ounce portions, buy smaller fillets. If menu calls for 4-ounce portions, buy larger fillets.

―――――― Stir-Fried Seafood or Shellfish ――――――

Yields: 4 servings
1 serving (3 ounces seafood, 1 cup vegetables):

calories	=	230
fat	=	9 gm
cholesterol	=	60 mg
exchanges	=	3 Meat +
		2 Vegetable

1 pound white fish fillets (red snapper, orange roughy, tuna, swordfish, sole, cod) **or**
1 pound medium shrimp
1 tablespoon olive oil
2 tablespoons soy sauce
Use any combination of vegetables:
4 medium carrots, julienne sliced
2 stalks celery
or
4 green onions, chopped
2 cups snow pea pods
or
2 cups broccoli florets
2 cups sliced fresh mushrooms

If cooking shrimp, peel, de-vein, and wash shrimp. Pat dry. Add 1 tablespoon olive oil to electric wok. Heat wok on MEDIUM-HIGH setting. Stir-fry seafood or shrimp 3 to 5 minutes. Toss every few minutes to assure all pieces brown evenly and don't stick to wok. If cooking fish, fillet will flake apart. Add cut-up vegetables of your choice. Stir-fry vegetables another 3 minutes. Add 2 tablespoons soy sauce during last 2 minutes of cooking.

Suggestion:
If menu calls for 2-ounce portions, buy smaller fillets. If menu calls for 4-ounce portions, buy larger fillets.

─────────────── Grilled Salmon ───────────────

Yields: 4 servings
1 serving (3 ounces cooked):

calories	= 180
fat	= 9 gm
cholesterol	= 60 mg
exchanges	= 3 Meat

4 4-ounce fresh or frozen salmon steaks
2 tablespoons lemon juice

Thaw salmon if frozen. Preheat gas grill on MEDIUM. Sprinkle steaks with lemon juice. Place on grill. For each inch of thickness, cook 10 minutes or until fish flakes easily with fork.

Suggestion:
If menu calls for 2-ounce portions, buy smaller steaks. If menu calls for 4-ounce or 5-ounce portions, buy larger steaks.

─────────────── Poached Salmon ───────────────

Yields: 4 servings
1 serving (3 ounces):

calories	= 180
fat	= 9 gm
cholesterol	= 60 mg
exchanges	= 3 Meat

4 5-ounce fresh or frozen salmon steaks
4½ cups water
⅓ cup lemon juice
⅛ teaspoon freshly ground pepper

Thaw salmon if frozen. In large skillet, combine water, lemon juice, and pepper. Bring to a boil. Add salmon. Simmer, covered, 7 to 10 minutes or until fish flakes easily when tested with a fork. Remove salmon from liquid with spatula. Chill or serve hot. Serve salmon with lemon wedges.

Suggestion:
If menu calls for 2-ounce portions, buy smaller steaks. If menu calls for 4-ounce or 5-ounce portions, buy larger steaks.

————————————— Shrimp Creole —————————————

Standard Recipe—Shrimp Creole #1

Yields: 2 servings
1 serving (1 cup):   calories   = 185
                       fat   = 1 gm
                       cholesterol = 79 mg
                       exchanges   = 2 Meat +
                                     1 Bread +
                                     1 Vegetable

NOTE: 5 shrimp = 1 Meat
        1 cup tomato sauce = 1 Bread
        ½ cup tomato sauce = 1 Vegetable
        ½ cup vegetables = 1 Vegetable

20 shrimp
2 cups (16-ounce can) tomato sauce
1 small onion, chopped
1 celery stalk, chopped
¼ green bell pepper, diced
¼ cup sliced mushrooms
2 tablespoons parsley
½ teaspoon pepper
1 to 1½ cups brown rice, prepared according to package directions in amount specified by menus

Peel, de-vein, and wash shrimp; set aside. (If shrimp are frozen, let them thaw first in refrigerator.) Simmer tomato sauce, onion, celery, green pepper, mushrooms, parsley and pepper in skillet for 30 minutes. Add shrimp and cook 10 to 15 minutes more, until shrimp are tender. Serve over brown rice.

Variations:

Shrimp Creole #2

Add 4 teaspoons olive oil to the Standard Recipe. Heat the oil in a skillet and add onion, celery, green pepper, and mushrooms and simmer 5 minutes. Add the tomato sauce, parsley, and pepper, then shrimp, as described in Standard Recipe.

Yields: 2 servings
1 serving (1 cup): calories   = 275
                    fat   = 11 gm
                    cholesterol = 79 mg
                    exchanges   = 2 Meat +
                                   1 Bread +
                                   1 Vegetable +
                                   2 Fat

Shrimp Creole #3

Add 2 teaspoons olive oil to the Standard Recipe. Follow instructions as listed for Shrimp Creole #2.

Yields: 2 servings
1 serving (1 cup): calories   = 230
                    fat   = 6 gm
                    cholesterol = 79 mg
                    exchanges   = 2 Meat +
                                   1 Bread +
                                   1 Vegetable +
                                   1 Fat

Shrimp Creole #4

Use only 10 shrimp in Shrimp Creole #3 recipe. Follow instructions as listed for Shrimp Creole #2.

Yields: 2 servings
1 serving (1 cup):   calories   = 200
                      fat   = 6 gm
                      cholesterol = 40 mg
                      exchanges   = 1 Meat +
                                     1 Bread +
                                     1 Vegetable +
                                     1 Fat

―――――――――――――――― Tuna Salad ――――――――――――――――

Yields: 3 servings
1 serving (¼ cup):   calories   = 120
                      fat   = 4 gm
                      cholesterol = 37 mg
                      exchanges   = 1 Meat +
                                     1 Fat

1 6½-ounce can tuna, water-packed
2 tablespoons diet mayonnaise
1 tablespoon lemon juice
Optional:
1 celery stalk, diced
1 green onion, diced
2 tablespoons apple, diced
3 small sweet pickles or 1 large

Combine all ingredients.

Variation:
Omit mayonnaise if fat-free recipe needed. Replace with 2 more tablespoons lemon juice and/or 2 tablespoons oil-free Italian Salad Dressing, pp. 218–219.

Yields: 3 servings
1 serving (¼ cup):   calories   = 80
                      fat   = 1 gm
                      cholesterol = 37 mg
                      exchanges   = 1 Meat

Shishkabob

Standard Recipe—Shishkabob #1

Yields: 4 servings
1 serving (3 ounces meat):

$$
\begin{aligned}
\text{calories} &= 235 \\
\text{fat} &= 12 \text{ gm} \\
\text{cholesterol} &= 80 \text{ mg} \\
\text{exchanges} &= 1 \text{ Vegetable} + \\
&\quad\;\; 3 \text{ Meat}
\end{aligned}
$$

1 pound lean meat (filet, sirloin, chuck), cut in chunks and
     trimmed of fat
½ cup commercial oil-free Italian Salad Dressing
½ cup red wine
8 cherry tomatoes
½ onion, cut into 8 chunks
½ green pepper, cut into 8 chunks
1 zucchini, cut into 8 chunks
4 skewers

Marinate meat overnight in salad dressing and wine, turning
once. On each skewer, alternate ¼ of the meat chunks, 2
cherry tomatoes, 2 chunks of onion, 2 chunks of green pepper
and 2 chunks of zucchini. On a charcoal grill or in an oven
broiler, cook shishkabobs 10 to 15 minutes each side, turning
as needed to cook evenly throughout.

Variations:

Shishkabob #2

Use ¾ pound lean meat.

Follow same directions as Standard Recipe.

Yields: 4 servings
1 serving (2 ounces meat):

$$
\begin{aligned}
\text{calories} &= 165 \\
\text{fat} &= 8 \text{ gm} \\
\text{cholesterol} &= 53 \text{ mg} \\
\text{exchanges} &= 1 \text{ Vegetable } + \\
& \quad 2 \text{ Meat}
\end{aligned}
$$

Shishkabob #3

Use 1¼ pounds lean meat. Marinate in ½ cup regular Italian Salad Dressing plus wine. Use 16 cherry tomatoes (4 per skewer). Follow same directions as Standard Recipe.

Yields: 4 servings
1 serving (4 ounces meat):

$$
\begin{aligned}
\text{calories} &= 490 \\
\text{fat} &= 36 \text{ gm} \\
\text{cholesterol} &= 105 \text{ mg} \\
\text{exchanges} &= 2 \text{ Vegetable } + \\
& \quad 4 \text{ Meat } + \\
& \quad 4 \text{ Fat}
\end{aligned}
$$

Shishkabob #4

Use 1 pound lean meat. Marinate in ¼ cup regular Italian Salad Dressing plus wine. Use 16 cherry tomatoes (4 per skewer). Follow same directions as Standard Recipe.

Yields: 4 servings
1 serving (3 ounces meat):

$$
\begin{aligned}
\text{calories} &= 330 \\
\text{fat} &= 22 \text{ gm} \\
\text{cholesterol} &= 80 \text{ mg} \\
\text{exchanges} &= 2 \text{ Vegetable } + \\
& \quad 3 \text{ Meat } + \\
& \quad 2 \text{ Fat}
\end{aligned}
$$

Shishkabob #5

Use ¾ pound lean meat. Marinate in ¼ cup regular Italian Sala
Dressing plus wine. Use 16 cherry tomatoes (4 per skewer).

Follow same directions as Standard Recipe.

Yields: 4 servings
1 serving (2 ounces meat):

> calories = 275
> fat = 18 gm
> cholesterol = 54 mg
> exchanges = 2 Vegetable +
> 2 Meat +
> 2 Fat

———————————— Easy Meat Sauce ————————————

Standard Recipe—Meat Sauce #1

Yields: 6 servings
1 serving (approximately ½ cup):

> calories = 165
> fat = 8 gm
> cholesterol = 50 mg
> exchanges = 2 Meat +
> 1 Vegetable

A 1-cup portion (as in the 2,200-calorie Basic menu) contains:

> calories = 330
> fat = 16 gm
> cholesterol = 100 mg
> exchanges = 4 Meat +
> 1 Bread

("1 Bread" denotes the extra carbohydrates in this portion)

½ pound (8 ounces) lean ground beef
½ pound (8 ounces) lean ground turkey
32 ounces (2 16-ounce cans) prepared spaghetti sauce
1 cup water
2 tablespoons Italian herb seasonings blend

Heat skillet on stove for 3 to 5 minutes. When hot, add ground meats and brown. Drain off fat. Add spaghetti sauce, water, and seasonings. Simmer 30 to 45 minutes.

Variations:

Easy Meat Sauce #2

Use half the beef and turkey (¼ pound of each) and follow the same directions as the Standard Recipe.

Yields: 6 servings
1 serving (approximately ½ cup):

calories	= 95
fat	= 3 gm
cholesterol	= 25 mg
exchanges	= 1 Meat +
	1 Vegetable

Easy Meat Sauce #3

Use ¾ pound (12 ounces) each of beef and turkey. Follow the same directions as the Standard Recipe.

Yields: 6 servings
1 serving (approximately 1 cup):

calories	= 280
fat	= 9 gm
cholesterol	= 75 mg
exchanges	= 3 Meat +
	1 Bread

Easy Meat Sauce #4

Use half the meat and double the sauce of the Standard Recipe, that is, ¼ pound each of beef and turkey and 64 ounces (2 32-ounce cans) of spaghetti sauce.

Yields: 6 servings
1 serving (approximately 1 cup):

                    calories   = 140
                    fat   = 4 gm
                    cholesterol = 25 mg
                    exchanges = 1 Meat +
                                   1 Bread

Homemade Meat Sauce

Yields: 6 servings
1 serving (approximately 1 cup):

                    calories   = 205
                    fat   = 9 gm
                    cholesterol = 44 mg
                    exchanges = 3 Meat +
                                   1 Vegetable

1 pound lean ground beef
1 cup diced onion
1 garlic clove, mashed
1 teaspoon cinnamon
¼ teaspoon black pepper
1 8-ounce can tomato sauce, unsalted
1 8-ounce can mushroom stems and pieces, drained
2 tablespoons Worcestershire sauce
1 teaspoon Italian seasoning

In skillet, brown beef and drain off fat. Steam the onion and garlic until tender. Add onion, garlic, cinnamon, pepper, tomato sauce, mushrooms, Worcestershire sauce, and Italian seasoning to skillet. Bring mixture to a boil, then simmer gently for about 15 minutes.

Note: This is an alternative recipe to the ones in the menus called Easy Meat Sauce #1, #2, #3, and #4.

Mexican Fajitas

Standard Recipe—Mexican Fajitas #1

Yields: 1 serving
1 serving (3 ounces cooked meat, 2 tortillas):

calories	= 350
fat	= 9 gm
cholesterol	= 75 mg
exchanges	= 3 Meat +
	2 Bread +
	1 Vegetable

4 ounces raw lean flank steak, cut into strips
3 tablespoons fajita sauce, bottled
2 tortillas, corn or flour
½ tomato, diced
¼ cup shredded lettuce
Optional:
2 tablespoons picante sauce

Pour fajita sauce over meat. Let stand for 10 minutes. Heat skillet on stovetop. When hot, add meat and cook quickly, about 5 minutes on each side. Remove from heat. Fill tortillas with meat, tomato, and lettuce. Top with picante sauce.

Variations:

Mexican Fajitas #2

Use 5 ounces of flank steak and 3 tortillas. Follow same directions as Standard Recipe.

Yields: 1 serving
1 serving (4 ounces meat, 3 tortillas):

calories	= 475
fat	= 12 gm
cholesterol	= 100 mg
exchanges	= 4 Meat +
	3 Bread +
	1 Vegetable

Mexican Fajitas #3

Use 4 ounces of flank steak and 3 tortillas. Follow same directions as Standard Recipe.

Yields: 1 serving
1 serving (3 ounces meat, 3 tortillas):

calories	= 415
fat	= 9 gm
cholesterol	= 75 mg
exchanges	= 3 Meat +
	3 Bread +
	1 Vegetable

―――――――――――――― Bean Chili ――――――――――――――

Standard Recipe—Bean Chili #1

Yields: 4 servings
1 serving (1 cup):

calories	= 330
fat	= 8 gm
cholesterol	= 25 mg
exchanges	= 2 Meat +
	2 Bread +
	1 Fat +
	1 Vegetable

Note: 1 ounce meat = 1 Meat
½ cup beans = 1 Meat + 1 Bread
1 cup tomato sauce = 1 Bread
1 teaspoon oil = 1 Fat
½ cup vegetables = 1 Vegetable

⅓ pound lean ground beef
4 teaspoons vegetable oil
1 medium onion, chopped fine
2 celery stalks, chopped fine
½ green bell pepper, chopped
2 cups cooked pinto or kidney beans
4 cups (32-ounce can) tomato sauce
½ teaspoon chili powder
½ teaspoon cumin
¼ teaspoon pepper

Brown ground beef in skillet and drain off fat (4 ounces of meat will remain). Add oil; then add onion, celery, and green pepper. Stir and heat thoroughly for 5 minutes. Add beans, tomato sauce, and seasonings. Simmer for 30 to 45 minutes, stirring occasionally.

Variations:

Bean Chili #2

Use less ground beef—3 ounces raw meat.

Yields: 4 servings
1 serving (1 cup):   calories   = 300
                     fat   = 7 gm
                     cholesterol = 12 mg
                     exchanges   = 1½ Meat +
                                   2 Bread +
                                   1 Fat +
                                   1 Vegetable

Bean Chili #3

Use less ground beef and less oil—3 ounces raw meat and 2 teaspoons oil.

Yields: 4 servings
1 serving (1 cup):   calories   = 275
　　　　　　　　　　　fat   = 2 gm
　　　　　　　　　　　cholesterol = 12 mg
　　　　　　　　　　　exchanges   = 1½ Meat +
　　　　　　　　　　　　　　　　　　2 Bread +
　　　　　　　　　　　　　　　　　　½ Fat +
　　　　　　　　　　　　　　　　　　1 Vegetable

———— Cajun Beans with Brown Rice ————

Standard Recipe—Cajun Beans #1

Yields: 2 servings
1 serving: calories   = 285
　　　　　　　　　　　fat   = 2 gm
　　　　　　　　　　　cholesterol = 0 mg
　　　　　　　　　　　exchanges   = 2 Bread +
　　　　　　　　　　　　　　　　　　2 Meat +
　　　　　　　　　　　　　　　　　　1 Vegetable

2 cups (16-ounce can) red beans, prepared
1 cup (8-ounce can) tomato sauce, unsalted
1 tablespoon Cajun seasoning

Combine and simmer ingredients on stove for 30 minutes.

Variations:

Cajun Beans #2

Add 4 teaspoons olive oil to Standard Recipe, and follow same directions.

Yields: 2 servings
1 serving:
                    calories   = 375
                    fat   = 12 gm
                    cholesterol   = 0 mg
                    exchanges   = 2 Bread +
                                    2 Meat +
                                    1 Vegetable +
                                    2 Fat

———————— Cajun-Style Red Beans and Brown Rice ————————

Yields: 8 servings
1 serving (1 cup beans, ¾ cup rice):
                    calories   = 365
                    fat   = 3 gm
                    cholesterol   = 0 mg
                    exchanges   = 3½ Bread +
                                    1½ Meat

1 pound dried pinto beans
2 cups chopped yellow onion
1 cup chopped green onion
1 cup chopped green pepper
1 clove garlic, finely chopped
¼ teaspoon red cayenne pepper
1¼ teaspoons black pepper
½ teaspoon salt
¼ teaspoon oregano
¼ teaspoon garlic powder
1 tablespoon Worcestershire sauce
3 dashes tabasco
6 ounces tomato paste (may use low-sodium)
¼ teaspoon thyme
1 teaspoon celery flakes
1 pound turkey ham, cut into bite-size chunks
6 cups brown rice, cooked according to package directions

Rinse beans and soak for 12 hours. Drain water. Fill stockpot
with water ½ inch above beans. Add remaining ingredients

except turkey ham and rice. Cook over low heat 1 hour, covered. Add ham and cook uncovered an additional 1 to 1½ hours. Serve over cooked brown rice.

Note: This is an alternative recipe to the ones in the menu called "Cajun Beans with Brown Rice #1 and #2."

——————————— Calico Bean Chowder ———————————

Yields: 12 servings
1 serving (1 cup):   calories   = 165
                       fat   = 3 gm
                       cholesterol = 3 mg
                       exchanges   = 1 Meat +
                                      1 Bread +
                                      ½ Milk

½ pound dried navy beans, great northern, or small white beans
2 cups dark or light red kidney beans, cooked or canned
1 teaspoon salt
1 cup chopped onion
1½ cups chopped celery
¼ cup diet margarine
¼ cup flour
¼ teaspoon pepper
3 cups skim milk
1 16-ounce can tomatoes (may use low-sodium)
1 package frozen whole-kernel corn
1 to 3 dashes tabasco sauce

Rinse dried beans and soak in 3 cups cold water for 6 to 8 hours. *Do not refrigerate.* Drain, rinse. In large stockpot, cook beans in 4 cups hot water with 1 teaspoon salt. Cook until tender—about 2 hours. *Do not drain.* Sauté onion and celery in diet margarine in saucepan. Blend in flour and pepper. Stir in skim milk and bring to a boil. Immediately add to bean mixture (if using canned kidney beans, add them at this time), then add tomatoes, corn, and tabasco. Heat to boiling. Cook for 10 to 15 minutes. Serve hot.

================================ Pinto Beans ================================

Standard Recipe—Pinto Beans #1

Yields: 4 servings
1 serving (½ cup):   calories   = 255
                       fat   = 10 gm
                       cholesterol = 0 mg
                       exchanges   = 1 Bread +
                                     1 Meat +
                                     1 Vegetable +
                                     2 Fat

Note: ½ cup beans = 1 Meat + 1 Bread

2 cups (16-ounce can) pinto beans, prepared
2 cups (16-ounce can) tomato sauce, unsalted
2 tablespoons and 2 teaspoons vegetable oil
2 teaspoons chili powder
Optional:
1 teaspoon Mexican seasonings

Combine all ingredients in saucepan. Heat and simmer on stovetop
20 to 30 minutes.

Variation:

Pinto Beans #2

Omit oil. Follow Standard Recipe directions.

Yields: 4 servings
1 serving (½ cup):   calories   = 165
                       fat   = 0 gm
                       cholesterol = 0 mg
                       exchanges   = 1 Bread +
                                     1 Meat +
                                     1 Vegetable

—————————————— Gumbo ——————————————

Yields: 7 cups
1 serving (1 cup):   calories   = 140
                      fat   = 1 gm
                      cholesterol = 78 mg
                      exchanges   = 1 Bread +
                                     1 Meat

½ pound chicken breasts, without skin
1 medium onion, chopped
1 medium green pepper, chopped
1 garlic clove, minced
1 tablespoon flour
1-pound can low-sodium whole tomatoes
½ pound fresh okra, sliced
1 tablespoon dried parsley
1 crushed bay leaf
½ teaspoon vinegar
½ teaspoon pepper
dash of red pepper
dash of thyme
½ pound crabmeat
½ pound cocktail shrimp, cooked

Trim excess fat from chicken breasts. Place in a saucepan with
water to cover. Bring to a boil. Cover, reduce heat, and cook
30 minutes. Drain chicken, and let cool to touch. Remove
chicken from bone, chop meat, and set aside.

Sauté onion, green pepper, and garlic with 1 tablespoon
water. Add flour and cook for 1 minute, stirring constantly.
Add 3½ cups water, chicken, and remaining ingredients except
crabmeat and shrimp. Cook until boiling, reduce heat, and
simmer 30 minutes. Stir in crab and shrimp. Cook 30 minutes.

Won Ton Soup

Yields: 6 servings
1 serving (1 cup):   calories   = 140
                                  fat   = 3 gm
                                  cholesterol = 34 mg
                                  exchanges = 2 Bread

1 package (1 pound) won ton skins
⅓ pound ground turkey
⅛ cup chopped cucumber
1 tablespoon shredded bamboo shoots
1 tablespoon chopped green onion
3 cups chicken broth
Seasoning for turkey:
¼ teaspoon ground ginger
1 teaspoon soy sauce
½ tablespoon vegetable oil
½ tablespoon cooking sherry
1 egg white
For garnish in soup:
1 tablespoon chopped green onion
¼ cup thinly sliced cucumber

Won ton filling:
Drain chopped cucumber, bamboo shoots, and green onion.
Mix ground turkey with seasonings. Add vegetables to turkey.

To fill won tons:
Place ½ teaspoon of filling in center of each won ton skin. Fold
one side of the wrapper over the filling, leaving ½ inch of
unrolled skin, and pull bottom corners of the folded tube gently
down until the ends overlap. Pinch ends together. In case of
dryness, use water to moisten bottom corners.

To cook won tons:
Bring 6 cups water to a boil. Place filled won tons in boiling
water. Return to a boil, add 1 cup cold water, and bring to a
boil again. Won tons will float on the surface of the water when
they are done. Remove with slotted spoon.
      Meanwhile, in saucepan bring chicken broth to a boil.

Garnish soup bowls with chopped green onion, sliced cucumber, and cooked won tons. Add chicken broth. Serve hot.

―――――――――― Vegetable Soup ――――――――――

Yields: 8 servings
1 serving (1 cup):   calories   = 70
                     fat   = 1 gm
                     cholesterol = 0 mg
                     exchanges   = 1 Bread

3 carrots, chopped
1 head cabbage, shredded
2 stalks celery, chopped
1 medium onion, chopped
1 cup frozen yellow corn
½ cup frozen green beans
2 teaspoons dried sweet basil
1 teaspoon dried parsley
1 28-ounce can tomatoes
6 low-sodium beef bouillon cubes, dissolved in 6 cups boiling
    water
½ teaspoon salt
¼ teaspoon pepper

Place vegetables and spices in a large pot with tomatoes and bouillon. Bring to a boil, and simmer, covered, until thick, about 45 minutes. Season to taste with salt and pepper.

―――――――――― Minestrone Soup ――――――――――

Yields: 10 servings
1 serving (1 cup):   calories   = 70
                     fat   = 0 gm
                     cholesterol = 3 mg
                     exchanges   = 1 Bread

½ cup dried white beans
8 low-sodium chicken bouillon cubes
½ cup shredded cabbage
2 carrots, sliced
1-pound can whole tomatoes, chopped
½ cup chopped onion
2 stalks celery, chopped
1 small potato, chopped
2 small tomatoes, chopped
1 ounce spaghetti noodles, uncooked and broken
½ garlic clove, minced
1 tablespoon dried parsley
¼ teaspoon pepper
½ teaspoon dried marjoram
½ teaspoon dried thyme
½ teaspoon dried oregano

Soak white beans overnight in water. The next day, in saucepan, dissolve bouillon cubes in 8 cups of boiling water. Add drained white beans to chicken broth. Add remaining ingredients. Reduce heat, cover, and simmer for 60 minutes or until beans are tender.

—————————————— Lentil Soup ——————————————

Yields: 8 servings
1 serving (1 cup):   calories   = 75
                        fat   = 4 gm
                        cholesterol = 0 mg
                        exchanges   = 1 Meat +
                                      1 Bread +
                                      1 Vegetable

1¼ cups dried lentils (approximately ½ pound)
1 quart cold water
1 cup chopped onion
1 garlic clove, crushed
½ teaspoon salt
¼ teaspoon pepper
1 stalk celery, chopped
2 tablespoons vegetable oil
1 16-ounce can tomatoes
1 bay leaf
1 teaspoon Worcestershire sauce

Wash lentils; drain well. Combine lentils with water, onion, garlic, salt, pepper, celery, and oil in large saucepan. Bring to a boil. Add tomatoes, bay leaf, and Worcestershire sauce. Reduce heat, cover, and simmer 45 minutes or until lentils are tender. Serve with lemon juice or wine vinegar if desired.

——————————— Sesame Broccoli ———————————

Yields: 6 servings

1 serving (1 cup):		
calories	=	70
fat	=	3 gm
cholesterol	=	0 mg
exchanges	=	2 Vegetable + ½ Fat

1 tablespoon sesame seeds, toasted
1 pound fresh broccoli, trimmed and cut into spears
1 tablespoon olive oil or safflower oil
1 tablespoon vinegar
1 tablespoon "lite" soy sauce
Optional:
1 teaspoon sugar

Toast sesame seeds on a cookie sheet in oven on low heat. Remove. Steam broccoli until tender-crisp. In saucepan, combine oil, vinegar, soy sauce, sugar, and sesame seeds. Heat until boiling. Pour sauce over broccoli, turning to coat evenly.

Variation:
Omit the oil to make fat-free.

Yields: 6 servings
1 serving (1 cup):   calories   = 50
                      fat   = 0 gm
                      cholesterol = 0 mg
                      exchanges   = 2 Vegetable

——————————— Carrot Raisin Salad ———————————

Yields: 2 servings
1 serving (½ cup):   calories   = 115
                      fat   = 5 gm
                      cholesterol = 1 mg
                      exchanges   = 1 Vegetable +
                                    1 Fruit +
                                    1 Fat
Note: 1 carrot (½ cup) = 1 Vegetable
         2 tablespoons raisins = 1 Fruit
         1 tablespoon diet mayonnaise = 1 Fat

2 carrots, grated
4 tablespoons raisins
2 tablespoons diet mayonnaise
pinch of salt (⅛ teaspoon)

Mix all ingredients. Chill 1 hour before serving.

——————————— Onion Stuffed Potatoes ———————————

Yields: 6 servings
1 serving (1 potato): calories   = 135
                       fat   = 2 gm
                       cholesterol = 0 mg
                       exchanges   = 1½ Bread +
                                     ½ Fat

6 long white potatoes
2 medium onions, pared and thinly sliced
2 tablespoons diet margarine
1½ teaspoons garlic powder
¾ teaspoon pepper
2 tablespoons grated Parmesan cheese
parsley, chopped, to taste
paprika to taste

Preheat oven to 400°F. Wash potatoes thoroughly. Slice cross-wise at ¼-inch intervals (*do not* cut all the way through). Place onion slices into slits in potatoes, then dot with margarine and sprinkle seasonings over top. Wrap potatoes in foil. Bake for 60 minutes.

―――――――――――――― Potato Salad ――――――――――――――

Yields: 4 servings
1 serving (½ cup): calories   = 115
                    fat   = 5 gm
                    cholesterol = 0 mg
                    exchanges = 1 Bread +
                                 1 Fat

2 medium red potatoes
5 green onions, chopped
2 celery stalks, chopped
1 tablespoon chopped parsley
⅛ teaspoon salt
⅛ teaspoon pepper
4 tablespoons diet mayonnaise

Wash and scrub new red potatoes, leaving skins on. Cut into small pieces. Steam 20 to 30 minutes or microwave 5 to 10 minutes, until firm, but cooked. Chill 1 hour. Combine potatoes, onion, celery, parsley, salt, pepper, and mayonnaise, and serve.

Pasta Salad

Standard Recipe—Pasta Salad #1

Yields: 2 servings
1 serving (approximately 2 cups):

calories	=	500
fat	=	20 gm
cholesterol	=	118 mg
exchanges	=	2 Bread +
		2 Vegetable +
		3 Meat +
		3 Fat

3 ounces dry pasta, choice of elbow macaroni, shells, or other
     (makes approximately 2 cups pasta cooked)
2 to 4 ounces chicken breasts, diced without skin or bone
½ cup chopped broccoli
½ cup sliced mushrooms
½ cup chopped yellow squash
½ cup diced green peppers
½ cup diced green onions
1 tablespoon olive oil
1 tablespoon corn oil

Prepare pasta according to package directions. Drain. Set aside
to cool. Steam chicken for about 15 minutes or until tender. Set
aside to cool. Steam broccoli, mushrooms, and yellow squash
separately until slightly tender (about 5 minutes). Set aside to
cool. Mix together pasta, chicken, and vegetables. Add uncooked green pepper and onion. Toss lightly with oils.

Note: per serving, 4 ounces raw chicken = 3 ounces cooked (3
Meat).

Variations:

Pasta Salad #2

Use 2 to 3 ounces chicken breasts. Use 2 teaspoons olive oil
and 2 teaspoons corn oil.

Follow same directions as Standard Recipe.

Note: per serving, 3 ounces raw chicken = 2 ounces cooked (2 Meat).

Yields: 2 servings
1 serving (approximately 2 cups):

calories	= 400
fat	= 14 gm
cholesterol	= 95 mg
exchanges	= 2 Bread +
	2 Vegetable +
	2 Meat +
	2 Fat

Pasta Salad #3

Use 1 to 3 ounces chicken breasts. Use 2 teaspoons olive oil and 2 teaspoons corn oil.

Follow same directions as Standard Recipe.

Note: per serving, 1½ ounces raw chicken = 1 ounce cooked (1 Meat).

Yields: 2 servings
1 serving (approximately 2 cups):

calories	= 350
fat	= 13 gm
cholesterol	= 73 mg
exchanges	= 2 Bread +
	2 Vegetable +
	1 Meat +
	2 Fat

Pasta Salad #4

Use 4 teaspoons olive oil and 4 teaspoons corn oil.

Follow same directions as Standard Recipe.

Note: per serving, 4 ounces raw chicken = 3 ounces cooked (3 Meat).

Yields: 2 servings
1 serving (approximately 2 cups):

calories	= 540
fat	= 24 gm
cholesterol	= 118 mg
exchanges	= 2 Bread +
	2 Vegetable +
	3 Meat +
	4 Fat

Pasta Salad #5

Use 4 ounces dry pasta (makes 2½ cups cooked pasta). Use 2 to 3 ounces chicken breasts. Use 4 teaspoons olive oil and 4 teaspoons corn oil.

Follow same directions as Standard Recipe.

Note: per serving, 3 ounces raw chicken = 2 ounces cooked (2 Meat).

Yields: 2 servings
1 serving (approximately 2½ cups):

calories	= 550
fat	= 24 gm
cholesterol	= 115 mg
exchanges	= 3 Bread +
	2 Vegetable +
	2 Meat +
	4 Fat

Pasta Salad #6

Use 4 ounces dry pasta (makes 2½ cups cooked pasta). Omit chicken breasts. Use 4 teaspoons olive oil and 4 teaspoons corn oil.

Follow same directions as Standard Recipe.

Yields: 2 servings
1 serving (approximately 2½ cups):

calories	= 440
fat	= 22 gm
cholesterol	= 70 mg
exchanges	= 3 Bread +
	2 Vegetable +
	4 Fat

———————————— Citrus Spinach Salad ————————————

Yields: 2 servings
1 serving (1 cup):

calories	= 65
fat	= 0 gm
cholesterol	= 0 gm
exchanges	= 1 Vegetable +
	1 Fruit

Note: 1 cup spinach = 1 Vegetable
      1 orange = 1 Fruit

2 cups fresh spinach leaves
2 oranges, sectioned

Wash and drain spinach. Section oranges. Combine spinach and fruit in bowl. Add dressing as menu suggests.

Variation:
For a change, try tangerine, tangelo, grapefruit sections, or a combination of fruits.

Spinach Lasagna

Standard Recipe—Spinach Lasagna #1

Yields: 6 servings
1 serving (4 × 4½-inch square):

calories	= 410
fat	= 11 gm
cholesterol	= 35 mg
exchanges	= 2 Bread +
	3 Meat +
	2 Vegetable

1 large onion, chopped
3 cloves garlic, minced
1 16-ounce can unsalted tomatoes, chopped
1 6-ounce can unsalted tomato paste
pinch of basil, oregano, and rosemary leaves
10 ounces uncooked lasagna noodles (6 cups cooked)
1 pound fresh spinach, lightly steamed and chopped, **or** 1 package (10 ounces) frozen spinach, chopped and thawed
1 cup skim ricotta cheese
3 tablespoons grated Parmesan cheese
2 cups low-fat cottage cheese
4 ounces part-skim mozzarella cheese slices
Optional:
½ cup sliced mushrooms

Lightly sauté onion and garlic. Add tomatoes, tomato paste, and herbs. Simmer for ½ hour. Cook noodles in unsalted water until tender and drain. Steam spinach and drain. Mix skim ricotta, Parmesan, and low-fat cottage cheese and mushrooms. Layer ingredients in a 9 × 13-inch baking dish in the following order:

    small amount of tomato sauce
    ⅓ of cooked noodles
    ½ of cheese mixture
    ½ of drained spinach
    ½ of tomato sauce
    repeat as above, ending with noodles and tomato sauce
Place mozzarella slices on top of casserole.

Preheat oven to 350°F. Bake for about 40 minutes until bubbly. Let stand about 15 minutes before serving.

Variations:

Spinach Lasagna #2

Use 1 cup low-fat cottage cheese and 2 ounces part-skim mozzarella slices. Follow same directions as Standard Recipe.

Yields: 6 servings
1 serving (4 × 4½-inch square):

calories	= 350
fat	= 9 gm
cholesterol	= 25 mg
exchanges	= 2 Bread +
	2 Meat +
	2 Vegetable

Spinach Lasagna #3

Use 2 16-ounce cans of tomatoes and 12 ounces uncooked lasagna noodles. Sauté onion and garlic in 3 tablespoons olive oil before following same directions as Standard Recipe.

Yields: 6 servings
1 serving (4 × 4½-inch square):

calories	= 575
fat	= 20 gm
cholesterol	= 35 mg
exchanges	= 4 Bread +
	3 Meat +
	1 Vegetable +
	2 Fat

Spinach Lasagna #4

Yields: 6 servings
1 serving (4 × 4½-inch square):

calories	= 425
fat	= 8 gm
cholesterol	= 25 mg
exchanges	= 4 Bread +
	2 Meat +
	1 Vegetable

Use 12 ounces uncooked lasagna noodles, 1 cup low-fat cottage cheese, and 2 ounces part-skim mozzarella slices. Follow same directions as Standard Recipe.

Zucchini Lasagna

Yields: 6 servings
1 serving (2½ × 2½-inch square):

calories	= 330
fat	= 16 gm
cholesterol	= 109 mg
exchanges	= 3 Meat +
	3 Vegetable +
	1 Fat

6 zucchini, sliced lengthwise
½ to 1 pound lean ground beef
1 6-ounce can tomato paste
½ teaspoon basil
½ teaspoon oregano
½ teaspoon salt
⅛ teaspoon garlic powder
1 cup cottage cheese
1 egg
¼ cup dry breadcrumbs
1 cup grated mozzarella cheese

Steam zucchini until translucent and tender. Set aside. In skillet, brown ground beef, drain excess fat. Add tomato paste, basil, oregano, salt, and garlic powder to beef. Set aside.

Combine cottage cheese and egg in small bowl. Preheat oven to 350°F. Layer ingredients in 8 × 8 × 2-inch baking dish in the following order:
    zucchini
    breadcrumbs
    meat mixture
    cottage cheese mixture
    mozzarella cheese
    Repeat as above.
    Cover. Bake until bubbly. Check and see if too "soupy"—if so, bake uncovered until consistency is firm, but not dry.

Optional:
Add layers of fresh mushrooms and/or add more meat, sauce, and cheese.

─────────────── Seasonal Fruit Salad ───────────────

Yields: 8 servings
1 serving (½ cup):   calories   = 40
                       fat   = 0 gm
                       cholesterol   = 0 mg
                       exchanges   = 1 Fruit

1 medium apple, chopped
1 banana, sliced
1 orange, sectioned
1 cup seasonal fruit of choice (seedless grapes, berries, melon, pineapple, pear)

Combine fruit and serve.

─────────────── Italian Salad Dressing ───────────────

Yields: 24 servings
1 serving (1 tablespoon):
                       calories   = 95
                       fat   = 10 gm
                       cholesterol   = 0 mg
                       exchanges   = 2 Fat

1 cup olive oil or safflower oil (or ½ cup each)
¼ cup lemon juice, fresh-squeezed
¼ cup herb vinegar
½ teaspoon dry mustard
1 teaspoon grated fresh onion or ½ teaspoon onion powder
½ teaspoon paprika
½ teaspoon dried oregano leaves
½ teaspoon dried thyme leaves
2 cloves garlic, crushed
Optional:
1 teaspoon salt
1 teaspoon sugar

Combine all ingredients, place in tightly covered jar, and shake thoroughly.

Note: Best if made several hours before serving. If olive oil is used, store at room temperature to prevent hardening.

―――――――――― Yogurt Dressing ――――――――――

Yields: 6 servings
1 serving (1 tablespoon):

$$\begin{array}{ll} \text{calories} & = 35 \\ \text{fat} & = 3 \text{ gm} \\ \text{cholesterol} & = 3 \text{ mg} \\ \text{exchanges} & = 1 \text{ Fat} \end{array}$$

2 teaspoons lemon juice
1 tablespoon oil
½ cup plain low-fat yogurt
½ teaspoon mint
½ teaspoon dill
Optional:
⅛ teaspoon garlic powder
⅛ teaspoon onion powder

Mix all ingredients together in a blender on medium speed for 5 seconds. Keep refrigerated in covered jar.

──────────────── Barbecue Sauce ────────────────

Yields: 12 servings
1 serving (2 tablespoons):

calories	= 45
fat	= 4 gm
cholesterol	= 0 mg
exchanges	= 1 Fat

¼ cup water
¼ cup vinegar
3 tablespoons olive oil
½ cup chili sauce or catsup
3 tablespoons Worcestershire sauce
1 tablespoon dry mustard
2 tablespoons chopped onion
freshly ground black pepper

Combine all ingredients in saucepan and simmer uncovered for 15 to 20 minutes.

Uses:
A good marinade for beef, pork, or chicken.

──────────────── Lime Ginger Sauce ────────────────

Yields: 4 servings

1 serving (¼ cup):	calories	= 25
	fat	= 0 gm
	cholesterol	= 0 mg
	exchanges	= 1 Vegetable

⅓ cup soy sauce
1 tablespoon lime juice
¼ teaspoon grated lime peel
¼ cup minced green onion
3 tablespoons water
1 garlic clove, minced **or**
½ teaspoon ginger root, minced **or**
½ teaspoon ginger powder

Combine all ingredients in small saucepan and heat until boiling; cook 1 minute.

Uses:
Can be used as marinade for poultry and fish and used to baste while baking, or can be used as dip for poached shrimp, fish, or chicken.

———————————— Marinara Sauce ————————————

Yields: 8 servings
1 serving (1 cup):   calories   = 70
                         fat   = 2 gm
                         cholesterol   = 0 mg
                         exchanges   = 1 Bread

Yields: 10 servings
1 serving (¾ cup):   calories   = 50
                         fat   = 1 gm
                         cholesterol   = 0 mg
                         exchanges   = 2 Vegetable

Yields: 16 servings
1 serving (½ cup):   calories   = 35
                         fat   = 0 gm
                         cholesterol   = 0 mg
                         exchanges   = 1 Vegetable

1 tablespoon olive oil
2 cloves garlic, minced
4 16-ounce cans low-sodium tomatoes, chopped
2 16-ounce cans low-sodium tomato sauce
2 teaspoons crushed oregano
1½ tablespoons dried parsley

Heat olive oil in skillet. When hot, sauté garlic. Do not brown garlic. Add chopped tomatoes and tomato sauce to skillet. Stir in oregano and parsley. Bring to a boil and simmer covered for 1½ hours, stirring occasionally.

Note: This sauce is virtually fat-free, due to the small amount of oil in such a large recipe. Each cup contains less than 2 grams of fat.

_____ Red Wine and Mushroom Sauce _____

Yields: 2 servings
1 serving (1 cup): | calories   = 125
                    | fat   = 2 gm
                    | cholesterol = 0 mg
                    | exchanges   = 1 Bread +
                    | ½ Fat

1 teaspoon diet margarine
2 tablespoons minced green onion
1 garlic clove, minced
3 cups sliced fresh mushrooms
½ cup red cooking wine
1 teaspoon cornstarch
½ cup low-sodium beef broth
freshly ground pepper

In large, nonstick skillet, over medium heat, heat margarine until bubbly. Stir in green onion and garlic; sauté 2 minutes. *Do not brown.* Add mushrooms; sauté until tender. Stir in wine; bring to a boil and cook 1 minute. Dissolve cornstarch in beef broth. Stir into mushroom mixture; bring to a boil and cook 1 minute, stirring constantly. Season to taste with pepper. Serve with poultry, fish, or veal.

Uses:
Add 1 15-ounce can low-sodium whole tomatoes, drained and chopped.

Yields: 2 servings
1 serving (1 cup): | calories   = 150
                    | fat   = 2 gm
                    | cholesterol = 0 mg
                    | exchanges   = 1 Bread +
                    | ½ Fat +
                    | 1 Vegetable

—————————— Teriyaki Sauce ——————————

Yields: 6 servings
1 serving (2½ tablespoons):

calories	= 45
fat	= 3 gm
cholesterol	= 0 mg
exchanges	= 1 Fat

1 tablespoon olive oil
¼ cup low-sodium ("lite") soy sauce
¼ cup pineapple juice
2 tablespoons vinegar
1½ teaspoons ground ginger
2 tablespoons finely chopped green onion
1 clove garlic, minced
1 tablespoon cooking sherry

Combine all ingredients and pour over chicken or fish. Marinate overnight for chicken and 1 hour for fish. Turn occasionally. When cooking poultry or fish, baste occasionally. Do not overcook.

Uses:
Marinade may be used for flank steak also.

—————————— Cornbread Muffins ——————————

Yields: 12 2-inch-square muffins
1 serving (1 muffin):

calories	= 110
fat	= 3 gm
cholesterol	= 20 mg
exchanges	= 1 Bread + 1 Fat

¾ cup flour, sifted
2½ teaspoons baking powder
1 tablespoon sugar
½ teaspoon salt
1¼ cups cornmeal, yellow or white water-ground
1 egg, beaten
2 tablespoons melted margarine
1 cup skim milk

Preheat oven to 425°F. Combine dry ingredients and set aside. Mix egg, margarine, and skim milk in second bowl. Pour liquid mixture into dry mixture. Blend with a few rapid strokes. Lightly grease a 6 × 8-inch pan with margarine or oil. Place pan by itself in the oven until sizzling hot. Pour muffin mixture into sizzling hot pan. Bake 25 minutes.

_____ Oat Bran Muffins _____

Yields: 24 small muffins
1 serving (1 muffin): calories   = 60
                        fat   = 1.5 gm
                        cholesterol = 0 mg
                        exchanges   = 1 Bread

2 cups oat bran
¼ cup sugar or brown sugar, firmly packed
2 teaspoons baking powder
1 cup skim milk
¼ cup egg substitute, or two egg whites, slightly beaten
¼ cup honey
2 tablespoons corn oil
1 tablespoon vanilla extract

Preheat oven to 425°F. Line 24 mini-muffin cups with paper baking cups or spray tins with vegetable oil cooking spray. Mix together all dry ingredients. Add skim milk, egg substitute, honey, oil, and vanilla extract. Mix just enough so dry ingredients are moistened. Divide mixture into muffin tins so cups are nearly full. Bake for 12 to 15 minutes or until lightly browned.

─────────── Homemade Cheese Danish Rolls ───────────

Yields: 1 serving
1 serving (2 halves): calories   = 260
                       fat   = 2 gm
                       cholesterol = 15 mg
                       exchanges   = 2 Bread +
                                     1 Meat +
                                     1 Fruit

1 whole wheat English muffin
4 tablespoons skim ricotta cheese
½ cup applesauce, unsweetened
1 teaspoon ground cinnamon

Preheat oven on BROIL. Toast whole wheat English muffin halves
lightly. Top toasted muffin halves with ricotta cheese and applesauce. Sprinkle with cinnamon. Broil 2 to 3 minutes until cheese
melts.

─────────────── Oatmeal Pancakes ───────────────

Yields: 12 small pancakes, each 5 inches across
1 pancake: calories   = 70
                      fat   = 0 gm
                      cholesterol = 1 mg
                      exchanges   = 1 Bread

1½ cups uncooked oatmeal
2 cups buttermilk
1 egg or 2 egg whites
1 cup whole wheat flour
2 teaspoons baking soda
1 banana, mashed

Combine oatmeal, buttermilk, and egg (or egg whites) and
let stand for at least ½ hour or refrigerate up to 24 hours.
Add remaining ingredients and stir the batter just until the
dry ingredients are moistened. Bake on a hot, lightly oiled
griddle.

———————— Whole Wheat Pancakes ————————

Yields: 12 small pancakes, each 5 inches across
1 pancake: calories   = 70
                          fat   = 1 gm
                          cholesterol = 0 mg
                          exchanges   = 1 Bread

⅔ cup whole wheat flour, preferably stone-ground
⅓ cup flour
¼ cup oats **or**
¼ cup more whole wheat flour
2 tablespoons wheat germ
2 teaspoons sugar
1 teaspoon baking powder
½ teaspoon baking soda
⅛ teaspoon salt (optional)
3 egg whites
1 cup buttermilk
¼ cup skim milk, more if mixture is too dry
1 tablespoon corn or safflower oil
Optional:
¼ teaspoon vanilla extract

Mix together all dry ingredients in a medium bowl. In a separate bowl, beat egg whites until fluffy. Set aside. In a third bowl, combine buttermilk, skim milk, oil, and vanilla (optional), folding in egg whites. Add to the dry ingredients, stirring just to combine them. Let the batter stand for about 10 minutes. Bake on a hot, lightly oiled griddle.

———————— Angel Food Cake ————————

Yields: 18 servings
1 serving (1½-inch slice):
                          calories   = 70
                          fat   = 0 gm
                          cholesterol = 0 mg
                          exchanges   = 1 Bread

1¾ cups egg whites (about 12)
1½ teaspoons cream of tartar
⅛ teaspoon salt
1 teaspoon vanilla
½ teaspoon almond extract
1¾ cups sugar
1¼ cups flour, sifted

Preheat oven to 375°F. Place egg whites, cream of tartar, salt, vanilla, and almond extract in a large *clean* mixing bowl. Beat the mixture until foamy. Gradually, 2 tablespoons at a time, add 1 cup sugar. Beat at least 10 seconds after each addition. Continue beating mixture until meringue is very firm and holds stiff straight peaks.

In a separate bowl, measure and sift together 3 times flour and remaining ¾ cup sugar. Divide flour/sugar mixture into fourths. Fold each fourth gently into meringue, just until flour/sugar mixture disappears. After all has been folded in, push batter *gently* into 10-inch *clean, ungreased* tube pan. Gently cut with a knife through batter in ever-widening circles to break air bubbles. Bake on the *lower* rack of the oven for 35 to 45 minutes. Remove from oven, invert pan on a bottle neck, and let cake hang until cold.

Apple Oatmeal Crisp

Yields: 8 equal servings per baking dish:
1 serving (⅛ of recipe):

calories	= 75
fat	= 2 gm
cholesterol	= 0 mg
exchanges	= 1 Bread

2 medium apples, cut into ¼-inch slices
1 tablespoon sugar
¼ teaspoon ground cinnamon
¼ teaspoon vanilla extract
1½ ounces oats (oatmeal)
3 tablespoons dry breadcrumbs
3 tablespoons whole wheat flour
1 tablespoon and 1 teaspoon margarine
1 tablespoon and 1 teaspoon light brown sugar, firmly packed

Preheat oven to 325°F. In a bowl toss apple slices, sugar, cinnamon, and vanilla. Transfer to 8 × 8-inch baking dish. In a separate bowl, blend the remaining ingredients with your fingers until crumbly but not overly mixed. Sprinkle over apples. Bake 45 minutes. Cool 10 minutes before serving.

—————————— Raisin Oatmeal Cookies ——————————

Yields: 24 cookies

1 serving (1 cookie): calories = 100
fat = 3 gm
cholesterol = 0 mg
exchanges = 1 Bread +
½ Fat

1 cup whole wheat flour, sifted
½ teaspoon baking soda
½ teaspoon salt
¼ teaspoon ground cinnamon
⅛ teaspoon ground cloves
⅛ teaspoon nutmeg
1½ cups quick-cooking oats
2 egg whites, slightly beaten
¼ cup brown sugar
¼ cup chopped dates
⅓ cup oil
½ cup skim milk
1 teaspoon vanilla extract
1 cup seedless raisins

Preheat oven to 375°F. In bowl, sift together flour, baking soda, salt, cinnamon, cloves, and nutmeg. Stir in oats. In a separate bowl, combine egg whites, brown sugar, dates, oil, skim milk, vanilla, and raisins. Add to flour mixture. Mix well. Drop batter a teaspoon at a time onto an oiled cookie sheet. Bake 12 to 15 minutes, depending on texture desired. Shorter baking time results in a chewy soft cookie, the longer time in a crisp cookie.

TEN

Alcohol and
the Cholesterol
Question

A recent spate of headlines and declarations in the popular press has proclaimed a similar message:

- "Drinking Beer or Liquor Can Cut Chances of Heart Attack in Half"—*The National Enquirer*

- "Drinkers Have Stronger Hearts"—*U.S.A. Today*

- ". . . two drinks a day appear to be healthful in combating arterial and heart disease . . ."—*The Wall Street Journal*

What does all this mean? Is it really true that a few drinks a day can provide some sort of panacea for atherosclerosis?

I wish to say this right at the outset: Alcohol is *not* a cure-all for cardiovascular disease! Some of the most recent studies on this subject do indicate that limited alcohol consumption *may* help with at least one risk factor associated with atherosclerosis—the raising of HDL levels. But for many people, the dangers of alcohol consumption far outweigh any possible benefits. As one researcher in this area, Dr. Kenneth W. Heaton of the University of Bristol in England, has said, "Heavy alcohol intake causes serious damage to the brain, liver, pancreas, stomach, nerves, and even the heart. It shortens or blights the life of millions." (*Executive Health Report*, vol. XXI, no. 11, August 1985)

In a similar vein, Dr. Roberta G. Ferrance and several colleagues have reported that "claims that moderate consumption of alcoholic beverages prevents coronary heart disease are exaggerated in the mass media and are less conclusive than is often suggested."

Their conclusion, based on the strength of available evidence, was that "it would be unwise to alter either the scientific or public focus on the damage caused by alcohol or to support changes in policy that might make drinking more socially acceptable and thereby encourage higher levels of consumption."*

So we mustn't rush to a favorable judgment about alcohol. The last thing anyone should do is stock up the liquor cabinet in the home with the expectation that we're going to wipe out heart disease in the family. Far from it! Any movement toward greater alcohol consumption may in fact kill us.

Still, it's important for us to understand what the effect of moderate alcohol consumption may be on cholesterol—and, by inference, on the risk of coronary artery disease. The final results are by no means in on this subject. But here are a few highlights, both pro and con, about the impact of alcohol consumption on one's arteries and heart:

• A study of 234 alcoholics in Pittsburgh beginning in 1983 showed that "alcohol consumption is associated with an increase in HDL cholesterol concentrations." Furthermore, this study established that the increase in HDL cholesterol was a "combination of an increase in both HDL-2 and HDL-3 cholesterol subclasses, mainly HDL-2 cholesterol." As you'll recall, many researchers today feel that HDL-2 cholesterol is the most protective subclass of HDL in combating cardiovascular disease.

• Others, however, have questioned whether moderate consumption of alcohol would really elevate the HDL-2, which is thought to be protective against atherosclerosis and coronary heart disease. (*Journal of the American Medical Association*, vol. 242, December 21, 1979, p. 2,746)

• A Harvard Medical School study showed that moderate consumption of beer, wine, or liquor ("moderate" being 2 ounces of alcohol per day) is "inversely correlated with death from *coronary heart disease.*" (*Journal of the American Medical Association*, vol. 242, December 21, 1979, pp. 1,973–74)

• A study in England showed that drinking half a bottle of white wine every day for six weeks—a potentially dangerous amount, I might add, for the average person—increased blood levels of HDL cholesterol significantly.

Using an index rather than the absolute value to compare the "before" and "after" levels of the HDLs, the researchers found that their average HDL cholesterol levels started at an index figure of 1.07. Then, with the wine-drinking, the levels rose to 1.25. Finally, when the participants began to abstain again, their HDL levels fell to 1.04.

One of those conducting the study concluded, "These changes suggest there is a reduction in the risk of coronary heart disease with moderate alcohol intake."

• A study of 12 patients at the Veterans Administration Medical Center in San Diego, California, under the supervision of Dr. Scott M. Grundy, showed that 630 calories of alcohol each day raised HDL levels in all patients studied, from an average of 34.8 mg/dl to 40.2 mg/dl. During this test, the triglyceride levels remained the same in 5 patients, rose temporarily in 5, and remained elevated in 2 others.

• Even as the researchers who are looking into this question report the increase in HDL concentrations, they tend to find that serious health problems and practices plague the individuals whom they're studying.

For example, "The Albany Study," done at the Albany Medical College in Albany, New York, investigated the cardiovascular condition of 1,910 employed men over a period of eighteen years. The men in the study who drank more alcohol, varying from 1 ounce to more than 90 ounces a month, had progressively higher levels of high-density lipoprotein concentrations. But they also had a higher incidence of cigarette use and higher blood pressure readings. Although the study found that there was no significant association between changes in the smoking and drinking habits, it seems that somehow the two habits do go together.

• A study from New Zealand (*American Journal of Epidemiology,* July 1987) showed that those who consume alcohol or perform physical activity have decreased risks of heart attacks and sudden coronary deaths. However, their conclusions were that leisure-time physical activity may be as important as other coronary heart disease risk factors, as alcohol consumption can explain only a minor proportion of coronary heart disease events.

What would I conclude from this seemingly contradictory evidence? Clearly, the jury is still out on this question. We have some indications that moderate consumption of alcohol may raise HDL levels and even reduce the possibility of heart disease. But the studies are scattered and, thus far, not definitive.

Because of the tremendous dangers of alcohol consumption, I would advise you *not* to take up drinking as part of your preventive health program. There are many other good ways to raise your HDL levels and lower your risk of cardiovascular disease. As we'll see in Chapter 12, aerobic exercise can raise your HDL levels as much as, if not more than, alcohol consumption will. Moreover, with this type of endurance activity, you can gain many other health benefits—but without all the other problems that go along with drinking.

In short, I think it's important to be aware of the studies done in this area. But it's also extremely important to weigh the dangers before extolling possible benefits.

ELEVEN

What's Wrong with Smoking?

Although the relationship between alcohol consumption and cholesterol remains somewhat vague, the situation with smoking is more definitive. Let me put this as bluntly as possible: *Without question, cigarette smoking increases your risk of heart disease and upsets your cholesterol levels.*

What's the evidence about smoking?

First of all, the famous Framingham Heart Study, which was conducted over the last several decades in Framingham, Massachusetts, reported back in the 1970s that cigarette smoking lowers blood levels of high-density lipoproteins (HDLs). As I have said many times in this book, HDLs are the component of cholesterol which, in the view of many people, acts as a protection against the development of atherosclerosis or coronary artery disease.

The Framingham Heart Study, an investigation of more than 2,000 women and nearly 2,000 men between 20 and 49 years of age, revealed a lower level of HDLs among smokers. Among a group which included heavy drinkers, the average decrease in HDL levels associated with smoking was 3 to 4 mg/dl in men and 5 to 6 mg/dl in women. When the researchers eliminated the heaviest drinkers from the sample—that is, those whose alcohol consumption would tend to raise the HDL levels—the average lowering in HDL levels was even greater: there was a decline of an average of 4.5 mg/dl for men and 6.5 mg/dl for women.

In this investigation, a key factor was the number of

cigarettes smoked per day, not the number of years a person had been smoking or whether filtered cigarettes were used. Also, the Framingham Study revealed that quitting smoking seemed to reverse the effect of the HDLs—although it took many months for this reversal to occur. Specifically, former smokers who had stayed away from cigarettes for *more* than a year had the same HDL levels as those who had never smoked. Apparently, it takes a year for beneficial effects to emerge: a group of 73 people who had stopped smoking for *less* than a year had lower HDL levels, which were similar to those of current smokers.

Another study involving 10,000 male civil servants in Israel, ranging from age 40 to 65, confirmed the basic Framingham findings. Once again, the HDL levels were lower for smokers than for nonsmokers, although the difference was not as great as in the Framingham Study. The lower HDLs among smokers in the Israeli investigation amounted to an average of only 2.5 mg/dl.

What about cigar and pipe smokers? The HDL levels of these people were about the same as for nonsmokers in the Israeli study. But in the Framingham Study, the cigar and pipe smokers who formerly had been cigarette smokers tended to have lower HDL levels than the average cigar smoker, pipe smoker, or nonsmoker. The reason, says Dr. Robert J. Garrison of the National Heart, Lung and Blood Institute, may be that "cigar and pipe smokers who formerly smoked cigarettes inhale to a greater extent and thus have a higher exposure level [to the negative effects of smoking]."

Other studies have fine-tuned the earlier findings about smoking and HDL levels. In the Lipid Research Clinics Program Prevalence Study, initiated in 1971 in thirteen clinics in four countries, the researchers have found that men who smoked twenty or more cigarettes per day had HDL levels 5.3 mg/dl lower (11 percent lower) than those of nonsmokers. Women who smoked twenty or more cigarettes per day had lower HDL levels than nonsmoking women. Those who used hormones had HDL levels 9.4 mg/dl lower (14 percent lower). Also, women who were not taking the hormones were 8.6 mg/dl lower (again, 14 percent lower) than nonsmokers who were not taking the hormones.

These researchers concluded, as we might expect, that cigarette smoking is associated with substantially lower levels of HDL cholesterol. But they went even further than this. They also said that they believe their evidence is consistent with a causal relationship between cigarette smoking and lower HDL levels. Furthermore, this causal relationship varies according to the number of cigarettes smoked.

They found, for example, that the greatest declines in HDL levels occurred among those smoking twenty or more cigarettes per day. But they also discovered that those who smoked fewer cigarettes—between one and nineteen cigarettes per day—had HDL levels which were at an intermediate level, between those of nonsmokers and those of heavy smokers.

Another area scientific researchers are exploring is the precise biological changes that occur in the vessels and heart as a result of smoking. One team of Wisconsin researchers has come to this conclusion: "Smoking increases the risk of heart attacks, in part by causing deposits which occlude [block] the arteries in the heart. But there also appears to be a second mechanism. Smoking may change certain components of the blood, making it more likely for a blood clot to form in the arteries."

For years it has been known that cigarette smoking has a temporary toxic effect on the heart. Also, we know that in a relatively short period of time, the ex-smoker can drop back into a much lower heart-attack risk category. Probably, though, smoking cigarettes isn't directly responsible for the development of atherosclerosis and plaque buildup. If it were, it's unlikely that this process could be reversed in as short a period of time as six to twelve months. Instead, smoking probably affects *some* of the clotting mechanisms in the body; this limited damage is much easier to reverse than full-blown plaque.

As with alcohol, the studies of the relationship between smoking and cholesterol are continuing. But the direction in which the evidence is taking us is quite clear. To sum up:

• Cigarette smoking lowers the "good" or HDL cholesterol, a result which ultimately is associated with a higher rate of atherosclerosis.

• Cigarette smokers are known to be more susceptible to developing atherosclerosis than are nonsmokers.

• The more cigarettes a person smokes, the more his or her HDL levels will decline.

• Female smokers tend to suffer greater declines in their HDL levels than do male smokers.

In short, the message from the scientific research is coming across loud and clear:

Don't smoke!

TWELVE

What Most People Don't Know About Cholesterol and Aerobic Exercise

"I'm just not very athletic . . . I don't have time to work out on a regular basis . . . My grandmother lived to 100, and the only exercise she ever did was her housework!"

The excuses for not exercising could fill a book. Yet, most people, nonexercisers and exercisers alike, are unaware that the reasons for regular endurance-promoting physical activity go far beyond just "keeping in shape" or building a beautiful body.

In fact, one of the most important purposes of exercise is to keep your cholesterol and blood lipids at normal levels. Exercise—more specifically, "aerobic" or endurance exercise—can do several important things for the state of your blood. First of all, for most people, aerobic exercise will elevate the level of HDL cholesterol, and especially HDL-2 cholesterol. And as we've seen, higher levels of HDL and HDL-2 are associated with a lower incidence of cardiovascular disease.

Also, endurance-type exercise, such as walking, jogging, or swimming, done on a regular basis, will tend to lower the triglycerides; and lower triglycerides, in turn, often accompany a lower risk of coronary artery disease.

Finally, this type of aerobic exercise will burn up more calories and help you to reduce fat and body weight. Remember: lower body fat is associated with lower LDL cholesterol.

But what exactly does aerobic exercise involve? The word *aerobic* means "living in air" or "utilizing oxygen." When it's applied to exercise, the word *aerobics* refers to "a method of physical exercise for producing beneficial changes in the respiratory and circulatory systems by activities which require only a modest increase in oxygen intake." (*Oxford English Dictionary*, 1986 edition.)

Aerobic exercise is usually contrasted with "anaerobic" exercise, which refers to sprinting or other types of physical activity which rapidly lead to exhaustion. Literally, these exercises are done "anaerobically" or "without oxygen."

It's easiest to understand these concepts in terms of specific exercises. Aerobic activities include such sports as walking, running, cycling, swimming, and cross-country skiing. Once you get in reasonably good shape and your endurance increases, you can do exercises of this type over a relatively long period—for many minutes, or even for hours at a time. As you participate in these activities, your breathing tends to be quite regular: you use oxygen at about the same rate that you take it in.

On the other hand, with anaerobic exercise, your body tends to use up more oxygen than it takes in. Sprinting, for example, will cause you to become "out of breath" rather quickly. Your respiratory mechanism will be out of balance for a time, as you push your body to its outer limits.

Generally, I recommend that those who are interested primarily in overall fitness—and maximum increase in their HDL levels—exercise aerobically twenty to thirty minutes a day, a minimum of three to four days a week. If you're a jogger and are in relatively good condition, this will translate into running approximately twelve to fifteen miles per week. For more detailed guidance on these and other sports, see the exercise recommendations at the end of this chapter.

The aerobic, endurance type of exercises are the kind that are most beneficial to the balance of cholesterol and other fats in your blood. Also, this is the best type of exercise to increase your general level of energy, your feelings of well-being, and probably your longevity.

To get an idea about what exercise can do for a person, consider the experience of one government official who came to the Aerobics Center for help. This man, who was in his mid-thirties, didn't have any symptoms of heart disease or any other physical problem. But he knew that he was "out of shape," and he wanted to recapture some of the high energy and harder muscle tone of his youth.

This man was quite sedentary when he enrolled in my program in July 1985. His lack of physical activity showed: He weighed in at 263 pounds, with 28 percent body fat. Moreover, the time that he could walk on the treadmill amounted to a relatively low 13:38 minutes. Given the fitness standards we've established for stress test performance at our clinic, this result indicated his general lack of an adequate aerobic capacity and his poor physical condition.

Perhaps most important of all, the components of his blood were abnormal—either elevated or imbalanced. Specifically, we found the following:

Total cholesterol	246 mg/dl
HDL cholesterol	31 mg/dl
LDL cholesterol	159 mg/dl
Total cholesterol/HDL Ratio	7.9
Triglycerides	281 mg/dl

Clearly, this man was setting the stage for a cardiovascular problem. His total cholesterol/HDL cholesterol ratio was particularly alarming. As we evaluated his nutritional habits, it became evident that at least part of his problem lay in what he was eating. Among other things, he consumed fried foods and red meat *daily*. Overall, his daily intake of fats exceeded 40 percent of the total calories he consumed, well above the recommended 20 to 30 percent level. Also, he tended to eat far more food than he needed, considering the minimal amount of physical activity in which he engaged.

Despite this man's physical condition and his abnormal blood picture, we were optimistic. We felt that we could achieve significant improvement by a straightforward exercise and diet program. First, our nutritionist encouraged him to eliminate all fried foods and substitute most of his red meat dishes with chicken or fish. Also, she placed him on a weight-loss regimen limited to 1,500 calories per day. Next, we placed him on a moderate but progressive jogging program. He responded rapidly and soon had worked up to running about thirty miles per week (five miles a day, six days a week). The results were dramatic!

When he came in for a checkup one year later, his weight had dropped from 263 to 219 pounds. His body fat was down from 28 percent to 18 percent. And the changes in his blood were even more striking. For purposes of comparison, here are the "before" and "after" values:

Lipids	Before	After (1 year later)
Total cholesterol	246 mg/dl	221 mg/dl
HDL cholesterol	31 mg/dl	56 mg/dl
LDL cholesterol	159 mg/dl	143 mg/dl
Total cholesterol/HDL ratio	7.9	3.9
Triglycerides	281 mg/dl	108 mg/dl

In addition, this man's treadmill time—which indicated his overall level of fitness and aerobic capacity—increased dramatically from 13:38 minutes to 25:10 minutes.

In short, in only one year's time, his blood had gone from a seriously abnormal state to one that was normal and in balance. The only possible remaining problem lay with a slightly elevated total cholesterol level. But this may in part have been the result of his relatively high HDLs. In any case, we encouraged him to stay on a low-fat, low-cholesterol diet to try to get his LDLs, and hence his total cholesterol, to decrease even further.

By any measure, this was a true cholesterol success story—with exercise playing a major role in the scenario. It was the exercise which brought the HDLs up. It was also diet and exercise which helped to lower his weight and body fat and, as a consequence, his total cholesterol and LDLs. These factors, along with a much lower cholesterol intake in his food, resulted in a very good ratio. Overall, he moved from a high coronary risk to the low category, all in less than one year.

Not everyone will experience comparable results. Some may see more dramatic increase in their HDLs and decreases in their ratios. Others may witness much more modest gains—or, in a few cases, no gains at all. What I'm talking about here is not some formula or surefire result that you can expect from one specific case, but rather a set of valid *general expectations*.

Taking certain steps with regard to exercise will do certain things for many people. But not everything works in quite the same way for each person. Every individual has peculiarities in his blood, metabolism, and other bodily mechanisms and organs. Those distinctive traits will determine how his physical system responds to exercise, diet, and a variety of other outside influences.

For example, one middle-aged man who came through one of our special two-week fitness and cholesterol-adjusting programs at the Aerobics Center embarked on a rather modest walking and jogging program. Within only a two-week period, his treadmill time went up from 12:13 minutes to 14:15 minutes. This performance was still low according to the standards of fitness we've established at the Aerobics Center for his age group, but it certainly reflected an impressive improvement in such a short period of time.

The real success story, though, lay in his cholesterol. How did his HDLs react? Before he began the program, we found that they were only 35 mg/dl. But within only two weeks, they had shot up to 47 mg/dl, for a total increase of 34 percent! This dramatic improvement, along with other changes in his blood which he had achieved through diet, brought his total cholesterol/HDL cholesterol ratio down from 6.0 to 3.8.

One woman who came through this same two-week program exercised sufficiently to increase her fitness and treadmill time slightly: she went from 16:00 minutes at the beginning to 16:19 minutes at the end of the two-week period. But her HDLs essentially stayed the same: they were 51 at the beginning and 50 after the two-week program. Nonetheless, her ratio dropped from a high-risk 6.5 to a near-normal 5.0.

How could this happen? The answer lies in the other cholesterol components in her blood. The combination of her LDLs and VLDLs dropped from 280 mg/dl at the beginning to 199 mg/dl at the end of the two-week program, for a 29 percent decline.

What happened here is probably that her HDLs dropped slightly, along with her LDLs, as a result of the very restrictive low-fat, low-cholesterol diet. But then her exercise, compensating for the dietary decline in the HDLs, brought them right back up again, almost to the same level they had been when she started. The overall result—especially in terms of her ratio—was that her blood was much better at the end than at the beginning.

In fact, all the people in this particular two-week program experienced an average drop in their HDLs of 6.0 mg/dl. For the most part, this was the result of their low-calorie, low-cholesterol diet. Yet, other important factors were at work: As a result of the exercise, their treadmill times went up an average of 13 percent. This improvement reflected an improvement in aerobic fitness—a condition which tends to raise HDL levels, or at least to limit their decline if a person is on a weight-loss diet. For the group on this two-week program, the exercise limited the drop of the HDLs. Also, the low-cholesterol diet and the loss of body fat through diet and exercise caused their total cholesterol levels to decline by a greater percentage than the HDLs. As a result, their total cholesterol/HDL cholesterol ratios dropped by an average of 17 percent.

Clearly, the relationship between exercise and cholesterol—and especially HDL cholesterol—is a complicated thing. Blood values will vary among individuals. Still, in light of the current research, it's possible to make some important generalizations about how exercise can affect your cholesterol.

I'll sum up some of these findings in the following "facts." You'll find specific guidelines for different types of aerobic activities at the end of the chapter.

Fact 1. Brisk walking over a period of just a few months can significantly increase your HDL levels.

Six young men, averaging 25 years of age and 217 pounds in weight, walked on treadmills over a period of sixteen weeks at the University of Minnesota's Laboratory of Physiological Hygiene. As a result, they experienced a 16 percent increase in their high-density lipoproteins.

The participants began at a walking speed of 1.5 mph on a 10 percent grade for fifteen minutes. Then, they gradually progressed over a two-week period to 3.2 mph for ninety minutes a day, five days a week. During this calorie-burning regimen, they lost more than 12 pounds each, even though they were not under any sort of dietary restrictions.

Note: The amount of exercise these young men were doing is much more than we at the Aerobics Institute have found necessary to achieve higher HDL levels. But certainly, the extra exercise helped them take off some of those extra pounds.

Fact 2. Very moderate exercise may result in a significant increase in HDL levels.

In one thirteen-week program of moderate exercise, consisting mainly of walking and slow jogging, 32 sedentary, middle-aged men with coronary artery disease increased their HDL cholesterol levels. They exercised twenty to thirty minutes per session, for an average of three sessions per week, and their average HDL levels went up from 35.8 mg/dl to 39.3 mg/dl.

Similarly, in a study reported by Dr. G. Harley Hartung, of the Baylor College of Medicine in Houston, some men who jogged eleven miles per week experienced dramatic increases in their HDLs. Apparently, such moderate exercise may be enough. Others, who ran as much as forty miles per week, experienced only modest increases. Dr. Hartung concluded that his "findings clearly show that the effect of endurance running on changes in HDL [cholesterol] is limited, at least in certain men."

Fact 3. Participation in a moderate exercise program can increase HDL cholesterol in survivors of a heart attack—and may also contribute to lowering their risk for subsequent heart attacks.

This was the conclusion of a group of researchers from the University of Washington School of Medicine who studied 83 heart attack survivors participating in a moderate, graded exercise program. Their program consisted of walking, jogging, and doing calisthenics for forty-five minutes a session, three times per week. The exercise participants were found to have HDL levels of 47.2 mg/dl, as compared with levels of 40.1 mg/dl in nonparticipants.

Fact 4. There's a direct correlation between increasing levels of physical fitness and healthier HDL levels and ratios of total cholesterol/HDL cholesterol.

In a study we did at the Institute for Aerobics Research involving 732 men who were without any symptoms and whose average age was 45 years, we came up with the following results:

Level of Fitness*	Cholesterol	HDL	Cholesterol/HDL Ratio
Very poor	224.5	37.0	6.06
Poor	226.6	40.0	5.66
Fair	213.5	41.5	5.14
Good	216.3	44.5	4.86
Excellent	211.2	49.3	4.28

*As determined by age-adjusted treadmill stress-test times formulated at the Aerobics Center in Dallas.

As you can see, these data suggest there are direct correlations between aerobic fitness and HDL cholesterol, and also aerobic fitness and the total cholesterol/HDL cholesterol ratio. On the other hand, the relationship between fitness and total cholesterol *isn't* completely consistent.

One other study has concluded that fitness levels, as measured by treadmill exercise tests, are *not* significantly related to HDL cholesterol levels for either men or women. The Lipid Research Clinics Program Prevalence Study reported on this test, which involved more than 2,300 men and more than 2,000 women, aged 20 years or older. The object was to determine the correlation of their HDLs to their physical activity, and also the correlation of their HDLs to their fitness, as measured by a treadmill exercise test.

According to this study, neither men nor women showed important differences in HDLs as far as their treadmill performances were concerned. But the active men and women did have higher HDL cholesterol levels than did their sedentary counterparts.

Why did this study conclude that there's no relationship between fitness levels and HDL concentrations?

In part, the reason may be that the study involved submaximal stress testing, in contrast to the maximal stress testing that we do at the Aerobics Center. In other words, those who were taking the stress test were allowed to get off the treadmill before they became fatigued. Consequently, they stopped before their heart rates reached their maximum capacity. So it was more difficult to identify who was really fit and who wasn't.

In contrast, in our tests the participants usually quit only after they reach their maximum heart rates. One reason we choose the maximal approach is that only when the heart is beating at its maximal or near-maximal level is it possible to ascertain true levels of aerobic fitness, *or* to identify many heart problems.

Fact 5. There seems to be a "plateau" effect in terms of how much a person's HDL cholesterol will rise with aerobic exercise.

Studies have shown that running up to eleven miles per week, for example, is associated with an average 35 percent increase in HDL cholesterol. At fifteen miles per week, the HDL cholesterol goes up even more. But beyond that level, the response of the HDL cholesterol isn't consistent. Some people do continue to experience an increase in their HDL cholesterol with increased mileage at twenty to twenty-five miles per week or even above. But others show a plateau effect, where the HDL level either holds steady or even declines slightly.

Fact 6. Being physically sedentary may significantly lower a person's HDL cholesterol.

Dr. William Haskell, of the Stanford Center for Research in Disease Prevention, recently said this:

> There is a very high probability that lipoprotein metabolism plays a central role in the etiology of coronary heart disease. In sedentary persons, one way to favorably alter lipoprotein metabolism and possibly delay the progression of coronary atherosclerosis is by an increase in habitual physical activity.
>
> More physically active persons tend to have lower plasma triglycerides and VLDL concentrations and a greater HDL mass due to higher concentrations of the subfractions HDL-2 and Apo A-I. Plasma LDL concentrations usually are not significantly reduced by exercise unless accompanied by weight loss. In healthy persons as well as in patients with ischemic heart disease, an increase in moderate-intensity endurance-type activity requiring an expenditure of approximately 1,000 kilocalories per week usually produces favorable lipoprotein changes.*

It would normally require about nine to ten miles of walking or jogging per week to burn up 1,000 calories and raise HDL levels, as suggested by Dr. Haskell. For more information on how to work up to this minimum level of exercise, see Exercise Recommendations, p. 250.

In a study at the University of Helsinki, in Finland, 30 patients who had been immobilized because of traumatic fractures of the spine were tested for their cholesterol levels. They were then compared with healthy people of similar age, sex, and relative body weight from the general population.

The study showed that the immobilized patients had much lower HDL cholesterol and lower levels of Apo A-I (the "good"

*Acta Medica Scandinavica, Vol. 711, pp. 25–37.

apolipoprotein) than did the uninjured people. Specifically, the
immobilized patients averaged high-risk HDLs of 32 mg/dl, as
compared with a normal average of 51 mg/dl in the mobile
group. As for the Apo A-I test, the immobilized group averaged
118 mg/dl, in contrast to 161 mg/dl in the healthy group. Also,
there was an increase in the ratios of immobilized patients in
comparison with those of the control group.

What can we conclude from this study? There's at least an
indication that, for the sake of improving your blood balance and
decreasing your risk of atherosclerosis, you should avoid sedentary living.

Fact 7. As you increase the intensity and duration of your
exercise, very complex interactions and changes begin to take
place in your body.

Among other things, as you lose body weight during exercise, your total cholesterol decreases and your HDL level
increases. Also, the pace at which these changes take place
depends on a number of factors, such as the levels at which you
begin exercise, your age, and the length and intensity of your
training.

One study, done at the University of Colorado, concluded
that physical training seemed to produce beneficial changes in
blood lipids and lipoproteins. But the investigators cautioned
other researchers to be careful when examining the relationship
between lipids, such as cholesterol, and physical training. Such
caution is warranted, they explained, because of the complex
interactions that occur with many other aspects of the body and
blood.

What does all this mean to you? You, as an individual,
must consider all of the cholesterol and other fatty components
in your blood as a whole. In the last analysis, it's up to you to
monitor yourself. In consultation with your physician, you must
design a lifestyle program that's appropriate for your needs.

Fact 8. For runners, there may be a threshold at about
eight miles per week, at which an established exercise program
will change your cholesterol balance for the better.

That was a conclusion of a study by Peter D. Wood,
William L. Haskell, Steven N. Blair (of our Aerobics Institute),
and others from an investigation of 81 sedentary but healthy
men, aged 30 to 55. In this study, 48 of the men were assigned
to a running program, while 33 remained as sedentary "controls" for comparison purposes. After one year of training, the

running group had become fitter and leaner than those who were not exercising. Also, the 25 men in the group who averaged *at least eight miles per week* of running increased their high-density lipoprotein levels by an average of 4.4 mg/dl. In addition, their HDL-2 subfractions *went up* by 33 mg/dl.

Fact 9. It's always best to choose aerobic exercise over increased alcohol consumption as a means to raise your HDL levels.

As we saw in chapter 10, drinking a moderate amount of alcohol each day may raise your HDL levels. But at this time it's not entirely clear what subfraction of the HDLs are affected by the alcohol intake. So, the potential benefits of the alcohol are not certain.

Also a report by Dr. G. Harley Hartung in *Sports Medicine* in 1984 noted that for people who are already active aerobic exercisers, alcohol consumption has no effect on HDL levels. It was only the inactive men in this study who experienced an increase in HDL levels with an alcohol intake equivalent to three beers a day.

Exercise, then, is clearly better than alcohol as a means to elevate your HDLs. In addition, it has other beneficial effects on your body and also, quite possibly, on your overall cholesterol balance. For one thing, exercise tends to *use up* calories, and a lower percentage of body fat is associated with lower levels of the "bad" LDL cholesterol. Alcohol, in contrast, may raise the levels of "good" HDL cholesterol. But it also tends to *put on* weight through increased calorie intake.

Fact 10. Smoking often negates the beneficial rises in HDLs which you achieve through exercise.

An English study was conducted with 40 men, including smokers and nonsmokers, 29 to 56 years of age, who had ischemic heart disease. They were put on an exercise program consisting of aerobic activities, which were designed to make them work at 80 percent of their maximal heart rate. The workouts consisted of twenty-minute periods each day for five weeks.

There was a big difference between the smokers and nonsmokers. The nonsmokers, and also those who gave up or reduced smoking during the course, experienced important increases in their HDL levels. But those who continued to smoke as much as they had before enjoyed only negligible changes in their HDL levels.

Again, the message comes across loud and clear: *Don't smoke!*

Fact 11. Aerobic exercise may have a more beneficial impact in raising the HDL levels in men than in women.

In one study of 24 men and 37 women, reported in *Circulation* in 1982, the participants embarked on a program involving three sessions of aerobic exercise each week. The workouts consisted of fifteen to twenty minutes of exercise at 70 percent of the maximal heart rate.

At the end of the study, the men showed a significant 5.1 percent average increase in HDL cholesterol levels and also beneficial changes in their ratios. The women, in contrast, experienced an average 1 percent *decrease* in their HDL cholesterol levels. Furthermore, they had no significant changes, on average, in their ratios.

Although the researchers concluded that moderate exercise may have different effects on men and women, it's necessary to exercise caution with studies of this type. For one thing, it's unclear whether other changes occurred in the participants' diets and activities. They did follow a self-reporting procedure to inform the researchers about their diets, smoking habits, and alcohol intake. But this kind of reporting tends to be imprecise.

In another study, conducted at the Department of Medicine in the University of Adelaide, in South Australia, 9 men and 15 women, averaging 31 years of age, were put on a mild exercise program. They jogged twice a week for a half-hour each session and also did calisthenics twice a week for twelve weeks.

As a result of this exercise program, the men experienced increases in their average HDL levels from 42 to 48 mg/dl. Also, their Apo As went up from 207 to 246 mg/dl—perhaps an even more beneficial change, as you'll recall from our previous discussions of this apolipoprotein.

The women, in contrast, had minor increases in their HDL levels, which went up only from 49 to 51 mg/dl. Also, their Apo A increases were relatively small, from 225 to 234 mg/dl. On the other hand, the women's total cholesterol and LDL cholesterol counts went down, and their ratios improved during the exercise.

To sum up, then, the present weight of the evidence suggests that there is a difference between the responses of men and women to aerobic activity. But there are sufficient benefits for both to warrant a recommendation of aerobic exercise for everyone.

Fact 12. "Power" sports—such as weight-lifting, shot-putting, discus-throwing, and even sprinting—do not increase HDL levels in blood, and may actually decrease them.

In one study conducted at the Center of Internal Medicine in Freiburg, West Germany, scientists examined the blood composition of 44 male power athletes and 52 sedentary male students. They found a remarkable difference in the HDL levels between these two groups, with the power athletes having much lower levels than the sedentary subjects.

The researchers concluded, "Intensive power training may produce specific adaptations in muscle metabolism. . . . The decrease of HDL-cholesterol levels in power athletes may be a . . . consequence of the adaptation to the specific training form."

In a related development, for several years some athletes have engaged in the dangerous practice of using anabolic steroids to build up strength and muscle mass. Many scientific articles have been written warning of the dangers of such an approach and strongly advising against their use.

In most cases, the concern has been about the future risk of developing cancer, such as cancers of the testicle or the prostate. But more recent studies have also shown that a dramatic decrease in the HDL cholesterol often accompanies anabolic steroid or androgen use. In the long run, in fact, the greatest potential risk may be in developing rampant atherosclerosis rather than cancer. Certainly this side effect should be enough to discourage the use of such products.

In short, those who use anabolic steroids, who concentrate on muscle building, or who limit their activity to anaerobic rather than aerobic or endurance-type activities, may find their HDL levels decreasing. As a consequence, they may be jeopardizing the overall balance of the cholesterol in their blood.

Fact 13. There seems to be *no* age limit on the beneficial impact of aerobic exercise in raising HDL levels.

Older people in our studies have enjoyed HDL increases as great as those in their younger counterparts. Also, even schoolchildren who are active aerobically can experience significant increases in their HDLs.

One study in Turku, Finland, evaluated 37 schoolchildren,

11 to 13 years of age. The group included 9 "trained" boys and 7 "trained" girls who had regularly participated in track-and-field athletics. Also, there were 12 boys and 9 girls who had not undergone such training. The study revealed that the children who had been athletically trained had higher HDL cholesterol levels than did the untrained children.

These are just a few of the facts you need to know about the relationship between aerobic exercise and blood lipids, including total cholesterol and HDL cholesterol levels. As you can see, the subject is extremely complex. Various cholesterol and lipid components interact with one another and also with the different lifestyles of those being tested. This complexity, once again, serves to emphasize this important point: You are an individual—and you must design your overall cholesterol-balancing program with your own special situation and bodily responses in mind.

Still, there are a number of things you can learn from others' successes with exercise. One of these things, as we've seen, is that it's important to embark on an aerobic exercise program such as brisk walking or jogging. This means exercising three to four times a week, for a minimum of twenty to thirty minutes for each session. For a runner, such a program should involve a minimum of eight to ten miles per week, and preferably twelve to fifteen miles per week. You needn't worry about doing any more exercise than this, however, unless you have some goals in mind other than fitness and establishing a healthy overall balance in your blood.

In the final analysis, then, a moderate amount of aerobic exercise is an absolutely essential part of any complete program for overall well-being, high-energy living—and well-balanced cholesterol. If you're not already on such a program, my best advice at this point is to get a medical checkup, and then get started—*today!* To help you begin an intelligent exercise program, I've included the following practical exercise recommendations.

Exercise Recommendations

In my book *The Aerobics Program for Total Well-Being* I list thirty-one exercises as being aerobic. That is, these are capable of producing beneficial changes in your cardiovascular and pulmonary systems—including elevation of your "good" HDL cholesterol levels. Collectively, these changes are usually referred to as "the training effect." To achieve the desired results of this training effect safely and effectively, it's important to understand and apply the following basic guidelines.

First, if you are over 40 years of age, it's advisable for you to undergo a thorough medical examination and a maximal performance treadmill stress test before you begin any vigorous exercise program. This recommendation becomes even more important if you have one or more of the following major coronary risk factors:

1. History of a heart attack or other major cardiovascular event in a family member less than 50 years of age

2. History of hypertension—that is, blood pressure consistently above 140/90 mmHg (millimeters of mercury)

3. Elevated total cholesterol, or total cholesterol/HDL cholesterol ratio (above the 75th percentile, according to your age and sex, as described on pp. 55 and 65)

4. Cigarette smoking, regardless of the number of cigarettes per day or the number of years you've smoked

5. Abnormal resting electrocardiogram

6. Diabetes mellitus, requiring either oral medication or insulin

If your treadmill stress test is normal, I recommend that you undergo repeat testing at three-year intervals. If the test is abnormal, you'll require close medical supervision and follow-up, with repeat treadmill stress testing at maximum intervals of twelve months. If you exercise after an abnormal stress test, the athletic activity should be done only under a physician's supervision.

Now, with your medical exam and stress test out of the way, you're ready to begin. The first essential step is to perform an adequate warm-up.

The Warm-Up

Each time you exercise, always spend a minimum of 3 to 5 minutes in a stretching type of warm-up. Appropriate exercises at this stage may include:

• Slow toe-touching

• Bending the torso from side to side, with the arms extended above the head

• Any other careful, measured movements which extend the spine and stretch the leg and back muscles

Such a warm-up will help you protect both your musculoskeletal and cardiovascular systems. In general, a muscle improperly stretched or warmed up is more prone to injury. Also, starting too vigorously into an exercise routine may be damaging to the cardiovascular system. Several studies have shown that starting too fast may result in irregularities of the heartbeat or an insufficiency of the blood supply to the heart muscle, even in the presence of completely normal coronary arteries. Many times I have tested patients with heart disease characterized by exercise-induced chest pain (angina pectoris). Almost invariably, when these people warmed up adequately before beginning to exercise, they could do greater physical work before chest pain occurred.

Finally, never engage in heavy calisthenics or weight training prior to the aerobic phase of the activity. If you engage in these exercises at all, they should be reserved until the end of the aerobic workout. In this way, you'll avoid an oxygen "debt," or anaerobic state, at the beginning of the aerobic phase.

Now, with your body properly warmed up, you're ready for the main event!

The Aerobic Phase

The aerobic phase of a workout, performed safely and effectively, is the key to success with any exercise program. Later, I'll provide detailed recommendations for individual programs. But first it's important to understand a little more about what is supposed to happen during this phase.

In general, remember the acronym FIT to determine whether the aerobic activity is sufficient to produce the "training effect":

"F" stands for frequency per week

"I" refers to the intensity or heart rate response

"T" stands for the time or duration of the activity

With one of the following combinations of the FIT concept, you can expect a "training effect" to occur. Also, remember that these are minimal levels, not maximums:

Frequency/week	Intensity (heart rate)	Time or Duration
4 times	Slightly above 140 beats/minute	20 minutes
3 times	Slightly above 130 beats/minute	30 minutes
4–5 times	Slightly above 110 beats/minute	45 minutes

Translated another way, the first combination of FIT, as summarized above, is consistent with jogging 2 miles in less than 20 minutes, 4 times a week. This is probably the most popular aerobic program in the world today.

The second example of FIT is consistent with aerobic dancing for 30 minutes, 3 times a week. The final example of FIT is consistent with walking 3 miles in 45 minutes, 4 to 5 times per week. Just about anyone, regardless of age or sex, can engage in safe and effective aerobic exercise by using one of these three approaches.

There is also another way to determine if your aerobic activity is effective. This involves using the concept of the target heart rate zone. The main idea is that you should exercise intensely enough to get your heart rate up to the target rate zone which will produce the training effect. To find your target heart rate zone, proceed with these steps:

First, find your predicted maximal heart rate as follows: For physically inactive men (and women regardless of activity), use 220 – age = Predicted Maximal Heart Rate (PMHR). For conditioned or physically active men, use 205 – ½ age = Predicted Maximal Heart Rate (PMHR). Then, multiply the PMHR by 65 to 80 percent, and that will be your target heart rate zone.

For example, a physically active man 40 years of age would have a PMHR of:

205 minus 40 divided by 2, or 185. Then he could find his target heart rate zone through his calculation:

65–80% of 185 (his PMHR) = 120–148 beats per minute.

For a woman 30 years of age, the PMHR would be:

220 − 30 = 190. Then, she would figure her target heart rate zone this way:

65–80% of 190 (her PMHR) = 124–152 beats per minute.

Recent studies have shown that young men trained at even lower intensity—that is, 45 percent of PMHR—showed a similar response to a group trained at higher intensity. Initially, their response to the training was slower. But after 12 to 18 weeks, the overall improvement in their cardiovascular fitness was not significantly different.*

Once you've determined your target heart rate zone, it's necessary to exercise within that zone for a minimum of 20 minutes, 4 times per week, or 30 minutes, 3 times per week.

Still another way to determine if your aerobic activity is adequate is to utilize the point system as described extensively in my aerobics books, particularly in *The Aerobics Program for Total Well-Being* (Bantam, September 1983). Using a single exercise or a combination of various exercises, women must work up to a minimum of 30 aerobic points per week and men to a minimum of 35 points per week. Studies conducted at the Institute for Aerobic Research here in Dallas have shown a high correlation between aerobics points earned per week and the level of cardiovascular fitness as determined by age and sex-adjusted treadmill times.

When you've finished the aerobic phase of your workout, however, that's not the end of the story! The cool-down which follows is crucial to your good health and fitness.

The Cool-Down

Without question, the most critical time of the exercise is during the cool-down or recovery, immediately after a very vigorous aerobic phase. As much as 60 percent of your blood might be pooled below the waist at that point, particularly after you've engaged in jogging or vigorous competitive sports. If you stop abruptly, the lack of adequate circulation to the brain and heart could produce severe consequences.

To avoid any danger, keep walking or moving around

---

*See Gaessar, G.A., and R.G. Rich, "Effects of High and Low Intensity Exercise Training on Aerobic Capacity and Blood Lipids." *Medical and Scientific Sports and Exercise*, vol. 16, 1984, pp. 269–74.

slowly for a minimum of 5 minutes after completing the exercise. Then, to determine whether the aerobic phase was beyond your physical capacity, check your recovery heart rate by counting your pulse for 15 seconds and then multiplying by 4 to get the rate per minute. If your pulse rate is below 120 beats per minute and you are under 50 years of age, or below 100 beats per minute and you are over 50 years of age, you can safely assume that the exercise in which you were involved was not too strenuous. But if your recovery heart rate response is above that level, don't exercise as long or as hard during your next session.

Caution: The worst possible thing to do immediately after vigorous exercise is to go directly into a sauna, steamroom, or whirlpool and sit down. If you happen to faint while in a sitting or upright position, the consequences could be disastrous.

Safety First!

Remember: If you run more than 15 miles per week or do aerobic dance longer than 4 hours per week, you are exercising for something other than cardiovascular fitness. Beyond that point, cardiovascular benefits are minimal, but muscular and skeletal problems accelerate. Your goal is to keep exercising for the rest of your life, and moderation and balance are the keys to the long-term success of any program.

To help you reduce injuries with any type of exercise, remember the acronym, "Four S's plus an O." They are:

S Stretch before you exercise.

S Shoes are key to injury-free exercise. An investment in a well-made shoe can save you a small fortune in doctor's bills.

S Style, including proper technique, is important in injury reduction. So learn how to pursue your sport safely and expertly.

S Surface determines the extent and damaging effect of the impact. Always try to avoid very hard surfaces such as concrete or macadam.

O Overuse of your body. That means more than 15 miles per week of jogging, or more than 4 hours per week of aerobic dancing.

Now, with these preliminary matters behind us, let's take a closer look at specific programs for specific aerobic activities. Even though there are thirty-one exercises which qualify as aerobic, the top five are:

1. Cross-country skiing

2. Swimming

3. Jogging or running

4. Cycling, either outdoors or indoors

5. Walking

Since cross-country skiing isn't readily available to most people, following are some suggestions for progressive exercise programs for the other four activities. In most cases I've included only one representative, standard program, designed especially for healthy but inactive men and women 30 to 50 years old. Certainly, healthy older people can also begin with these programs. For those older than 50 who are healthy but sedentary, I've included special programs for stationary cycling and walking. Remember, too, the importance of the warm-up and cool-down in every exercise program.

Swimming

The advantages of swimming include the utilization of many muscle groups and therefore a total body conditioning program. Also, the buoyancy involved in swimming helps protect participants from muscle and bone problems. Swimming is particularly good for people with arthritic or musculoskeletal problems, such as those involving the back. For the healthy but totally inactive man or woman 30 to 50 years of age, I'd recommend the following program:

Week	Distance (yards)	Time Goal (minutes)	Frequency/Week
1	300	12:00	4
2	300	10:00	4
3	400	13:00	4
4	400	12:00	4
5	500	14:00	4
6	500	13:00	4

Week	Distance (yards)	Time Goal (minutes)	Frequency/Week
7	600	16:00	4
8	700	19:00	4
9	800	22:00	4
10	900	22:30	4

Use whatever stroke enables you to swim the required distance in the prescribed time. Rest as often as you like during the first few weeks. Then, by the tenth week, you should achieve adequate aerobic fitness and be able to swim longer or faster without rest periods.

Running or Jogging

The advantage jogging or running has over other aerobic activities is the ease with which it can be done. I myself have jogged all over the world in a variety of circumstances and conditions.

For people who have no orthopedic problems, running or jogging may be the exercise of choice. Remember, too, if your only goal is cardiovascular conditioning, running "long and slow" is always preferable to "short and fast."

For the healthy but inactive man or woman 30 to 50 years of age, I suggest the following program:

Week	Activity	Distance (miles)	Time Goal (minutes)	Frequency/Week
1	walk	2.0	34:00	3
2	walk	2.5	42:00	3
3	walk	3.0	50:00	3
4	walk/jog	2.0	25:00	4
5	walk/jog	2.0	24:00	4
6	jog	2.0	22:00	4
7*	jog	2.0	20:00	4
8	jog	2.5	26:00	4
9	jog	2.5	25:00	4
10	jog	3.0	31:00	4
11	jog	3.0	29:00	4
12	jog	3.0	27:00	4

*By the seventh week, you'll achieve a minimum aerobic fitness level. By the twelfth week of this program, you'll reach an excellent level of aerobic fitness.

Cycling

Some very highly conditioned people with whom I have had the opportunity to work are strictly outdoor cyclists. Cycling is less traumatic to the joints than running. Many of those people are past 60 years of age and a few are past 70—yet they deny any major musculoskeletal problems.

Admittedly, cycling outdoors is potentially more dangerous than other types of physical activity. Also, it's difficult, at times, to maintain a satisfactory speed due to traffic, stoplights, or weather. Still, this activity can be effective, and that is why I classify it in my top five.

A suggested program for the healthy but inactive man or woman 30 to 50 years of age is as follows:

Week	Distance (miles)	Time Goal (minutes)	Frequency/Week
1	4.0	20:00	3
2	4.0	18:00	3
3	5.0	24:00	4
4	5.0	22:00	4
5	5.0	20:00	4
6	6.0	26:00	4
7	6.0	24:00	4
8	7.0	30:00	4
9	7.0	28:00	4
10	7.0	27:55	4

By the tenth week, an adequate level of aerobic fitness has been reached and can be maintained with a four-day-a-week exercise program. If desired, cycling faster, farther, or more frequently each week will increase the fitness level.

Stationary Cycling

Various injuries may occur with jogging or running, and there are other risks such as accidents which may happen when cycling outdoors. As a result, stationary cycling has become immensely popular in recent years.

The enthusiasm has increased with the addition of various electronic incentives, such as computerized resistance which simulates different types of terrain, heart rate monitoring, and caloric expenditure determinations. Also, the combination of arm and leg activity is a big plus for many people.

For the healthy but inactive man or woman 30 to 50 years of age, I recommend the following program. During the first 6 weeks, warm up by cycling for 3 minutes, at 17.5 to 20 mph, with no resistance, before beginning the actual workout. At the conclusion of the exercise period, cool down by cycling for 3 minutes with no resistance.

Week	Speed (mph/rpm)	Time Goal (minutes)	PR After Exercise*	Frequency/Week
1	15/55	6:00	<140	3
2	15/55	8:00	<140	3
3	15/55	10:00	<140	3
4	15/55	12:00	<150	4
5	15/55	14:00	<150	4
6	15/55	16:00	<150	4
7	15/55	18:00	<150	5
8	15/55	20:00	<150	5
9	17.5/65	18:00	>150	5
10	17.5/65	20:00	>150	5
11	20/75	18:00	>150	5
12	20/75	20:00	>150	5
13	20/75	22:30	>150	5
14	25/90	25:00	>150	5

> = "more than"
< = "less than"

*Add enough resistance so that the pulse rate (PR), counted for 10 seconds immediately after exercise and multiplied by 6, equals the rate specified. If the pulse rate is higher, lower the resistance before cycling again; if it's lower, increase the resistance.

Stationary Cycling for Age 50 and Over

Since this type of exercise has the potential of being performed safely by people of any age, I'd recommend the following program for the healthy but inactive man or woman age 50 and over.

Week	Speed (mph/rpm)	Time Goal (minutes)	PR After Exercise*	Frequency/Week
1	15/55	4:00	<100	3
2	15/55	4:00	<100	3
3	15/55	6:00	<100	3
4	15/55	6:00	<110	4
5	15/55	8:00	<110	4
6	15/55	10:00	<110	4
7	15/55	12:00	<110	4
8	15/55	14:00	<110	4
9	15/55	16:00	<110	4
10	15/55	16:00	<120	5
11	15/55	18:00	<120	5
12	15/55	20:00	<120	5
13	17.5/65	18:00	<120	5
14	17.5/65	20:00	<120	5
15	20/75	20:00	<130	5
16	20/75	22:30	<130	5
17	20/75	25:00	<130	5
18	20/75	30:00	<130	4

*Add enough resistance so that the pulse rate (PR) counted for 10 seconds immediately after exercise and multiplied by 6 equals the rate specified. If your pulse rate is higher, lower the resistance before cycling again; if it is lower, increase the resistance.

During the first 6 weeks, warm up by cycling for 3 minutes, at 17.5 to 20 mph, with no resistance, before beginning the actual workout. At the conclusion of the exercise, cool down by cycling for 3 minutes with no resistance. From the tenth week on, the exercise periods can be divided into two equal periods, performed twice daily.

Walking

Without question, walking is one of the best all-around physical activities, especially for older people and anyone who is just starting an exercise program. It can be done anywhere, indoors or outdoors, and no special equipment other than a good pair of shoes is required. The only disadvantage of walking is that it takes two to three times as long as running to achieve the same cardiovascular benefit.

I suggest the following walking program for the healthy but inactive man or woman, 30 to 50 years of age:

Week	Distance (miles)	Time Goal (minutes)	Frequency/Week
1	2.0	36:00	3
2	2.0	34:00	3
3	2.0	32:00	4
4	2.0	30:00	4
5	2.5	39:00	4
6	2.5	38:00	5
7	2.5	37:00	5
8	3.0	46:00	5
9	3.0	45:00	5
10	3.0	43:00	4

By the tenth week, you'll reach an adequate level of aerobic conditioning which can be maintained with a 4-times-per-week schedule.

Walking for Age 50 and Over

Since walking is an effective program for people even past 50 years of age, I recommend the following program for the healthy but inactive man or woman over 50 years of age:

Week	Distance (miles)	Time Goal (minutes)	Frequency/Week
1	1.0	20:00	4
2	1.5	30:00	4
3	2.0	40:00	4
4	2.0	38:00	4
5	2.0	36:00	4
6	2.0	34:00	4
7	2.5	42:00	4
8	2.5	40:00	4
9	2.5	38:00	4
10	3.0	47:00	4
11	3.0	46:00	4
12	3.0	45:00	4

By the twelfth week, you'll achieve an adequate level of aerobic conditioning, which can be maintained with 4 exercise periods each week.

If you prefer to participate in another aerobic exercise, or want more information about these activities, look at my book *The Aerobics Program for Total Well-Being* for more specific age-adjusted guidelines and recommendations.

To complete your exercise prescription, you also have to consider total body conditioning. Far too many times I have encountered runners, for instance, who develop a problem with the back, upper body, or extremities. The reason? Their programs did not include adequate stretching or conditioning exercises.

As I mentioned earlier, slow toe-touching and leg-stretching is advisable before you begin the aerobics phase of a workout. After the aerobic workout or on alternate days, weight-lifting, using light weights and high rapidity, can be an effective way to achieve muscular strength and some aerobic conditioning. Very heavy weights and slow movements are usually more appropriate for anaerobic muscle-building programs.

Remember, too, it's possible to become "overmuscled," just as it is possible to become "overfat." Either way, the heart will suffer. So, my advice is that you stick with an aerobic exercise program supplemented by workouts with light weights or calisthenics.

THIRTEEN

The Wisdom and Risk
of Drug and
Vitamin Therapy

If you have a problem with your cholesterol level, it's always best to treat it with changes in diet, exercise, or other aspects of lifestyle. But sometimes these "natural" approaches simply don't work.

You may cut your cholesterol-carrying foods far down. You may jog fifteen miles a week. You may quit smoking. You may do a variety of other things designed to lower your cholesterol. But sometimes, with some people, this just isn't quite enough. As a result, it may be necessary to turn to prescriptive means to correct the abnormalities in your cholesterol and blood lipids—and that may mean drugs, vitamin therapy, or a combination of both.

But when should you consider using medications to treat your cholesterol?

First, let me state unequivocably that you should embark on a drug or vitamin program *only* under the supervision of a physician who is experienced in the application of such therapy. *Under no circumstances should you experiment with this sort of treatment by yourself!*

Still, even though the ultimate guidance for going on a drug regimen must be in the hands of a qualified physician, it's important for you, as the person being treated, to understand the principles behind such drug therapy. I'm a great believer in the idea that each patient should be as informed as possible about his condition and about available treatments for it.

There may be times when you are in the best position to

call a problem or issue to your doctor's attention. But you'll be much better qualified to do this if you know what's going on inside your body. It's also important for each person to be knowledgeable enough to ask intelligent questions when physicians prescribe various forms of treatment. If you know what to inquire about and are not satisfied with the answers, you'll be better able to select another physician who is more appropriate for your needs.

So, what exactly do you need to know about drug and vitamin therapy?

What You Need To Know

At the outset, it's wise to have some idea about when to begin to take drugs or vitamins. Assume that you discover you are in one of the higher-risk categories with any of the components of your cholesterol or other blood fats. The first thing you should do is to try diet therapy of the type that we've described in chapter 9 of this book. Your doctor will let you know if there is some pressing need for you to skip this step and go directly on drugs. If the diet therapy doesn't work, drugs or vitamins may be in order.

A "consensus conference" published in the *Journal of the American Medical Association* in 1985 suggested that those in moderate-risk and high-risk categories with relatively high total cholesterol levels should first double-check their blood values with a second blood test. If the first test is confirmed, the experts suggest trying diet therapy.

"Drug therapy should be used only after a careful trial of diet modification, using the most rigorous diet appropriate for the particular individual," the conferees said. "Even when use of drugs seems appropriate, it is important to stress that maximal diet therapy should be continued."*

There are many drugs, and also combinations of drugs and vitamins, which may be used to control cholesterol or lipid problems. In fact, the list of acceptable treatments seems to grow longer almost every month. So it's important to check

Journal of the American Medical Association, vol. 253, no. 14, April 12, 1985, p. 2,084.

with your physician to ascertain the latest thinking on the subject before you decide on a particular drug therapy. Here is an overview of some key drugs—and one vitamin, niacin—which are commonly used to treat various cholesterol problems.

Cholestyramine, also known by the brand name Questran. This drug tends to have a strong effect in lowering total cholesterol and LDL cholesterol levels. It may slightly elevate triglycerides and VLDLs, but usually it has no effect on HDL cholesterol.

This substance is what is known as a "bile acid sequestrant." This means it reduces LDLs by encouraging their removal after they have been released into the bloodstream. Also, a bile acid sequestrant stimulates LDL receptor activity. The receptors, as we know, enable the body's cells to "rescue" the loose LDLs and their accompanying Apo B partners by pulling them into the cell tissues, away from dangerous accumulations in the vessel walls.

Bile acids contain cholesterol that has been removed from the body's cells and deposited in the liver. By helping to get rid of the bile acids, this drug prevents the reabsorption of the cholesterol into the body and the blood vessels.

The typical dosage of cholestyramine is one packet or one scoopful—9 grams of Questran contain 4 grams of cholestyramine resin—three or four times daily. The side effects from this drug may include constipation, nausea, bloating, and inhibition of the body's ability to absorb fat-soluble vitamins, such as A, D, and K.

Colestipol HCL, also known by the brand name Colestid. This drug, also a bile acid sequestrant, tends to have a significant impact in lowering total cholesterol and LDL cholesterol levels. To a lesser extent, it may raise triglyceride levels, though the effect on HDLs tends to be negligible.

The usual dosage for colestipol is 15 to 30 grams per day, divided into two to four separate doses.

Like cholestyramine, colestipol may cause nausea, constipation, bloating, and a decreased ability of the body to absorb vitamins A, D, and K, along with certain other drugs.

Probucol, also known by the brand name Lorelco. This drug lowers total cholesterol. LDL cholesterol usually goes down significantly with this drug, as it enhances the transportation of cholesterol remnants and "garbage" back for final disposal in the liver. This drug also may *lower* HDL levels—obviously *not* a good thing for those concerned about maintaining a healthy total cholesterol/HDL cholesterol ratio.*

Probucol has been proved highly effective in lowering total cholesterol by reducing both the LDL and HDL fractions. Yet, in rabbits, the addition of the drug pantetheine to probucol blocked the HDL-lowering effect, and the only decrease was in the LDL cholesterol. These results suggest that such combination therapy may prevent the HDL-lowering effect of probucol.

The usual prescription of this drug is 500 mg. twice a day.

The side effects include diarrhea, nausea, abdominal pain, headache, rashes—and, as I've indicated, a lowering of HDL cholesterol levels.

Clofibrate, also known by the brand name Atromid-S. This drug tends to have a significant impact in lowering triglycerides and VLDL levels. It also can lower total cholesterol levels slightly in some patients. The impact on LDLs may involve either an increase *or* a decrease, depending on the individual's response. HDL levels may go up or stay about the same.

Generally, physicians prescribe 2 grams per day in more than one dose.

The side effects may include upset stomach, pancreatitis, gallbladder problems (including gall stones requiring surgery), nausea, diarrhea, and symptoms approximating those of flu. At least one study (WHO) demonstrated an increased mortality due to noncardiovascular causes in a cloribrate-treated group.

Gemfibrozil, also known by the brand name Lopid. This drug can be used to bring about an increase in HDLs, and relatively great decreases in triglycerides and VLDLs. To a lesser extent, gemfibrozil tends to lower total cholesterol and LDL levels. This particular substance can be quite helpful in enabling people with naturally low HDL levels or out-of-balance total cholesterol/HDL cholesterol ratios to get their blood in better shape.

The usual dose is two 300 mg. capsules twice a day.

Side effects may include abdominal pain, nausea, vomiting, and diarrhea.

Niacin, or nicotinic acid (one of the B-complex vitamins, B-3), also known by the brand names Nicolar and Nicobid. This

---

*The International Symposium on Drugs Affecting Lipid Metabolism in Florence, Italy (October 22–25, 1986), included extensive discussions of the beneficial effects and the problems associated with probucol.

is not Nicotinamide or Niacinamide which is an amide of nicotinic acid. This vitamin tends to have a significant effect in
lowering triglycerides and VLDL levels. It may also lower total
cholesterol and LDL cholesterol. In my practice, I've found
with a number of people that nicotinic acid tends to be the only
treatment which can raise the HDL levels.

In general, it's best to start off with low doses of niacin,
say up to 100 mg. per day. Then it can be increased gradually
over a period of several weeks to 1 to 2 grams three times a
day, for a total of 3 to 6 grams daily.

Increasing amounts of this vitamin, especially if large doses
are taken all at once, tend to produce severe overall flushing in
the body, dry skin, intestinal disorders, and, sometimes, abnormal functions of the liver. In fact, in doses above 4.5 grams per
day, it is common for most patients to have abnormal liver
function studies and some patients may have these abnormalities noted even at doses of 2.5 grams per day.

New Drug Therapies

One of the most exciting recent developments in the prevention of heart disease is the development of a new drug to lower
blood cholesterol. This drug is Lovastatin, formerly called
Mevinolin. It may eventually be a key ingredient for the prevention of heart attacks in hundreds of thousands of Americans.

A related drug called Compactin was discovered several
years ago in Japan, but those who discovered it didn't recognize
its potential. Subsequent studies by Drs. Joseph L. Goldstein
and Michael S. Brown at the University of Texas Health Science Center at Dallas demonstrated that Compactin increased
the number of LDL receptors. Obviously, a drug that increases
the number of LDL receptors could significantly reduce blood
cholesterol. Another metabolic product of Compactin (CS-S14)
recently has been shown to have a potent cholesterol-lowering
effect by inhibiting the enzyme HMG-CoA-Reductase. (JAMA
1987; 257:3088–3093).

About this same time, Merck and Company in the United
States developed an analog of Compactin that was at first called
Mevinolin, and later Lovastatin. Dr. Scott M. Grundy approached
Merck and Company and asked them to let his staff use the
drug in patients with high cholesterol levels. Merck supplied

the drug, and the Food and Drug Administration (FDA) granted permission to test the drug in patients.

Lovastatin proved to be extremely potent for lowering the LDL cholesterol in patients with high cholesterol levels—without affecting the HDL levels. The drug not only increased the LDL receptors but inhibited the formation of cholesterol in the liver by interacting with the enzyme HMG-CoA-Reductase. The results were so good that in 1987, Merck and Company launched a $100 million development program to make Lovastatin available for all patients with very high cholesterol levels.

At this time, the only side effects from the drug have been minimal: they include slight reversible changes in some liver enzymes and an occasional eye problem, lenticular opacities, which has *not* been shown to be a precursor to cataracts. If the results continue to be so good and the side effects so minimal, the drug should be available for public use by this printing.

In addition to these developments, another study conducted by Dr. Scott M. Grundy and Dr. Gloria Lena Vega at the University of Texas Health Science Center at Dallas has shown that Lovastatin taken with colestipol is even more effective in lowering the LDL cholesterol levels.

This practice of using a *combination* of drugs or drugs and vitamins in treating cholesterol balances has been an important development in the field of cholesterol and blood lipid treatment. At least one study, reported in the *American Journal of Cardiology* in 1986, has indicated that combining probucol and colestipol can both (1) increase the cholesterol-lowering effect of the drugs *and* (2) decrease the uncomfortable side effects in the stomach and intestines, which may be produced by either drug when used alone.

Another combination which works with a number of patients involves combining colestipol with nicotinic acid. For some people this treatment can both lower total cholesterol levels and raise the levels of "good" HDL cholesterol.

One physician on the staff at the Cooper Clinic, Dr. Keller Greenfield, found after a considerable amount of testing and experimentation on himself that this particular combination worked extremely well. Dr. Greenfield had had relatively high cholesterol from the time he was first tested back in 1971. At that time, it was 255 mg/dl, and the next year it was up to 315. By going on a very strict low-fat, low-cholesterol diet, he lowered his cholesterol level by 30 to 50 points, so that by 1975 it was down to 232 mg/dl. But then his total cholesterol count began to move up and down again, sometimes reaching up into the 300s.

In the early 1970s, Dr. Greenfield also went on a more extensive exercise program. When he first was tested for cardiovascular fitness on the treadmill in 1971, he walked for 18 minutes. With his fitness program under way, he made it up to 22 minutes by 1972. His times steadily increased until he reached a personal record in March 1983 of 25:05 minutes.

But even as his times on the treadmill were going up, the results of his exercise electrocardiogram during the tests began to get worse. They were normal up until 1976, but then were classified as "equivocal" beginning in 1976. "Equivocal," by the way, means that there is some slight indication of advancing atherosclerosis or clogging in the coronary arteries, which control the blood flow to the heart.

By December 1981 his stress test was clearly "positive." This means that there was definitely an indication of coronary heart disease—and a need for more serious treatment.

At the same time, his total cholesterol was far too high—313 mg/dl. Even fourteen months later, in March 1983, despite strenuous efforts on his part to lower it by diet, his total cholesterol still stood at 280.

Dr. Greenfield was in such good shape at this time that he had actually run a marathon three weeks before his stress test. But clearly he needed to do something to correct his progressive hardening of the arteries and the excess cholesterol in his blood.

As a result of the positive stress test, Dr. Greenfield underwent coronary arteriography, in which dye was injected into his blood system through an artery in his groin. X-rays then were taken of the coronary arteries, which fed blood to his heart. This test, which was done in May 1983, showed he had significant three-vessel heart disease—a "scary" amount of blockage of blood flow to the heart, as he put it.

One surgeon recommended that Dr. Greenfield have a bypass operation, but he said no, he didn't want to try that just yet. Instead, he opted for more conservative treatment— continuing with his low-cholesterol diet and also trying to see if some sort of drug treatment might work for him.

He tried several types of drugs and combinations of drugs

until he finally settled on a combination of colestipol and nico-tinic acid. Colestipol, you'll recall from the earlier discussion, tends to have a significant impact in lowering total cholesterol and LDL cholesterol levels. Nicotinic acid, on the other hand, may help somewhat in lowering total cholesterol levels. But its main impact lies in lowering triglycerides, and also, sometimes, in raising HDL levels.

In Dr. Greenfield's case, this combination worked like a charm. For the next few years his total cholesterol dropped steadily through the low 200s and even into the mid-100s. The count once went as low as 140 mg/dl!

At the same time, his HDL cholesterol, which had always been relatively high, probably because of his running, began to go up even more. He was consistently showing HDL readings between 60 and 74 mg/dl—a result which gave him total cholesterol/HDL cholesterol ratios that plummeted. The ratios went from a range of about 5.9 to 6.8 during 1983 to a consistent level of an incredibly low 2.2 to 2.6 by 1986. At the same time, his triglyceride levels, which had been moderately elevated in the 141 to 156 mg/dl range, dived down to much lower levels of 53 to 81 mg/dl.

I include all these cholesterol and lipid values because by now you have a good idea of what they mean in relation to one another. Clearly, Keller Greenfield's cholesterol balance had gone from a dangerous area to levels which, according to all the information available, gave him excellent protection.

But was this really the case? Was there really a connec-tion between the improvement in his cholesterol through drug and vitamin treatment and what was happening with his atherosclerosis?

The answer is a resounding "yes"—there was definitely a connection between the two! His treadmill stress test went from a 1983 result of "positive," which indicated the presence of coronary heart disease, back to "equivocal" in 1985. Since his coronary arteriogram, he has undergone several MUGA scans, which involve injection of a radioactive material into the bloodstream after exercising nearly to exhaustion. Then, the heart is "scanned" with a nuclear monitoring device.

As a result of this MUGA scan, Dr. Greenfield was found in December 1985 to have a heart condition which was "sug-gestive but not diagnostic of myocardial ischemia at high work-loads." This means that if he had any blockage in his coronary arteries at all, it was minimal. What had happened here? In 1983, his coronary arteriogram had showed significant, three-vessel blockage. But by the end of 1985, a significant improvement had apparently taken place in the vessels which fed blood to his heart. It seems that the combination of colestipol and nicotinic acid had begun a process of *reversal* of his atherosclerosis!

Drugs, singly or in combination, can at times do wonders to bring the cholesterol levels of certain individuals into a healthy balance. But again, let me emphasize that these are *individual* experiences. What worked for Dr. Keller Greenfield might work for someone else; then again, it might not. He had to experiment with different types of drugs before he finally found the right combination. If you find yourself in a situation similar to his, you'll probably have to experiment as well.

But remember: Dr. Greenfield is a physician and an expert in this field. So, if you do decide to experiment, you'll have to do so under the guidance of a physician.

But the good news is that an increasing variety of drugs and other prescription treatments are coming on the market to help with cholesterol problems. So the odds are greatly increasing that your doctor can do something to help you if you're confronting a difficulty with your blood cholesterol levels.

Drugs (including nicotinic acid) can be powerful tools to correct problems with progressive atherosclerosis and to increase a person's chances to live a longer, healthier life. At the same time, we must all be very careful in using this approach. I didn't hesitate to mention the side effects of most of these drug treatments because it's absolutely essential that you understand the risks and drawbacks. You should be very careful to monitor your body if you find that you have to go on one of these drugs. That way, you'll be in a more knowledgeable position to consult with your doctor—and even to suggest possible alternative treatments.

Sometimes, as we've seen, if you report a bad reaction to a particular prescription, a combination of drugs may lower the negative effects. Or it may help you to switch from one type of medication to another in order to minimize discomforts. Or, if you are experiencing a problem with your cholesterol, your difficulty may be caused or aggravated by some other unrelated type of medication that you're taking. For example, certain types of medications that are prescribed for hypertension may lower the HDL cholesterol or throw other blood lipids out of balance. Studies have shown that the use of diuretic drugs to lower high blood pressure may also elevate cholesterol and triglyceride levels. As a result, those on some types of hypertensive medications may be at an increased risk of atherosclerosis and heart attacks.

What all this adds up to is that drugs are often a two-edged sword. They may help in one area, but they may do some damage in another. Therefore, it's essential that you stay in close touch with your doctor. Keep him informed of any changes or problems you experience in your body and blood mechanisms.

The dangers inherent in many drugs almost always make it advisable for a person with a cholesterol problem to try first the "natural" approaches, such as diet and exercise. It's only when these don't work that we should consider moving on to drug treatment.

FOURTEEN

Coffee and the Cholesterol Question

Coffee occupies a peculiar position in our society. On one hand, when many of us get up in the morning we absolutely have to have it. We swear we can't open our eyes without it! On the other hand, as much as we love the brew, drinking coffee tends to make many people uncomfortable. This litany, which I've heard over the years, probably reverberates through your experience:

- "Coffee makes me nervous—I can feel my anxiety levels rising as I finish the second cup."

- "Coffee changes my personality—I actually became a nice person after I stopped drinking it."

- "I can't drink a cup of coffee alone—I have to have a cookie or pastry or something to go along with it. And that's where my extra pounds are coming from!"

There may be an even more ominous reason to worry about America's favorite after-meal drink: A number of studies have suggested a relationship between coffee consumption and higher levels of cholesterol—and even cardiovascular disease. Tea, including herbal tea, by the way, has not been implicated in this indictment.

What's the evidence? A classic study on this subject is the Tromsø Heart Study, conducted at the University of Tromsø in Norway and reported in the June 16, 1983, issue of the *New England Journal of Medicine*. This investigation involved an

examination of the relationship between (1) coffee consumptio
and (2) levels of total cholesterol, high-density lipoprotein
(HDLs), and triglycerides. The study was conducted in a popu
lation of 7,213 women and 7,368 men between the ages of 2
and 54 years.

The Tromsø researchers found that drinking boiled coffe
was associated with higher total cholesterol levels and highe
triglyceride levels in people of both sexes. Also, the coffe
consumption was associated with lower levels of HDL choles
terol in the women. Furthermore, with both men and women
total cholesterol levels tended to go up as those participating i
the study consumed additional cups of coffee.

In later research, the Tromsø Heart Study reported tha
cholesterol concentrations fell significantly among those wh
abstained from drinking coffee for five weeks. The levels con
tinued to fall for those who continued to abstain for a total o
ten weeks. Cholesterol levels rose in the participants wh
returned to drinking boiled coffee after abstaining for five weeks
But those who returned to *filter-made* coffee after a five-wee
period of abstinence experienced no increases in their cholestero

"We conclude that a daily intake of six or more cups o
boiled coffee increases the serum cholesterol concentration i
healthy subjects," the researchers said.

They concluded that abstention from heavy coffee drinkin
is "an efficient way of reducing serum cholesterol concentra
tions in men with hypercholesterolemia." But they also sai
that further study was needed to determine how a particula
brewing method may affect the relationship between coffee an
cholesterol.

Other medical experts, responding to these findings, o
fered some words of caution:

• The researchers didn't give specific information on th
diets of the people they studied. Consequently, it may be tha
heavy coffee drinkers may be on a different diet from the ligh
drinkers.

• Most coffee drinkers add cream or milk to their coffee
These dairy additions could be significant in increasing choles
terol levels.

• These studies do not control for stress. It may be tha
coffee consumption increases during times of stress. The cho

lesterol increases may be more closely related to the stress factor than to the coffee.

• Other studies have yielded conflicting results: One group of researchers has found no relationship between drinking more than six cups of coffee per day and subsequent heart attacks. Also, the Framingham Study reported no relationship between the amount of coffee consumed and the development of cardiovascular disease.

Clearly, the medical community is not unanimous on the Norwegian study. But, more recently, other evidence has emerged which also points to a coffee-cholesterol connection.

A study at the Stanford University Medical School has suggested that sedentary and mildly active middle-aged men who drink more than two cups of coffee a day are more likely to have high levels of cholesterol. One statistician who helped conduct the study said that his team had found a "risk threshold" at two and one-quarter cups of coffee per day.

To put this in other terms, the study analyses revealed that concentrations of both Apo B and LDL cholesterol—the two major villains in the atherosclerosis scenario—are unrelated to drinking up to two cups of coffee per day. Above two cups, however, the problems with the LDLs and Apo B's begin.

In another study, involving Japanese men in Hawaii, researchers at the Honolulu Heart Program determined that there was a significant relationship between coffee consumption and higher levels of total cholesterol. During the six years of the study, the average coffee consumption was 3.4 cups per day and the average tea consumption was 1.8 cups per day. Those consuming no coffee had an average cholesterol level of 210 mg/dl, while those who drank 9 or more cups of coffee per day had levels of 220 mg/dl. There was no such relationship between cholesterol levels and tea or cola consumption.

There may be a link between coffee and cardiovascular disease. A recent report from the Johns Hopkins Medical School, in which 1,130 male medical students were followed for nineteen to thirty-five years, found that a person who drinks five or more cups of coffee per day is almost three times as likely to develop heart disease as is the person who drinks no coffee at all.* Some observers have suggested that the link between

*New England Journal of Medicine, vol. 315, no. 16, October 16, 1986, pp. 977–82.

coffee and cholesterol may provide a possible explanation for the cause of the heart disease in this study.

These and other studies have also turned up some other provocative facts about the relationship between cholesterol and coffee:

• So far, scientific researchers have been unable to establish any relationship between the caffeine in coffee and rising cholesterol levels. Studies of other drinks with caffeine, such as tea and cola, have shown no elevation of cholesterol. So, apparently there is something else in the makeup of coffee which triggers the rise of cholesterol levels.

• Even extremely small amounts of coffee may increase total cholesterol levels. In a study at the Kaiser Permanente Medical Center in Oakland, California, investigators found that cholesterol levels began to move up steadily, even for those who consumed less than one cup of coffee per day.

In this study of more than 40,000 people, average cholesterol levels stood at 216.3 mg/dl for the men who drank no coffee at all, and they moved up to 219.5 mg/dl for those who drank less than one cup per day. The amounts of cholesterol continued to climb up steadily, to 225.9 mg/dl, for those who drank more than six cups per day.

As for women, their average cholesterol levels stood at 219.6 mg/dl for nondrinkers. They were higher, at 222.6 mg/dl, for those who drank less than one cup; and the average total cholesterol was 225.4 mg/dl for women who consumed more than six cups of coffee per day.

• Some studies have suggested that the cholesterol levels in women tend to go up more than in men. But other studies have shown the opposite. Still others have reported similar reactions in the two sexes. Obviously, more research needs to be done on this subject.

Your Personal Approach to Coffee

What should your approach to coffee be?

As I've said, the growing weight of evidence suggests that drinking coffee, even in small amounts, may throw your cholesterol components out of balance. Still, each person's body tends to respond differently to coffee, as well as to other substances or influences.

So you might do well to test yourself: If you're a coffee drinker, get your blood tested during a period when you're drinking your average number of cups per day. Then, go "cold turkey." Quit drinking coffee completely for four to six weeks; then schedule another blood test. If your cholesterol levels have dropped during this period of abstention—and you haven't done anything else to alter your total cholesterol count—then you may very well be one of those people whose body is sensitive to coffee consumption. You may conclude that it's best to stay away from the brew, now that you've broken the habit!

I myself have only a swallow or two of coffee in the morning when I get to the office. That's my entire quota for the day! My schedule is so frenetic and packed with appointments that I feel I don't really need the extra "zip" from coffee to keep me going.

However, you may feel that you simply can't stay away from your coffee each day. If that's the case, I urge you to ascertain as best you can what impact the coffee is having on you and your cholesterol levels, and whether it may be contributing to a medical problem or serious imbalance in your blood.

You may be in great need of lowering your cholesterol so as to balance your total cholesterol/HDL cholesterol ratio. In such a case, if I were you, I'd stop drinking coffee immediately. If your cholesterol is basically at healthy levels, even with a low to moderate level of coffee drinking, then perhaps you can be a little more relaxed about your approach to this drink.

In any event, try to limit your total daily caffeine intake in mg. to no more than double your body weight in pounds. For example, a 150-pound person should consume no more than 300 mg. of caffeine per day. Remember, a cup of coffee has about 140 mg. per cup, and a cup of tea 68 mg. Colas usually have 38 to 40 mg. per bottle or can, unless they are decaffeinated.

No matter how good that cup of coffee may taste or smell, never assume that it's the same thing as drinking a glass of water. There's every indication that for many people coffee does change the cholesterol balance in the blood—that's a fact that every health-conscious person must keep in mind.

FIFTEEN

Lessons from
the Eskimos

It's long been known that the Eskimos, and also Japanese who consume large quantities of fish, tend to have a very low incidence of coronary heart disease. In recent years, some explanations have been offered for this phenomenon. One of the most intriguing—and scientifically substantiated—is that their secret of protection lies in the fatty fish which is a major component of their diet.

The Eskimos' diet is high in the flesh of certain deep-water fish which contain an important Omega-3 fatty acid, known by the tongue-twisting name "eicosapentaenoic acid," or EPA. Some good sources of this fatty substance are bonito, herring, mackerel, pompano, common salmon, whitefish, shad, albacore, Chinook salmon, and trout. These deep-water fish are especially good sources of EPA because they have access to plankton, which is rich in EPA. Other fish which tend to be good sources of the Omega-3 EPA are bluefish, sardines, bass, and halibut.

In brief, the Omega-3 fatty acids seem to be able to do three things:

1. They tend to "thin out" the blood. Through this process, there is less tendency for the blood to develop clots which could clog vessels and cause a heart attack.

In more scientific terms, EPA is a precursor for prostaglandin-3, a hormonelike substance in the blood which controls clotting and artery spasms. A unique quality of EPA seems to be its ability to prevent the rapid collection of blood platelets at the site of plaque accumulations in the vessels, which are building up through atherosclerosis. When the blood platetlets collect, a blood clot may form, and a heart attack may result.

2. The Omega-3 fatty acids tend to lower triglyceride levels in the blood. As we've seen, high triglyceride levels may be associated with dangerously low levels of "good" HDL cholesterol and with other high-risk factors in the development of heart disease.

3. Fish oil, at least in large doses, can lower serum lipid concentrations, but there is no acceptable evidence that it can prevent heart disease. In addition, the fish oil capsules now on the market are labeled for a maximum dosage of 3 grams or less daily. This is the equivalent of about 8 ounces of salmon. There is considerable speculation as to whether this amount of the oil would have any important effect on serum lipids. And in some people, fish oil may actually increase the LDL cholesterol levels!

So, what is the evidence that eating this type of fatty fish really works? It's one thing to look at the Eskimos and see that they have a low rate of cardiovascular disease. But what's the exact connection between fish consumption and lower cholesterol? To answer these questions, let's look at a few of the studies.

The Dutch Study. Researchers from the Institute of Social Medicine at the University of Leiden in the Netherlands noted that a low death rate from coronary heart disease exists among Greenland Eskimos. The researchers acknowledged that this low rate has been attributed to the Eskimos' high consumption of fish. So the Leiden team decided to explore this matter more fully.

After choosing the town of Zutphen in the Netherlands, they selected 852 middle-aged men with coronary heart disease as participants. Over the twenty-year period of the study, 78 of the men died from coronary heart disease. The investigation focused on the dietary habits and family histories of all the men—and the results tended to support the "fish interpretation" of the Greenland Eskimos' low death rates from coronary heart disease.

Specifically, the researchers found that deaths from coronary heart disease were "more than 50 percent lower among those who consumed at least 30 grams of fish per day, than among those who did not eat fish." This amounts to as little as 1 ounce of fish a day, or the equivalent of two or three fish meals per week.

Furthermore, those doing the study concluded that "the consumption of as little as one or two fish dishes per week may be of preventive value in relation to coronary heart disease."*

The Oregon Study. Another research team, from Oregon Health Sciences University, studied a group of people who had a genetic inability to metabolize fat. They discovered that those who ate a diet rich in fish oils had much lower levels of cholesterol and triglycerides than did those who ate vegetable oils.

Three diets were tested on each patient. One was high in fish oil, mostly from salmon. The second diet included equivalent amounts of safflower and corn oil. The third diet was a very low-fat diet, which is usually given to patients, such as those involved in the study, who have an inherent problem metabolizing fat.

The final results were that when the participants were on the fish oil diet they experienced drops in their total cholesterol levels ranging from 27 percent to 45 percent. Their triglycerides declined 64 to 79 percent.

Both the other diets were considerably less effective than the fish oil diet in achieving these results. It's interesting that both fish which tend to be high in fat, such as salmon and tuna, and those low in fat, such as cod and flounder, were equally effective.

The first results of research in this area are thus quite encouraging. But still, a great deal more needs to be done before we seize upon fish as the be-all and end-all of prevention in cardiovascular disease.

One nagging problem which must confront any fish eater is the problem of pollution. It may be that a certain type of fish can help lower your cholesterol and otherwise put your blood lipids in better balance. But if that fish happens to be part of a group which has been tainted by certain toxins, the dangers of eating that fish may far outweigh the benefits. So it's important

*The New England Journal of Medicine, vol. 312, no. 19, May 9, 1985, pp. 1,205–09.

to keep abreast of the condition of seafood in your particular area if you expect to eat more fish.

With these cautionary words in mind, my advice is to weight your weekly diet more heavily in favor of fish. But don't rely on the use of supplemental fish oil capsules. Even though these capsules have been heavily advertised in the lay literature, their long-term benefit has not yet been proved. In fact, there may be something else in fish *other than* the Omega-3 acids which provides some protection from heart disease. In any event, the capsule dosage would have to be enormous to measure up to the regular dietary consumption of fish.

So, I am unable to recommend the routine consumption of fish oil capsules as protection against heart disease until more research data is available. Instead, I suggest that you try to eat fish as a regular part of your diet at least once or twice a week. The diets in chapter 9 have been designed with this principle in mind.

SIXTEEN

Obesity Is
Never Benign

Americans tend to be an overweight people—and this tendency is causing problems with our blood vessels and our hearts.

The problem, however, lies not so much in a person's heaviness or body weight as in *obesity*. Obesity refers to an excessive amount of body fat—defined as more than 19 percent for males and more than 21 percent for females. You don't measure body fat by stepping on a bathroom scale. Rather, it's necessary to use medical calipers, or pinchers, which measure skin-fold thicknesses in different parts of the body. Or, in certain clinics, you can be weighed under water to determine your percentage of body fat. This procedure involves sitting on a platform in a tank of water and then being dipped under the water briefly so that a technician can measure how much water is displaced by your body. From this measurement, the technician uses a standard formula to determine your percentage of body fat.

You can sometimes get a rough idea about whether you have too much body fat just by weighing yourself. But to do this it's important for you already to have been measured for your percentage of body fat in a clinical setting so that you're aware of how your body weight corresponds with a healthy level of body fat.

But in general, total body weight, or poundage, is not a very good way of comparing the obesity of different individuals. Why is this?

Each of us is made differently, with different sets of

muscles and bone structures. So, one man may be 5 feet 6 inches tall and weigh 190 pounds—yet have only a 15 percent level of body fat, simply because he's heavily muscled or heavy-boned. Another man may be exactly the same height and weight and yet have 30 percent body fat because he has a lighter build and perhaps eats too much for his frame and metabolism.

To evaluate yourself properly, you must have your percentage of body fat measured at a proper clinic. In this way, you'll know better whether or not you're obese—and thus at greater risk for cardiovascular disease.

The Risks of Obesity

What exactly are the risks if you have too high a percentage of body fat?

A major area of risk with obesity involves the way body fat affects the condition of your blood. A variety of studies have shown that those with higher percentages of body fat tend to have higher levels of total cholesterol, of the "bad" LDL cholesterol, and of triglycerides than do those who are leaner. For example:

• The Tecumseh Study in Tecumseh, Michigan, examined more than 4,000 adults in an attempt to identify correlations between their dietary habits and cardiovascular disease. The researchers found that there was definitely a relationship between total cholesterol and triglyceride levels and obesity: the higher the body fat, they concluded, the higher the lipid values.

• In another study, at the University of Pennsylvania, 73 obese men and women were measured before and after a sixteen-week weight reduction program. Among other things, the researchers discovered significant differences between the men and the women.

In the men, a 10.7-kilogram weight loss was associated with a 15.8 percent decrease in the "bad" low-density lipoprotein cholesterol (LDL). Also, there was a 5 percent increase in the "good" HDL. In the women, in contrast, an 8.9-kilogram weight loss resulted in only a 4.7 percent decrease in the LDL cholesterol levels and a 3.3 percent decrease in HDLs. The ratios improved significantly in the men, but not in the women.

These researchers concluded, "These differences suggest that weight reduction may be an important means of improving plasma lipoprotein patterns in men, but may be of more limited values in women."

• Another study indicates that reductions in total cholesterol and LDL levels are greatest when a weight loss program is combined with exercise training. The researchers, from the University of Colorado and the University of Virginia, found that when body weight decreased in conjunction with exercise, the average total cholesterol values went down 13.2 mg/dl, and the LDL levels declined 10.1 mg/dl. The drops were less dramatic when people lost weight without exercise.

In many cases, the major link between obesity and cardiovascular disease is a tendency among obese people to have higher total cholesterol levels, and especially higher LDL levels. In fact, obesity should probably be regarded as an independent risk factor when evaluating a person's likelihood of suffering from cardiovascular disease.

Obesity as an Independent Risk Factor?

Sometimes, obesity seems to operate in an almost mysterious way, all by itself. That was the situation with a case involving a close friend of mine.

This man was 47 years old when he first came to see me in 1971. He had never been in particularly good shape. His treadmill stress test times varied between about 15 and 17 minutes, which placed him in relatively low fitness categories for his age. Also, his percentage of body fat varied from about 24 to 28 percent of his total body weight, when he should have been below 19 percent. In other words, his body fat was far too high and definitely in a range which increased his risk of cardiovascular disease. In addition, he was constantly under pressure with his business, which was on the verge of bankruptcy.

But when I looked at his cholesterol blood values, nothing seemed particularly amiss. His total cholesterol levels ranged from a low of 195 to a high of 224 over the fifteen years that he had been under our care. Also, his HDL levels were in a healthy range, from 44 to 53 mg/dl. These values gave him total cholesterol/HDL ratios which varied from about 3.8 to 4.7—not bad for a man of his age. His LDLs ranged from the low to the moderate risk range and his triglycerides were relatively low.

But finally, a warning signal flashed with a result of "equivocal" on a treadmill stress test he took in the mid-1980s. This meant there was some possibility he could be developing atherosclerosis, with blood being increasingly blocked from reaching his heart through the coronary arteries. Also, his total body weight began to creep up even more, as did his percentage of body fat.

In a case of this type, a change in diet and lifestyle is usually sufficient to correct the problem—and that's what we attempted. I recommended that he lose weight on a low-cholesterol diet, that he embark on a regular aerobics fitness program, and that he take steps to reduce the stress in his life. On this last point, we suggested that he could reduce the stress in his life through (1) an aerobic exercise program; (2) the rearrangement of his daily schedule and work commitments; and (3) the use of some relaxation techniques. But he resisted on all counts.

The final result was tragic. He died suddenly, at 62 years of age, of a massive heart attack. I analyze his case this way: As far as his physical profile was concerned, one big problem that I could identify was his level of obesity. Apparently, his total cholesterol levels were slightly elevated, up in the low 200s, and his LDLs sometimes placed him in a moderate risk category. But his HDLs were high enough to keep his total cholesterol/HDL cholesterol ratio in balance much of the time.

In this case, there may have been something in the obesity itself which contributed to the heart problem. Or perhaps this man's obesity interacted in some way with his relatively moderate cholesterol values to produce deadly changes which would never have occurred in a leaner man.

Another factor which may have contributed to this man's heart attack was the amount of stress he was under. He had been facing considerable business anxieties. This tremendous pressure—though it didn't show up in any dramatic way in his lipid profile—may also have been operating independently to create additional problems for his heart.

As his stress stayed high and his body weight increased, his level of fitness, as measured by his treadmill times, steadily decreased. Apparently he didn't realize what I have said so many times before—that "exercise is nature's best tranquilizer." Remember, too, that obesity is a very common manifestation of stress.

To sum up, then, three important independent factors were at work here: (1) the man's percentage of body fat, or his obesity, was far too high, a fact which may have been reflected ever so slightly in his lipid profile; (2) his stress levels added an undetermined amount of pressure on him; (3) his level of fitness was gradually deteriorating.

As this man's experience shows, not all the cases I encounter can be neatly packaged and explained. But there were in a sense some clear risk indicators, such as obesity, inactivity, and stress. In contrast to this man, many people who have come through our clinic have listened and acted when the presence of such risk indicators was pointed out to them. And they have lived longer and more energetic lives as a result.

For example, one 52-year-old man who came into our clinic about eight years ago could only be described as monstrously overweight. He tipped the scales at nearly 350 pounds, and his body fat was 56 percent of his total weight.

As you might expect, the excess poundage he was carrying around reduced his energy level severely. He could hardly walk two blocks without getting winded, and he performed very poorly on the stress test that we gave him.

On the other hand, his cholesterol levels were in the high normal range, and in general he seemed to be in fairly good health—except for his excessive weight. Specifically, his total cholesterol level was 220, and his total cholesterol/HDL cholesterol ratio was a little high at 5.1.

Knowing that such gross obesity could operate as an independent risk factor on the condition of his heart—and perhaps even eventually threaten his life—I urged him to begin a strict diet and exercise program. The exercise regimen would consist mostly of walking.

At first he resisted, primarily because it was painful for him to think about giving up the extra helpings and sweets that he loved so much. Also, the prospect of using his body more vigorously wasn't particularly to his liking.

But finally he agreed to try the suggested program, and I'm happy to report that now, about a year later, his weight has gone down significantly. Also, his energy level and outlook on life have improved dramatically. Specifically, he has lost about 70 pounds; his percentage of body fat has dropped to about 45 percent; and he's now walking more than a mile a day. As a result, the risks he faces from overweight are declining practically by the day.

If this man continues to lose weight and increase his exercise in the same way he's done in the past, he'll soon completely eradicate obesity as a risk factor in his life. I might add that as he diets and exercises, his cholesterol levels—which were reasonably normal and healthy to begin with—have gotten even better. His total cholesterol is now hovering right at 200 and his total cholesterol/HDL cholesterol ratio is below 5.0.

Unfortunately, the first time that we can usually identify obesity as an independent risk factor in any individual is when that person has a heart attack. For that reason, most of the stories that we can tell about the problem of overweight have a sad ending. But many times, as in this man's case, we've been able to head off problems with obesity before they get started. And that, in large part, is what a personal preventive medicine program is all about.

SEVENTEEN

The Stress Connection

Anxiety. Tension. Pressure.

These terms characterize much of modern-day society, and it's likely that they will continue to be our cultural bywords well into the future. We want to succeed, achieve, and win. So we keep pushing ourselves harder and faster, in an effort to snare some gold ring that always seems to elude us.

Amid this pressure, we hear experts warning, "Stress is a killer!" And we may even agree—at least intellectually—that they're right. But in practice, we don't seem really to believe that stress is so bad, because we continue to live our lives at the same frenetic, uncontrolled pace.

But that's a dangerous attitude to have. Medical research into the question of stress keeps piling up evidence which should make us believe wholeheartedly in the dangers of stress—and in the need to reduce our pressures and find a little more relaxation and peace in our lives. Some of the most interesting research of this type relates to the issue of how stress can act as a trigger to raise cholesterol and other lipid levels.

A number of studies have shown that cholesterol values rise during different types of emotional stress. These include academic examinations, occupational problems, job loss, difficulties in underwater demolition training, surgery, difficult childbirth, and other stressful experiences and activities. To give you an idea about how certain situations may elevate your total cholesterol levels—and put your lipids out of balance—let's take a brief look at a few of the studies in a little more detail.

• In a Norwegian study, 9 female medical students experienced a one-fifth increase in their total cholesterol levels during an important examination.

These young women, aged 22 to 30 years, were studied during their most important preclinical exam, a test known to impose considerable mental stress on most students. Blood samples were drawn immediately after the exam; forty-eight hours later; and finally, two months later, during a time when there wasn't any particular academic pressure. The total cholesterol levels in all the students were higher on the exam day—by an astounding 20 percent—than on either of the other two days.

• Researchers at the Johns Hopkins Medical School examined a number of medical students who suffered from genetically high cholesterol, or hypercholesteremia. The investigators found that the students were thirty times more likely to have heart attacks at an early age than were their classmates with normal cholesterol. Furthermore, those who suffered heart attacks *also* as a group had a personality profile "denoting sensitivity and vulnerability to stress."

• Cholesterol levels of men who lost their jobs went up, but then dropped later when they found new jobs. These were the findings of a longitudinal study, conducted at the University of Michigan, on the cholesterol levels of 200 married men with stable occupational histories. They had all lost their jobs because of a plant shutdown. Those in the study, which was reported in the *Journal of the American Medical Association* in November 1968, were evaluated over a period of two years. During this time, the researchers also discovered that depression levels of the men correlated directly with their total cholesterol counts.

• An investigation of students in a navy underwater demolition team (UDT) training program showed that the 24 young men who failed the course experienced a significant rise in their total cholesterol levels during the final two weeks of the program. In contrast, the 27 who passed the course had stable cholesterol levels throughout their training.

• A study was conducted in India on 65 patients of different age groups who were in a surgical ward. All the patients experienced "statistically significant" rises in their total cholesterol just before their operations were performed. In particular, their preoperative rise in cholesterol varied from 39 percent to 56.9 percent. The researchers concluded, "These findings support previous reports of the effect of mental tension on serum cholesterol level."

• Even newborn babies are not immune to this stress-cholesterol connection. In a study conducted in Helsinki, Finland, researchers found that triglycerides went up and HDL cholesterol went down in the infants who were born during the longest periods of labor.

The experts' conclusion: "The results suggest that intrapartum stress raises . . . triglycerides, and induces qualitative and quantitative changes in the . . . high-density lipoprotein . . . in the newborn."

What Can You Do About Stress?

The precise mechanism by which increased stress is linked to a rise in cholesterol levels isn't yet clear. Various studies have been conducted testing the changes in uric acid and other bodily chemicals and secretions, along with cholesterol levels, during stressful times. But any definitive word on the reasons for the rise in cholesterol at times of stress must await further research.

But there's no reason for *you* to wait to reduce the stress in your life! There are at least four things you can do to lower your stress:

Stress Antidote 1. First, you can embark on a regular aerobic exercise program of the type I've described in chapter 12. Research has shown that this type of endurance activity triggers the release of endorphins, a morphinelike chemical in the brain which acts as a natural tranquilizer. Most regular runners report that after a workout they experience a tremendous sense of relaxation and well-being.

I'm certainly an example of this phenomenon. Most afternoons, after a long, stressful day at work, my body feels tight and my mind is full to the brim of the day's pressures and concerns. So I put on my running gear, head for the track at the Aerobics Center if I'm in Dallas—or the open road if I'm out of town—and jog for three miles.

The end result is consistently pleasurable and relaxing.

The pressures of the day melt away during this aerobic activity, and I'm soon ready for several more hours of family time, socializing, or even work.

Stress Antidote 2. Another possible avenue for you to take is to develop relaxation techniques, which have been shown to be good treatments for hypertension and various anxiety-related ills. One proven approach has been developed by Dr. Herbert Benson, a cardiologist and professor at the Harvard Medical School, who advocates the elicitation of what he calls the "Relaxation Response."* In brief, he recommends a widely used generic approach to inducing measurable physiologic responses usually associated with relaxation techniques. These include reduced blood pressure, reduced heart rate, lower speed of the body's metabolism, slower brain waves, and a slower rate of breathing.

How do you elicit this Relaxation Response? Dr. Benson recommends that you follow these steps**:

1. Sit comfortably in a quiet environment and concentrate on relaxing all your major muscle groups.

2. Focus for ten to twenty minutes, twice a day, on some word or phrase. Say the word to yourself on each exhalation. Any word or phrase will do, though clinical work has demonstrated that terms associated with a person's deepest beliefs— such as a Bible passage—tend to have the most beneficial effect.

3. Assume a passive attitude when intrusive thoughts come into your mind. In other words, don't aggressively try to push the thoughts away; rather, when they appear, just say "oh, well," and return to your focus word or phrase.

"Several investigations have demonstrated that stress elevates serum cholesterol levels," Dr. Benson told me. "So it is not surprising that preliminary studies have shown that the regular elicitation of the Relaxation Response lowers serum cholesterol."

*See Dr. Benson's *The Relaxation Response* (New York: Avon Books, 1976), and his *Beyond the Relaxation Response* (New York: Berkley, 1985).
**The preceding description, which can be found in other formats in Dr. Benson's books and research reports, comes from an interview conducted with him for this book.

Stress Antidote 3. It's quite helpful to be involved in solid, supportive relationships.

One investigation, done at the Departments of Medicine and Psychiatry at the University of New Mexico School of Medicine, examined 256 healthy elderly adults who had "good social support systems." These were defined as "satisfying relationships with trusted individuals in whom [they] could confide." The study found that these people had lower cholesterol levels and also more effective functioning of their immune systems.

Stress Antidote 4. You can rearrange your daily life, including your schedule and environment, with the goal to reduce your stress level. If you feel under excessive pressure because of too much work, either reduce your involvements and responsibilities, or find another job! I know this may seem easier to say than to do. But after all, what's more important—your present job commitments, or your life?

Sometimes, a simple shift or change in your living and working environment may significantly reduce the stress you feel. One man I know, who conducted his business out of his home, found himself getting into an increasing number of arguments with his wife. Both spouses consistently experienced high levels of anxiety, though they often couldn't identify the source of their discomfort.

Then the husband moved his office out to another location and took with him all the furniture, files, books, and other equipment he used in his work. As a result, the physical environment in their home became relatively uncluttered, with many more open spaces than before.

Almost immediately, both husband and wife experienced a greater inner serenity than they had known for years. They felt more relaxed and certainly under considerably less stress. Perhaps most important of all, they now rarely got into arguments with each other. The key to this improvement in the quality of their lives—and the lowering of their stress levels—had clearly been the change in their physical environment.

Stress remains a mysterious subject in the health field. But even though there's a great deal about this insidious influence that we still don't know, one thing is clear: too much anxiety and pressure in your life can have a negative and even dangerous impact on your psychological and physical well-being, including the state of the components of your blood. So my advice is to take the stress in your life seriously—and feel free to be creative as you do what you can to eliminate it!

EIGHTEEN

The Connection Between Age and Cholesterol

We've known for years from the scientific literature that you can expect an increase of total cholesterol with increasing age. Many people have assumed that this is just an inevitable part of what's involved in "getting older."

But is this really true? Is a rise in your total cholesterol—and the possibility of an increasing imbalance in your blood lipids—an irreversible part of aging? Or can you do something about it?

Questions like these led us to study complete cholesterol data on some 2,000 healthy men at the Cooper Clinic in Dallas. As a result of this investigation, we discovered the following:

Age vs. Cholesterol*

Age (years)	under 30	30–39	40–49	50–59	60 +
Total cholesterol	179	191	205	208	208
HDL	43	42	43	43	44
LDL	136	149	162	165	164
% body fat	18.1	22.0	23.5	23.8	23.0

*From Kenneth H. Cooper, *The Aerobics Program for Total Well-Being*, p. 87.

As you can see from this study, men do indeed experience an increase in total cholesterol with advancing age. At the same time, however, their HDL levels, or "good cholesterol," remain nearly constant. The factor that accounts for the increase in total cholesterol is the "bad" LDL cholesterol, which tends to go up as people get older, for reasons I'll explain shortly.

We discovered with these men that their ratios of total cholesterol/HDL cholesterol increased from 4.1 to 4.8, from the beginning to the end of the age range.

We've also studied 589 women, of an average age of about 40, to see if there is any relation between their age and total cholesterol levels. The results came out as follows:

Age	under 30	30–39	40–49	50–59	60 +
Total cholesterol	179	186	194	219	221
HDL	53	57	58	60	62
LDL	126	129	136	159	159
% body fat	26	26	27	30	29

As the facts demonstrate, there are some differences in the responses to aging among men and women—notably that HDLs stay about the same for men, but go up to some extent for women. But with both sexes, the total cholesterol and "bad" LDLs tend to increase at a much faster rate.

What's the reason for the rise in LDLs and total cholesterol as people get older?

There are growing indications that increasing age may be accompanied by a decrease in activity of LDL receptors. Receptors, you'll recall, are those "rescuers" on the body's cells which pull in the LDL and process it for the cells' use, rather than allow it to float freely in the body's blood. The LDLs which are not pulled out of the bloodstream by the receptors may begin to accumulate with their Apo B partners as plaque on the walls of the blood vessels. Progressive atherosclerosis, complete blockage of a blood vessel, and a heart attack may eventually result.

Some researchers feel that the blood of older people has more LDLs simply because the body naturally produces more LDLs as age increases. But this tendency could be related to increasing obesity or percentage of body fat in older people. As you can see from the above chart, the body fat of the men we studied tended to go up as age increased. Finally, the tendency toward obesity plateaued and then decreased slightly after age 60.

In our study, the younger men were relatively lean, with

only 18 percent body fat. Men past 40, on the other hand, had a relatively high percentage of body fat, which on average was nearly 24 percent. We found that the correlation between a person's percentage of body fat and his total cholesterol and LDL cholesterol was much stronger than the correlation between his cholesterol levels and his age.

Some of these people whose percentage of body fat went up with age nevertheless remained at the same weight throughout their lives. From chapter 16, you can probably guess why this happens. In other words, a person might weigh the same at age 40 as he did at age 21, yet his waist measurements could be considerably larger! This is simply a reflection of the fact that his muscle mass may be decreasing with a sedentary lifestyle, while his body fat is increasing.

In general, people in this category may be eating the same or fewer calories than they used to but may not be burning them as rapidly or maintaining their muscle mass because they're getting less exercise. So, their weight may stay the same, but their percentage of body fat may begin to increase, as it did with a number of the men whom we studied.

But none of this is inevitable. By maintaining a high level of physical fitness, with a moderate but regular program of aerobic exercise—and perhaps some calisthenics to increase your upper body strength—you can lower your percentage of body fat and increase your muscle mass. And the chances are that you can maintain your body at about the levels you enjoyed when you were younger. By keeping active, exercising, and watching your diet, you can actually retard the effects of aging— and succeed in keeping your total cholesterol levels in healthy balance.

NINETEEN

The Difference
Between
Men and Women

Women tend to have less of a problem than men with heart disease, at least before they go through menopause. Why is this?

In large part, it's probably because of their naturally higher levels of HDL cholesterol. Among other things, their higher HDLs give them lower—and healthier—total cholesterol/HDL cholesterol ratios than those of men. This lower ratio probably helps protect them from hardening of the arteries more than their male counterparts.

In more concrete terms, a normal HDL level in men tends to be 45 or higher, while in women it's 55 or higher. In one of our studies at the Aerobics Center, women aged 40 to 49 had an average total cholesterol of 194 mg/dl and an HDL cholesterol count of 58, for a ratio of 3.34. In contrast, men aged 40 to 49 had an average total cholesterol of 210 and an HDL reading of 44, for a ratio of 4.77.

Other studies we've done with people across all age ranges have confirmed this important difference between men and women. Consider the comparison between men and women as far as HDL levels and ratios are concerned (see chart p. 298).

You'll note in these charts that although there are decided differences in the cholesterol balance between the men and women, the ratios for both groups are relatively healthy. You'll recall from chapter 6 that men with ratios below 4.6 and women below 4.0 usually tend to face little risk of heart disease from their cholesterol. Largely, our participants did rather well

Age Ranges	Median HDL (mg/dl)	Median Ratio, Total Cholesterol/ HDL Cholesterol
Males		
under 30	43.0	4.1
30–39	42.0	4.5
40–49	43.0	4.8
50–59	43.0	4.8
60 & over	44.0	4.7
Females		
under 30	51.0	3.2
30–39	54.0	3.3
40–49	57.0	3.2
50–59	59.0	3.5
60 & over	55.0	3.7

on these exams, probably because they tended to be involved in regular aerobic exercise and good nutrition programs.

But in the general population, where there are also considerable differences between the HDL levels and the ratios of men and women, many people pay little attention to exercise and diet. As a result, their ratios may creep up, and the differences between men and women can become more a matter of life or death.

To put this another way, total cholesterol levels in sedentary people who are not diet- or exercise-conscious are usually higher than in those who follow preventive medicine principles. Their ratios are more likely to move up into high and even critical risk ranges. This means that for many men especially— even more than for women, who tend to start out at higher HDL levels—there can be a great risk cf heart disease.

Some other important gender-related differences, several of which I've mentioned in previous chapters, have also emerged in recent research:

• Women who use birth control pills have at times been found to have slightly elevated total cholesterol levels, marked elevations in their triglycerides, slightly higher LDLs, and lower levels of the "good" high-density lipoproteins (HDLs).

In other cases, however, the opposite occurs: the HDL cholesterol increases and the LDL cholesterol decreases. The effect of birth control pills on the serum cholesterol level is dependent on the ratio of estrogen to progesterone. In women, it's the estrogen that increases the HDL levels and reduces the LDLs. In postcoronary men, however, supplemental estrogen has not been associated with any decrease in mortality.*

• As women age, their HDL levels usually increase; as men age, their HDLs stay about the same.

• As men lose weight, their ratios of total cholesterol/HDL cholesterol generally improve; as women lose weight, their ratios stay about the same.

• Women who smoke cigarettes experience greater declines in their HDL cholesterol than do men who smoke.

Although women start off with a decided advantage by having higher HDL levels and lower ratios, that's no reason for them to become complacent. For one thing, cardiovascular disease is on the rise among women, largely because they're smoking more, eating improperly, failing to exercise, and otherwise not taking advantage of their natural protection. In the younger female population especially, smoking has been increasing, and that can only bode ill for their future health.

Many important findings—and warnings—about keeping cholesterol in balance apply to one degree or another to women, much as they apply to men. For example, women who engage exclusively in weight-training tend to have lower HDL levels than do women who participate in aerobic exercise. And the same point applies to men.

So, even though there are many differences between the sexes on the cholesterol issue, there are also a number of important similarities—including the ongoing need to take preventive steps to keep cholesterol components at healthy levels. Women do have reason to feel fortunate about their natural tendency to have well-balanced blood, including healthy levels of the various cholesterol components. But, like men, they

*See Walace, R.B.; J. Hoover; E. Barrett-Connor; et al: "Altered Plasma Lipid and Lipoprotein Levels Associated with Oral Contraceptives and Estrogen Use." *Lancet*, vol. 2, 1979, pp. 111–115.

must continue to pay close attention to their diets, exercise commitments, and lifestyles, especially as they get older. That may be the only way that the initial benefits they enjoy will stay with them and enable them to age happily and energetically.

TWENTY

"Mono" Fats and Oats: Are These Effective "Natural" Treatments for Cholesterol?

Nutritionists are constantly searching for ways to fine-tune our diets so as to put our cholesterol and lipids in better balance. The ultimate goal is to identify "natural" approaches—which may involve changes in diet or lifestyle, but which don't require drugs or other types of medical intervention.

Two concepts which have recently appeared as a way to improve our cholesterol picture are monounsaturated fats, including such foods as olive oil, and oat products. But what is the evidence that these foods can really help us? To answer this question, let's take a closer look at some recent research and reports on these topics.

Is Olive Oil the Solution?

In the past, attempts to lower cholesterol in the diet have centered on foods which contain polyunsaturated fats, such as various vegetable oils. But more recent research, much of which has been conducted by Dr. Scott M. Grundy, has shown that monounsaturated fats, such as olive oil, may be a better alternative.

Dr. Grundy had noted that in the Mediterranean basin—and particularly in Greece, Crete, and southern Italy—there tended to be low rates of coronary heart disease. Furthermore, the traditional diet in those areas was high in olive oil, which contains relatively large quantities of monounsaturated fats. But despite this intake of fat, the levels of cholesterol, as well as of coronary disease, were relatively low.

"The interesting thing about olive oil is that it's rich in oleic acid, which is a monounsaturated fatty acid," Dr. Grundy said. Yet, olive oil is also low in polyunsaturates.

So Dr. Grundy decided to conduct a study to see how well a diet rich in monounsaturated fatty acids compared with a diet high in polyunsaturates or other types of fats.

In one study, Dr. Grundy and Dr. Fred H. Mattson, of the Department of Medicine of the University of California at San Diego, formulated three liquid diets, which differed from one another only in the kinds of fats they contained: one contained saturated fats; another contained monounsaturated fats; and the third contained polyunsaturated fats. The fats in these diets made up 40 percent of the participants' total calories. (Although the average American diet contains about 40 percent fat, you'll recall that I recommend in this book that fats be kept below 30 percent of total daily calories.)

The 20 patients involved in the study consumed the three diets one after the other, devoting four weeks to each diet. After each diet routine, their blood was tested for total cholesterol, total triglycerides, HDLs, LDLs, and VLDLs.

As everyone expected, when the patients were on the saturated-fat diet, their total cholesterol levels tended to be highest. When they were on the polyunsaturated-fat diet, their total cholesterol levels dropped—and that included *both* their "bad" LDLs *and* their "good" HDLs.

As for the monounsaturated-fat diet, the researchers found that this regimen lowered the total cholesterol and the LDLs as effectively as the polyunsaturated-fat diet had done. But the mono diet didn't lower the HDLs as often. In effect, the mono-fat diet tended to "target" the LDLs for reduction, but not the HDLs.

"This area of the study was not conclusive, but it was very promising," Dr. Grundy said.

As a result of such evidence, Dr. Grundy recommends that monounsaturated fats, such as olive oil, be worked in to our diets more, while polyunsaturated fats should be reduced. He notes that animal experiments have indicated some possible negative side-effects of polyunsaturates, including the development of cancer, the suppression of the immune system, and drastic changes in the cell membranes.

Dr. Grundy is not saying that polyunsaturates should be eliminated completely from the diet, because, as he notes, a small amount of this fat is necessary for the body's system as what's called an "essential fatty acid." But he believes that it's wise to follow these guidelines:

• Keep saturated fats below 10 percent of total calories

• Keep monounsaturates at a level of 10 to 15 percent of total calories

• Keep polyunsaturates at 5 to 10 percent of total calories

In fact, these are approximately the levels which we've recommended in chapter 9 of this book.

In another study, Dr. Grundy investigated the impact of different types of fats on 11 patients during three dietary periods, each of which lasted four weeks. The average cholesterol levels of the patients at the beginning of the investigation were 251 mg/dl.

One of the diets included liquid foods, prepared in a laboratory according to a special formula, which were rich in monounsaturated fatty acids. This was clearly a "high-mono" type of diet. The second set of liquid diets was low in all fats; and the third was high in saturated fatty acids.

The diets which were high in monounsaturated fats and high in saturated fats contained 40 percent of their total calories as fat and 43 percent as carbohydrates. The low-fat diet, in contrast, had 20 percent fats and 63 percent carbohydrates. Finally, the body weight of all the participants was kept steady by adjusting the amount of calories they consumed each day.

The final results, once again, suggested some definite benefits for a high-mono-fat diet. Specifically, the high-mono diet lowered average total cholesterol 13 percent. In contrast, the low-fat diet lowered total cholesterol only 8 percent. The high-mono diet also seemed to "attack" the levels of LDLs, or "bad" cholesterol, more effectively than the low-fat diet did. To put this more precisely, the high-mono diet lowered the LDLs 21 percent, while the low-fat diet lowered the LDLs only by 15 percent.

Just as important, the high-mono diet had *no effect* on the level of triglycerides or on the all-important high-density lipoproteins (HDLs). Conversely, the low-fat diet tended to raise the triglyceride levels and also *reduce* the HDL levels—two results which can jeopardize a healthy balance of cholesterol and other blood fats.

What Can We Conclude?

What can we conclude from these studies?

It seems that diets which are rich in monounsaturated fats, such as olive oil, can be at least as effective and perhaps even more effective in lowering total cholesterol levels than diets which are low in fat and high in carbohydrates. As I've already indicated, the high-mono-fat diets seem able to "target" the type of cholesterol which most needs to be reduced—that is, the LDL cholesterol. These insights have been incorporated in the diets in chapter 9 in that I've emphasized the use of various foods that are relatively high in monounsaturated fats.

In other words, as the total cholesterol decreases with a high-mono-fat diet, it's the "bad" LDLs which go down, while the "good" HDLs stay fairly constant. As a result, those on high-mono-fat diets tend to improve their total cholesterol/HDL cholesterol ratios and their overall cholesterol picture more than do those who are on regular low-fat diets or diets high in polyunsaturates.

Dr. Grundy, who has done much of the major work in this area, is cautious in making generalizations about the precise long-term benefits of a "Mediterranean-type" diet, which is relatively high in monounsaturated fats. But he does believe—and I agree—that in light of the present evidence, it would be wise to begin including an increasing percentage of monounsaturated fats in your overall fat consumption.

The Fiber Factor

In recent years there have been suggestions and theories about the healthful effects on cholesterol of various natural foods. The popular press has been flooded with accounts of the great benefits of brewer's yeast, pectin (which is found in apples and some other fruits), and a variety of other fiber-related substances. But perhaps the most promising findings involve the effects of oat products on total cholesterol levels.

The first thing to understand about this topic is that not all bran is the same. There's a difference between water-soluble fiber, which reportedly helps remove cholesterol, and insoluble fiber, which does not. Oats and dried beans are among the foods which contain water-soluble fiber, while wheat bran has insoluble fiber. Still, I don't want to give insoluble fiber any "bad press" because wheat bran, vegetables, fruits, and other such foods containing insoluble fiber may help prevent colon cancer by assisting the body in cleaning out the intestines on a regular basis.

For our present purposes, however, we're mainly concerned about the benefits of water-soluble fiber, and especially oats. Why oats? Increasing numbers of studies are indicating that oats can be a useful supplement to your diet in helping to balance cholesterol levels.

During a recent investigation done at the Northwestern University Medical School in Chicago, 208 healthy men and women, aged 30 to 65, participated in a twelve-week program designed to show the effect of eating oat products on cholesterol and other blood lipid levels. In the first six weeks, all the participants followed the American Heart Association's recommended diet, which limits fat intake to 30 percent of total calories. The meals contained an equal distribution of saturated, monounsaturated, and polyunsaturated fats. The dietary cholesterol in their meals was limited to 250 mg. per day—considerably below the average of 450 mg. per day of the general public. But during this first six weeks, those involved in the study didn't consume any oat products.

By the end of the first six weeks, the average cholesterol levels for all volunteers had dropped by 5 percent. At that time, they were divided at random into three groups, and all continued to follow the fat-modified diet. But group 1 was instructed to include 2 ounces of oat bran in their menus; group 2 was told to include 2 ounces of oatmeal; and group 3, serving as the "control" against which the other two groups would be compared, didn't eat any oat products at all.

Group 1 reported later that they ate an average of 39 grams of oat bran per person per day, and group 2 said that they consumed an average of 35 grams of oatmeal per day. In each case, this amounted to about 1 ounce per person per day.

By the end of the study, after a full twelve weeks had elapsed, both groups 1 and 2, who had been eating the oat products, experienced further reductions of 3 percent in their total cholesterol levels. The control group, in contrast, had practically no additional cholesterol reduction.*

Other studies involving individuals with high cholesterol levels have reported even greater drops in total cholesterol. For example:

• One 1980 study focused on 4 men who ate 100 grams a day of oat bran (in the form of hot cereals and muffins) over a ten- to thirteen-day period. The result was significant reductions in total cholesterol levels.

• In 1981, 8 men, aged 35 to 62, consumed 100 grams of oat bran daily over ten days. They reported 13 percent decreases in their total cholesterol levels.

• A third study, involving 20 men, aged 34 to 66, reported experiencing a 19 percent drop in total cholesterol levels over three weeks. They consumed 100 grams of oat bran daily.

How Do Oats Work?

What's the mechanism by which these declines in cholesterol levels apparently occur?

Early researchers suggested that loss of cholesterol through bile acids in daily bowel movements might have been enhanced by increased consumption of water-soluble fibers in foods such as oats. But later studies have indicated that not that much cholesterol is lost through the feces. According to another theory, oat bran may act as a kind of resin which binds bile acids and accelerates the clearance of LDL cholesterol from the blood. But considerably more research is needed in this area before we can hope to understand the exact impact that oat products have on our bodies and blood.

Despite this lack of understanding, however, it seems reasonable to include increasing amounts of oat products in your diet, especially if you have a problem with high total cholesterol levels. It may be that your body won't respond to

*See *Journal of the American Dietetic Association*, vol. 86, no. 6, June 1986.

these foods in such a way that your cholesterol goes down. But then again, you may be pleasantly surprised to find that a bowl of oatmeal daily can produce some beneficial changes in your body and your blood.

TWENTY-ONE

Children
and Cholesterol

Considerable controversy has swirled around the question of whether children should be fed the same low-cholesterol diets as are recommended for adults.

One view held by the American Academy of Pediatrics has said that there is "no compelling new evidence to make recommendations concerning modification of the diet during the first two decades of life."

In other words, they're saying that there's no reason for youngsters to go on low-fat, low-cholesterol diets—unless there's some clear medical evidence for doing so, such as inherited high cholesterol. The Academy suggests a fat intake of 30 to 40 percent of a youngster's calories. The pediatricians worry that, among other things, cutting down on fats might eliminate nutrients which are important to overall growth and physical development.

But an important objection is raised by the American Heart Association and a panel of experts convened by the National Institutes of Health, which have recommended that children older than two years of age, like adults, should reduce their intake of fat and cholesterol. Their goal is to limit the daily fat intake of children and adults to no more than 30 percent of daily calories. The objective, these groups say, is to help prevent the buildup of fatty deposits in vessels, which may lead later to heart attacks and strokes.

Which position is right? What's the evidence to support one view or the other?

One point that tends to uphold the view of those who want to limit cholesterol-laden foods for children is the fact that some youngsters begin to develop the fatty deposits of atherosclerosis in their blood vessels at a very young age. A variety of studies have revealed that there may be fatty streaks in the aortas (the largest artery leading from the heart) of eight- to ten-year-olds! Researchers also have discovered fatty streaks in the coronary arteries of some youngsters at about the age of puberty.

One of the most famous, landmark articles documenting the early onset of coronary atherosclerosis in American men was published in the *Journal of the American Medical Association* in 1953. It was entitled "Coronary Disease Among U.S. Soldiers Killed in Action in Korea," and was written by Major William F. Enos and colleagues. They focused on some 200 soldiers whose ages ranged from 18 to 48 years, with an average age of 22.1.

In evaluating the hearts of these young men killed in combat, Dr. Enos and his colleagues showed that 35 percent had coronary lesions which didn't cause significant obstructions. Another 39 percent had narrowing of the coronary arteries ranging from 10 percent to 90 percent. Finally, in 3 percent, plaque deposits had completely closed one or more vessels. In other words, only 23 percent of these young men had no visible signs of any coronary artery disease!

As a part of the Bogalusa Heart Study in Bogalusa, Louisiana, investigators checked risk factors for cardiovascular disease in young people from birth through age 26. The study was a biracial investigation, with approximately two-thirds of the subjects being white and one-third black. Researchers observed the youngsters between 1973 and 1983 and collected data from more than 8,000 people.

Among other things, the Bogalusa Study has revealed that there were fatty streaks in the aortas and coronary arteries (those which lead *to* the heart) of 35 young people who died untimely deaths—mainly from accidents, homicides, or suicides. Their average age at the time of death was 18. The fatty streaks in the young people's blood vessels were strongly related to their levels of both total cholesterol and LDL cholesterol.

The researchers concluded that their "data suggest that a rational approach to the prevention of cardiovascular disease should begin early in life."

An article in *The New York Times* (October 29, 1986), summing up the impact of studies like this, says that by age 4, the average American child has already reached a total cholesterol level that's as high as it should be in adulthood. Moreover, it seems that about 30 percent of the nation's children have cholesterol levels that most experts regard as "abnormally high." Yet there is some encouraging news: Young children have one-half of their total cholesterol in the HDL form. Adults have approximately one-fifth in that form.

Despite this situation, however, it's important not to be hasty in prescribing adult diets for very young children. Children *are* different from adults! Their blood balances are still developing through puberty. This means that, for *most* children, it may be appropriate to use a distinctively child-oriented approach to controlling cholesterol.

Examinations in the Bogalusa Heart Study of the lipid profiles of children at birth have shown that the basic biochemical relationships in the human body are already established at that time. In other words, we start off with certain "givens," or tendencies toward certain cholesterol and blood-fat levels that we inherit from our forebears.

Then, as children get older, their cholesterol levels usually continue to go through certain predictable but distinctive developmental changes. One Dutch study of 458 youngsters, aged 5 to 19 years, has demonstrated that during a child's growth and maturing years, the factors that influence cholesterol levels differ from influences later in life.

For one thing, average total cholesterol levels in this study decreased in both boys and girls between the ages of 10 and 16 years. Also, average levels of "good" HDL cholesterol stayed the same for boys and girls until age 17. They then increased for the females and decreased for the males. That is, it's only at puberty that the differences between men and women, which we discussed in chapter 19, become apparent.

Another investigation, the Lipid Research Clinics Program Prevalence Study, focused primarily on changes in the HDL levels of youngsters and came up with some fascinating results. They found that from ages 6 to 10, the average HDL levels were lower in girls than in boys—a complete "flip-flop" of later adult blood values. But then the HDL counts for boys began to decrease and the counts for girls increased, until by ages 18 to

25 the young women had HDL levels that averaged 10.5 mg/dl higher than those of the young men.

The researchers in this study concluded that the most important influence on HDL cholesterol levels in adolescent boys was the change in their sex hormone levels. Further documentation of this fact was published in the *Journal of the American Medical Association,* January 23, 1987. A three-phase study tested the hypothesis that the decrease in the HDL cholesterol observed in boys at puberty is related to an increase in their testosterone levels. In the first phase, 57 boys aged 10 to 17 years were categorized into four stages of puberty based on their physical appearance and their blood testosterone levels. These four groups showed increasing testosterone levels and decreasing HDL levels. In the second phase, 14 boys with delayed puberty were treated with testosterone and the same effect on the HDL was noted. In the third phase, 13 boys with delayed adolescence demonstrated increasing plasma testosterone levels and decreasing HDL levels during puberty. In all cases, levels of HDL cholesterol and Apo A-I were affected in the same way.

Higher HDLs for women are inevitable because of hormonal differences. But the levels of HDLs and the overall cholesterol balance can certainly be influenced by such measures as not smoking, eating a proper diet, and participating in aerobic exercise.

In addition to these sex-related considerations, another factor underlying the cholesterol condition of every youngster is what might be called the *inheritance factor*. To a great degree, your blood balance depends on the genes you've inherited—or haven't inherited—from your mother, your father, or various ancestors.

For example, a few children have a rare genetic disease called homozygous familial hypercholesterolemia (FH). This disorder—which involves a lack of cell receptors to pull the "bad" LDL cholesterol and their Apo B "partners" out of the bloodstream—may cause heart attacks in children or adolescents because of rapid buildup of plaque in the arteries.

The little elementary-school girl whose situation I described in chapter 2 had this problem. As a result, she had to undergo a dual heart and liver transplant, an operation which saved her life. But there are also places like the General Clinical Research Center at the University of Texas Health

Science Center at Dallas, where such children can be treated in less radical ways.

Many of us have certain inherited traits which may be cause for concern—though they're probably not as serious as the problem which confronts youngsters who have serious genetic flaws. Our family histories can be an important predictive tool, as we try to decide on a way of life that will minimize our risks for cardiovascular disease.

In a study conducted by the University of Michigan and the Mayo Clinic with 98 healthy children in Rochester, Minnesota, the cholesterol levels of the youngsters were compared with the cardiovascular health histories of their relatives. The researchers noted that earlier studies have indicated that cholesterol levels at birth aren't good predictors of family heart disease. But by age 6, the study found, both HDL and LDL cholesterol become predictors of heart disease in older relatives.

As a result, the researchers said, "We can infer from our study that children between the ages of 6 and 16 years with elevated LDL or low HDL are probably at increased risk for [coronary heart disease] in adulthood."

But even though family history and inherited traits will influence your cholesterol values and those of your children, there's no reason to become complacent and say, "What will be, will be." On the contrary, countless studies—even of those with serious cases of elevated cholesterol—have indicated that diet, exercise, lifestyle, and drugs can be crucial elements in programs designed to counter a dangerous family history.

In practical terms, what approach should you take to trying to control your youngster's cholesterol? Here are a few steps which you may find helpful in formulating your own distinctive family program:

Step 1. First, get your child's blood values checked. That means learning the five major lipid components—total cholesterol; LDL; HDL; total cholesterol/HDL ratio; and triglycerides.

When should you have this done? The American Heart Association suggests that regular testing for cholesterol should begin by age 20. But in light of the Bogalusa findings and similar studies, I believe you should have a complete blood test done when your child is between the ages of 6 and 10. Of course, it would be wise to have a blood test done even earlier if you have a family history of genetically high cholesterol or other lipid problems.

Step 2. Understand the meaning of the cholesterol and lipid values in your child's blood test.

One simple set of guidelines to follow has been suggested by the *Journal of the American Medical Association.* There, a "consensus conference" of medical experts says that if a child aged 2 to 19 years has total cholesterol levels of about 170 mg/dl, further blood tests and consultations would be appropriate. If the total cholesterol is between 170 and 185, diet counseling and changes are definitely in order.

If the levels are higher than 185, close supervision and strict dietary instructions may be necessary. Children with total cholesterol counts higher than 200 mg/dl may have one of the hereditary lipid problems, such as hypercholesterolemia. In such a case, parents should definitely seek the advice of a medical specialist and should be prepared not only for dietary changes but for drug treatment.

Step 3. Decide on a proper diet for your child.

In general, I agree with those who recommend waiting until a child is at least 2 years of age before placing him or her on a low-fat or low-cholesterol diet such as those followed by many adults.

As a "Commentary" in the *Journal of the American Medical Association* has put it, "for the diet of the infant, it seems reasonable to consider breast milk the standard until some convincing evidence is presented to indicate something better for most of the first year of life." The average breast milk contains 40 to 50 percent of the calories as fat, and about 150 mg/dl as cholesterol.

But after about age 2, you should start cutting down on cholesterol-carrying foods. At least by elementary-school age, you should have the child essentially on a healthy low-cholesterol adult diet. Refer to the diets for adults in chapter 9 to get appropriate menus and recipes for your older children. Of course, the degree to which you will need to limit cholesterol-carrying foods will depend on the results of your youngster's blood tests.

Step 4. Encourage your child to develop an aerobic exercise program.

As we've seen, the lipid balance of young children differs markedly from that of adults, primarily because of the hormonal changes that occur during puberty. But still, it's wise to get your child started on an active exercise program as early as possible—for a number of reasons:

• Habits that are formed at a young age will tend to stick with your child into adulthood. By getting your boy or girl accustomed to endurance sports which tend to raise the "good" HDL levels, you'll be providing that youngster with an inheritance which could well mean a long and healthy life.

• Obesity at a young age can pave the way to a lipid profile that can increase your child's risk of atherosclerosis.

A study done at the Louisiana State University Medical Center in New Orleans found a direct correlation between (1) relatively high body fat in children 5 to 12 years old, and (2) elevated levels of total cholesterol and LDLs. Remember, the higher the body fat, the lower the "good" HDLs tend to be.

Here are some specific guidelines to keep in mind as you design an aerobic exercise program for your child:

• Start your child "exercising," in the sense of staying active, playing vigorously, and walking, from the earliest possible age. Good physical habits will develop strong bones and muscles and lay a solid groundwork for later, structured exercise.

• *Don't* begin extensive, structured, long-distance aerobic activity until your youngster is at least 10 years old. Of course, organized sports such as soccer or informal activities like hiking are fine. I become concerned mostly when parents start their children running for miles at a very young age. Their muscles and bones just haven't developed enough until about age 10 for serious aerobic efforts.

• By the junior-high years, all children should be involved in vigorous aerobic exercise, either at home or as part of a school athletic program. If your child isn't interested in school sports or if the endurance workouts there seem inadequate, you should get your child started with one of the aerobic programs described in chapter 12. To begin, just have him or her follow the suggested programs for healthy adults, 30 to 50 years of age. Before you know it, your youngster will probably advance far beyond these levels and will be ready for the more rigorous regimen in my book *The Aerobics Program for Total Well-Being.*

For most people, the major problems with out-of-balance cholesterol don't develop until at least middle age. But why make your child wait to correct a problem which he or she can begin to remedy right now? Why wait until your youngster's life is in jeopardy before you tell him what his cholesterol outlook is?

Remember, heart disease is characterized by years and years of incubation, and then by only seconds required for the fatal event. If the epidemic of heart disease in this country is ever going to be controlled, it must start with an aggressive preventive approach with our children.

So *now* is the time to instill those healthy habits in your children, while they're still young and their minds, appetites, and exercise patterns are still malleable. One of the greatest gifts parents can pass on to their offspring is a more complete knowledge of how their bodies operate—and an understanding of what they can do to increase their chances of living out their full life span in good spirits and good health.

TWENTY-TWO

Can Cholesterol Cause Cancer?

The connection between cholesterol and cancer is controversial and has given rise to enough recent medical articles to paper your living room wall. To get a handle on this topic, it's helpful to divide our discussion into two separate parts:

1. The experts and studies that say there's an *inverse* relationship between cancer risk and cholesterol levels (that is, low cholesterol—below 180 mg/dl—tends to be associated with increased cancer risk).

2. The experts and studies that say there's a *direct* correlation between cholesterol and cancer (that is, the higher your cholesterol, the greater your risk of cancer).

In the Framingham Heart Study, scientists identified an inverse statistical relationship between cholesterol levels in the blood of men and their cancer risks. It was found that those with lower levels of cholesterol had higher deaths from cancer of the colon, as well as at other body sites. At least seven other studies over the years have also reported some connection between low cholesterol and cancer risk.

But more recently, medical researchers have questioned these findings. Some say that some people with low cholesterol may have cancer; but they deny there's necessarily a *causal* connection; instead of low cholesterol triggering cancer, it could be that malignancies which are *already present* are causing the cholesterol levels to decline.

Very convincing data regarding this subject were published

in the *Journal of the American Medical Association* on February 20, 1987. The study focused on blood cholesterol levels and cancer deaths in 361,662 men, 35 to 57 years of age.* During a seven-year follow-up, mortality studies revealed a significant excess of cancer in those people with the lowest serum cholesterol levels—but only during the early years of follow-up. In later years of the follow-up, the researchers found less cancer.

These findings are consistent with the inference that the association between low serum cholesterol level and cancer is at least in part due to an effect of *preclinical* cancer on serum cholesterol levels. In other words, low cholesterol didn't appear to cause cancer in these cases. Rather, the cancer caused the cholesterol levels to be lower.

Another line of argument centers on recent studies which report a connection between high cholesterol levels and increased cancer risk. In the December 25, 1986, issue of the *New England Journal of Medicine*, a medical team from Sweden found that men with high cholesterol levels—above 250 mg/dl—were about 60 percent more likely than those with normal cholesterol levels to get rectal and colon cancer.** Another study in that same *NEJM* issue by a West German group connected high cholesterol levels with colon polyps which often become cancerous.

But this is not the end of the story. At least one other recent study—done at the Kaiser Permanente Medical Care Program in Oakland, California, and reported in 1986 in the *American Journal of Epidemiology*—found *neither* a direct *nor* an inverse relationship between total cholesterol levels and large-bowel cancer! They also said there was no evidence of a "threshold value" for cholesterol, below which the risk of cancer increases.

So, where do we stand? I would conclude it's best to set as your target that middle range of total cholesterol which we've advocated throughout this book—180 to 190 mg/dl. And

---

*Sherwin, Roger W.; Jeremiah Stamler; et al, "Serum Cholesterol Levels and Cancer Mortality in 361,662 Men Screened for the Multiple Risk Factor Intervention Trial." *Journal of the American Medical Association*, vol. 257, no. 7, February 20, 1987, pp. 943–48.
**New England Journal of Medicine*, vol. 315, no. 26, December 25, 1986, pp. 1629–33.

of course, always remember the principle of balance. *All* the components of your cholesterol and lipids must be working harmoniously together if you hope to maintain a healthy, low-risk profile.

TWENTY-THREE

Can Atherosclerosis Be Reversed?

It's fitting, I suppose, that we deal with this topic at the end of the book. Like the cancer question, a great deal remains to be discovered about the extent to which the deadly work of out-of-control cholesterol can be reversed. Yet, in many ways, for many people, this is the most important question of all.

Despite the uncertainties, I'm ready to be much more definite and optimistic on reversibility than I am on the cancer question. Why? I think the growing weight of evidence, both in various clinics and in certain limited studies, supports the belief that atherosclerosis—the deadly clogging of the arteries from excess LDLs and Apo Bs—can be stopped *and* even reversed.

The possibility of reversal has been established in recent reports in the *Journal of the American Medical Association* (June 19, 1987), by Dr. David H. Blankenhorn and several colleagues at the University of Southern California School of Medicine in Los Angeles. Their Cholesterol-Lowering Atherosclerosis Study (CLAS) involved 162 non-smoking men, aged 40 to 59 years, who all had undergone coronary by-pass surgery. The men, who were treated with colestipol hydrochloride and niacin over two years, experienced an average 26 percent reduction in their total cholesterol; a 43 percent drop in their LDLs; and a 37 percent increase in their HDLs. Most significant of all, angiograms done before and after the study showed conclusively that 16.2 percent of the patients experienced clear regression or reversal of their atherosclerosis, as compared with only 2.4 percent of participants who were placed on a placebo.

In my practice, I've seen some rather dramatic turn-arounds as a result of diet, exercise, and drug therapy. Earlier in this book, we considered the case of one of our staff physicians, Dr. Keller Greenfield. He evidently experienced some regression of his atherosclerosis as a result of taking a combination of colestipol and nicotinic acid (the same combination of drugs used with the CLAS study). A comparison of a coronary arteriogram of his coronary arteries with later MUGA scans indicated that his arteries were apparently becoming "unclogged."

There's other evidence as well: Finnish researchers followed the progression of coronary atherosclerosis by using repeated angiography in 28 patients and 20 "controls," or participants not undergoing scientific treatment. The serum cholesterol levels of all those in the study either exceeded 278 mg/dl, or their triglyceride concentrations were greater than 177 mg/dl, or both. They also had symptoms of coronary artery disease in two or three vessels.

The 28 patients, consisting of 26 men and 2 women, were treated with diet and drugs—clofibrate (Atromid-S) or nicotinic acid, or both. The purpose of these medications was to lower the blood fat concentrations. The 20 controls, all men, received only medical treatment for coronary artery disease, but no special treatment to reduce the level of blood fats.

In the 28 patients, the total cholesterol levels decreased 18 percent; the triglycerides, 38 percent; and the LDL cholesterol, 19 percent. Also, their HDL cholesterol increased by an average of 10 percent. There were no such significant beneficial changes in the lipid levels of the controls. The patients and controls were followed for seven years with the same ongoing treatments.

What were the results on the development of atherosclerosis in these participants? By all criteria, there was less progression of the coronary lesions in the patients than in the controls. Furthermore, the increase in coronary obstruction was inversely related to the HDL cholesterol levels. Surprisingly, though, progression of the disease was not related to the LDL cholesterol concentration during treatment. Cardiac survival was 89 percent after seven years in the patients, compared with 65 percent after five years in the controls.

The conclusion of this study was that it's possible to retard progression of even advanced coronary atherosclerosis. How? By reducing high blood-fat concentrations, including cholesterol, and increasing HDL cholesterol concentrations.*

Studies of rhesus monkeys by Dr. Robert W. Wissler of the University of Chicago School of Medicine have demonstrated reversal of atherosclerosis as well. The monkeys were given a combination of cholestyramine and probucol—and they experienced major regressions in fatty deposits in their blood vessels within one year.

Dr. David T. Nash of the University of New York Upstate Medical Center in Syracuse has reported stopping cholesterol deposits in humans—and even reversing them in some cases. In his two-year study of 17 patients, he put 9 on drug and diet therapy for two years. He used the other 8 as "controls" for purposes of comparison.

All the patients underwent coronary arteriograms, which showed they had 50 percent or greater narrowing of a major coronary artery. Also, all the patients had total cholesterol levels above 250 mg/dl.

Of the 9 who were on therapy, 8 showed no changes in their fatty-cholesterol deposits: their disease was halted. One patient experienced some reversal of his blocked arteries. Moreover, these patients on therapy experienced a drop of 23 percent in their cholesterol levels, from 270 mg/dl to 209 mg/dl.

Of the 8 "controls," 1 went on a diet and exercise program on his own, dropped his cholesterol level, and experienced a regression in his disease. Five of the other "controls" experienced progression of their cholesterol deposits, and 2 experienced no change.

Obviously this was a small study but it stands as a contribution to the growing body of evidence that atherosclerosis is reversible. Much more research remains to be done before we know all we need to know about how lowering cholesterol levels and otherwise putting your cholesterol and lipids in balance will reverse atherosclerosis. But still, the outlook is definitely encouraging.

The main message that should come across to all of us is

*Nikkila, Esko A., et al, "Prevention of Progression of Coronary Atherosclerosis By Treatment of Hyperlipidaemia: A Seven Year Prospective Angiographic Study." British Medical Journal, vol. 289, July 28, 1984, pp. 220–23.

that, to an important degree, *we can control our cholesterol.* And that means—with proper diet, exercise habits, and knowledge of the potentials of modern medicine—we can greatly increase our chances for much longer, more productive, and far happier lives.

Or, as the *Journal of the American Medical Association* has put it: "In the coming decades, the most important determinants of health and longevity will be the personal choices made by each individual."

Selected References

Chapter One

Bosler, Tommy Joy. "Getting a Grip on Cholesterol." *BioLogue*, vol. 6, no. 1.

Brody, Jane E. "Choosing Prudently to Avoid Cholesterol." *The New York Times*, November 5, 1986.

"Facts about Blood Cholesterol." U.S. Department of Health and Human Services, National Institutes of Health.

Fenley, Bob. "Trail of Discovery." *BioLogue*, vol. 6, no. 1.

"Fish Oils and Colon Cancer." *Nutrition Research Newsletter*, July 1986.

"Fish Oils and Lipoproteins." *Nutrition Research Newsletter*, July 1986.

Levy, Robert I., M.D., and Basil M. Rifkind, M.D. "The Structure, Function and Metabolism of High-Density Lipoproteins: A Status Report." *Circulation*, vol. 62, suppl. IV, November 1980.

Lyon, Pamela. "The Great Adventure." *BioLogue*, vol. 6, no. 1.

"Reducing Cholesterol the International Way." *Nutrition & Health News*, vol. 3, summer 1986.

Rutherford, Susan. "When Diet Isn't Enough." *BioLogue*, vol. 6, no. 1.

"Test Your Knowledge of Nutrition." *Patient Care*, January 30, 1986.

Thompson, Paul D., M.D. and Amby, Burfoot. "Eat to Live." *Runner's World*, September 1986.

Chapter Two

"A Cholesterol Primer." *The Aerobics News*, vol. 1, no. 1, May 1986.

"Campaign Seeks to Increase US 'Cholesterol Consciousness.' " "Medical News," *Journal of the American Medical Association*, vol. 255, no. 9, March 7, 1986.

"Cholesterol: 1769–1982." A Mini-course in Lipids, Six pack Times.

"Cholesterol: The Villain Revealed." *Discover*, Time-Inc., 1985.

Goldstein, Joseph L., and Michael S. Brown. "The Low-Density Lipoprotein Pathway and Its Relation to Atherosclerosis." *Annual Review of Biochemistry*, vol. 46, 1977, pp. 897–930.

Chapter Three

Castelli, William P., M.D., et al. "Incidence of Coronary Heart Disease and Lipoprotein Cholesterol Levels—The Framingham Study." *Journal of the American Medical Association*, vol. 256, no. 20, November 28, 1986.

"Cholesterol Complication." *New York Daily News*, March 3, 1986.

"Down with Cholesterol." Taste, *Dallas Times Herald*, January 15, 1986.

Glueck, Charles J., M.D. "Nonpharmacologic and Pharmacologic Alteration of High-Density Lipoprotein Cholesterol: Therapeutic Approaches to Prevention of Atherosclerosis." *American Heart Journal*, vol. 110, no. 5, November 1985.

————. "Role of Risk Factor Management in Progression and Regression of Coronary and Femoral Artery Atherosclerosis." *American Journal of Cardiology*, vol. 57, no. 14, May 30, 1986.

Gotto, A.M., Jr., M.D., Ph.D. "Classification and Structure of Lipoproteins." *American Journal of Cardiology*, vol. 56, December 31, 1985, pp. 2J–4J.

Grundy, Scott M., M.D., Ph.D. "Cholesterol and Coronary Heart Disease." State of the Art/Review, *Journal of the American Medical Association*, vol. 256, no. 20, November 28, 1986.

Harper's Review of Biochemistry, twentieth edition. California: Lange Medical Publications, chapters 17 & 18, 1985.

Schlierf, Gunter, M.D. "Symposium on High-Density Lipoproteins and Coronary Artery Disease: Effects of Diet, Exercise, and Pharmacologic Intervention." Opening Remarks, *American Journal of Cardiology*, vol. 52, no. 4, August 22, 1983.

Stamler, Jeremiah, M.D., et al. "Is Relationship between Serum Cholesterol and Risk of Premature Death from Coronary Heart Disease Continuous and Graded?" *Journal of the American Medical Association*, vol. 256, no. 20, November 28, 1986.

"Status and Perspectives on the Role of Cholesterol." *American Journal of Cardiology*, vol. 54, no. 5, August 27, 1984.

Sullivan, Walter. "Converging on a Nobel Prize." *The New York Times*, October 15, 1985.

"Unusual Lipid Profile in an Asymptomatic Patient." Questions and Answers, *Journal of the American Medical Association*, vol. 256, no. 20, November 28, 1986.

Wynder, Ernst L., et al. "Population Screening for Cholesterol Determination." *Journal of the American Medical Association*, vol. 256, no. 20, November 28, 1986.

"Your Heart and Dyslipidemia—It's More Than 'High Cholesterol.'" Parke-Davis, Warner-Lambert Company, 1986.

Chapter Four

Arntzenius, Alexander C., M.D., et al. "Diet, Lipoproteins, and the Progression of Coronary Atherosclerosis—The Leiden Intervention Trial." *New England Journal of Medicine*, vol. 312, no. 13, March 28, 1985.

Beckles, A. L. G., et al. "High Total and Cardiovascular Disease Mortality in Adults of Indian Descent in Trinidad, Unexplained by Major Coronary Risk Factors." *The Lancet*, June 7, 1986.

Bishop, Jerry E. "Cholesterol Link to Cancer is Emerging from Studies on Way to Avert Coronaries." *The Wall Street Journal*, October 14, 1980.

———. "Heart Attacks: A Test Collapses." *The Wall Street Journal*, October 6, 1982.

———. "Scientists Are Firming Link to Cholesterol with Coronary Disease." *The Wall Street Journal*, January 10, 1984.

Brensike, John F., M.D., et al. "Coronary Artery Disease—Effects of Therapy with Cholestyramine on Progression of Coronary Arteriosclerosis: Result of the NHLBI Type II Coronary Intervention Study." *Circulation*, vol. 69, no. 2, February 1984.

Brody, Jane E. "Panel Suggests Many in U.S. Need to Reduce Cholesterol." *The New York Times*, December 13, 1984.

———. "Personal Health." *The New York Times*, December 19, 1984.

Brown, W.V., M.D. "Some Ounces of Prevention that Lower Heart Risk." Questions & Answers, *The New York Times*, August 31, 1986.

"Cholesterol: the Stigma is Back." Medicine, *Time*, January 19, 1981.

Cooper, Kenneth H., M.D. "The National Lipid Research Study—Part I." *Inside Aerobics*, vol. 5, no. 4, April 1984.

———. "The National Lipid Research Study—Part II." *Inside Aerobics*, vol. 5, no. 5, May 1984.

———. "The National Lipid Research Study—Part III." *Inside Aerobics*, vol. 5, no. 6, June 1984.

———. "Less Disease or Better Treatment." *Inside Aerobics*, vol. 6, no. 6, June 1985.

Crouch, Michael, Ph.D., et al. "Personal and Mediated Health Counseling for Sustained Dietary Reduction of Hypercholesterolemia." *Preventive Medicine*, vol. 15, 1986, pp. 282–91.

Englebardt, Stanley L. "New Light on Cholesterol." *Reader's Digest*, February, 1978.

"Heart Disease Deaths Are Dropping, but Why?" *The New York Times*, November 18, 1984.

Helgeland, Anders, M.D. "Treatment of Mild Hypertension: A Five Year Controlled Drug Trial—The Oslo Study." *American Journal of Medicine*, vol. 69, November 1980.

"High-Density Lipoprotein Cholesterol and Antihypertensive Drugs: The Oslo study." *British Medical Journal*, August 5, 1978.

"Hold the Eggs and Butter." *Time*, March 26, 1984.

Kannel, William B., M.D., M.P.H. "Lipids, Diabetes, and Coronary Heart Disease: Insights from the Framingham Study." *American Heart Journal*, vol. 110, November 1985.

Karr, Albert R. "Cholesterol Risks Cited by National Institutes of Health." *The Wall Street Journal*, December 13, 1984.

Levy, Robert I., M.D. "Primary Prevention of Coronary Heart Disease by Lowering Lipids: Results and Implications." *Journal of the American Medical Association*, vol. 255, no. 7, February 21, 1986.

"The Lipid Research Clinics Coronary Primary Prevention Trial Results." Lipid Research Clinics Program, *Journal of the American Medical Association*, vol. 251, no. 3, January 20, 1984.

"Lowering Blood Cholesterol to Prevent Heart Disease." National Institutes of Health Consensus Development Conference, December 10–12, 1984.

"Lowering Cholesterol and the Incidence of Coronary Heart Disease." Letters, *Journal of the American Medical Association*, vol. 253, no. 21, June 7, 1985.

"Mass Intervention vs. Screening and Selective Intervention for the Prevention of Coronary Heart Disease." *Journal of the American Medical Association*, vol. 255, no. 16, April 25, 1986.

Newman, William P., III, M.D., et al. "Relation of Serum Lipoprotein Levels and Systolic Blood Pressure to Early Atherosclerosis—the Bogalusa Heart Study." *New England Journal of Medicine*, vol. 314, no. 3, January 16, 1986.

Randal, Judith. "Tag Cholesterol as Heart Risk." *New York Daily News*, January 13, 1984.

Schorr, Burt. "Anti-Cholesterol Treatment Can Cut Risk of Heart Disease Up to 50%, a Study Shows." *The Wall Street Journal*, January 13, 1984.

Spain, David M. "Atherosclerosis." *Scientific American*, August 1966, pp. 48–56.

Tyroler, H.A., M.D. "Total Serum Cholesterol and Ischemic Heart Disease Risk in Clinical Trials and Observational Studies." *American Journal of Preventive Medicine*, vol. 1, no. 4, 1985.

Yaeger, Deborah. "Cardiologists Focus Efforts on Prevention of Heart Attacks." *The New York Times*, July 2, 1984.

Chapter Five

"Apolipoprotein Levels." *Medical World News*, May 24, 1982.

Criqui, Michael H., M.D., M.P.H. "Epidemiology of Atherosclerosis: An Updated Overview." *American Journal of
Cardiology*, vol. 57, no. 5, February 12, 1986, pp.
18c–23c.

Kottke, Bruce A., M.D., Ph.D. "Lipid Markers for Atherosclerosis." *American Journal of Cardiology*, vol. 57, no. 5,
February 12, 1986, pp. 11c–17.

"Lowering Plasma Cholesterol by Raising LDL Receptors."
Editorials, *New England Journal of Medicine*, vol. 305, no.
9, August 27, 1981.

Chapter Six

"Apolipoprotein Levels Predict Coronary-Artery Disease." *Medical World News*, May 24, 1982.

Berg, Aloys, and Joseph Keul. "Influence of Maximum Aerobic
Capacity and Relative Body Weight on the Lipoprotein
Profile in Athletes." *Atherosclerosis*, vol. 55, 1985, pp.
225–31.

Bishop, Jerry J. "Scientists Are Learning How Genes Predis-
pose Some to Heart Disease." *The Wall Street Journal*,
February 6, 1986.

Blackburn, Henry, M.D. "The Meaning of a New Marker for
Coronary-Artery Disease." *New England Journal of Medicine*, vol. 309, no. 7, August 18, 1983.

"Does Assay of Cholesterol in High-Density Lipoprotein Subclasses Give Clinically Useful Information?" Letters, *Clinical Chemistry*, vol. 32, no. 1, 1986.

Gidez, et al. "Determination of HDL Subclasses in Human
Plasma." *Journal of Lipid Research*, vol. 23, 1982, pp.
1206–23.

"The HDL: The Good Cholesterol Carriers?" "Research News,"
Science, vol. 205, August 17, 1979.

Heiss, Gerardo, M.D., Ph.D., et al. "Plasma High-Density
Lipoprotein Cholesterol and Socioeconomic Status." *Circulation*, vol. 62, suppl. IV, November 1980, pp. 108–15.

Kannel, William B., M.D., M.P.H. "High-Density Lipoproteins: Epidemiologic Profile and Risks of Coronary Artery

Disease." *American Journal of Cardiology*, vol. 52, no. 4, August 1983.

Kottke, Bruce A., M.D., Ph.D., et al. "Apolipoproteins and Coronary Artery Disease." *Mayo Clinic Proceedings*, vol. 61, Rochester, Minnesota, May 1986.

Laakso, Markku, et al. "Association of Low HDL and HDL2 Cholesterol with Coronary Heart Disease in Noninsulin-Dependent Diabetics." *Arteriosclerosis*, vol. 5, no. 6, November/December 1985.

Lewis, Barry, M.D., Ph.D., FRCP, FRCPath. "Relation of High-Density Lipoproteins to Coronary Artery Disease." *American Journal of Cardiology*, vol. 52, no. 4, August 22, 1983.

Maciejko, James J., Ph.D., et al. "Apolipoprotein A-I as a Marker of Angiographically Assessed Coronary-Artery Disease." *New England Journal of Medicine*, vol. 309, no. 7, August 18, 1983.

McQuade, Walter. "Good News from the House on Lincoln Street." *Fortune*, January 14, 1980.

"New Cardiovascular-risk Markers: Common Genetic Protein Abnormalities." *Medical World News*, February 15, 1982.

"Ratios and Risk of Coronary Heart Disease." Questions and Answers, *Journal of the American Medical Association*, vol. 255, no. 7, February 21, 1986.

Schierf, Gunter, M.D., et al. "Influence of Diet on High-Density Lipoproteins." *American Journal of Cardiology*, vol. 52, August 22, 1983.

Swanson, John O., M.D., et al. "Serum High Density Lipoprotein Cholesterol Correlates with Presence but Not Severity of Coronary Artery Disease." *American Journal of Medicine*, vol. 71, August 1981.

Witztum, Joseph, and Gustav Schonfeld. "High Density Lipoproteins." *Diabetes*, vol. 28, April 1979.

Chapter Seven

Enger, Sven Chr, et al. "High-Density Lipoproteins (HDL) and Physical Activity: The Influence of Physical Exercise, Age and Smoking on HDL-Cholesterol and the HDL-/Total Cholesterol Ratio." *Scandinavian Journal of Clinical and Laboratory Investigation*, vol. 37, no. 3, 1977, pp. 251–55.

Hopkins, Paul N., M.S.P.H., and Roger R. Williams, M.D. "A Simplified Approach to Lipoprotein Kinetics and Factors Affecting Serum Cholesterol and Triglyceride Concentrations." *American Journal of Clinical Nutrition*, vol. 34, no. 11, November 1981, pp. 2560–90.

Lapidus, Leif, et al. "Triglycerides—Main Lipid Risk Factor for Cardiovascular Disease in Women?" *Acta Medica Scandinavica*, vol. 217, no. 5, 1985, pp. 481–89.

Richards, E. Glen, Ph.D., Scott M. Grundy, M.D., Ph.D., and Kenneth Cooper, M.D. "Influence of Plasma Triglycerides Within the Normal Range on Particle Size and Heterogeneity of Low Density Lipoproteins." Unpublished.

Sauar, Jostein, et al. "The Relation Between the Levels of HDL Cholesterol and the Capacity for Removal of Triglycerides." *Acta Medica Scandinavica*, vol. 208, no. 3, 1980, pp. 199–203.

Schaefer, E.J., et al. "Plasma-Triglycerides in Regulation of H.D.L-Cholesterol Levels." *Lancet*, August 19, 1978.

"Treatment of Hypertriglyceridemia." The National Institutes of Health Conference, September 27–29, 1983.

"Triglycerides and Coronary Heart Disease." Letter to the Editor, *New England Journal of Medicine*, vol. 303, no. 18, October 30, 1980.

Vega, Gloria Lena, Ph.D., and Scott M. Grundy, M.D., Ph.D. "Gemfibrozil Therapy in Primary Hypertriglyceridemia Associated with Coronary Heart Disease." *Journal of the American Medical Association*, vol. 253, no. 16, April 26, 1985.

Witztum, Joseph L., M.D., et al. "Normalization of Triglycerides in Type IV Hyperlipoproteinemia Fails to Correct Low Levels of High-Density-Lipoprotein Cholesterol." *New England Journal of Medicine*, vol. 303, no. 16, October 16, 1980.

Chapter Eight

Bates, Harold M., Ph.D. "The Laboratory in Prevention: HDL-Cholesterol and Coronary Heart Disease." *Lab Management*, April 1980.

"Body Position Is Found to Affect the Accuracy of Heart Disease Tests." *The New York Times*, June 24, 1986.

Cholesterol Counts. U.S. Department of Health and Human Services, National Institutes of Health Publication No. 85-2699, June 1985.

Cooper, Kenneth H., M.D., and William H. King, M.D. "Age, Body Weight, Percent Body Fat and Cholesterol." Unpublished. September 1980.

Fazen, Marianne, MT(ASCP). "A Special Report—Accurate Lipid Measurements in the Clinical Laboratory." Unpublished. February 28, 1986.

————. "The Question of Clinical Measurements of HDL Subfractions and/or HDL Apolipoprotein A-I." Unpublished. April 3, 1986.

Friedewald, William T., et al. "Estimation of the Concentration of Low-Density Lipoprotein Cholesterol in Plasma, without Use of the Preparative Ultracentrifuge." *Clinical Chemistry*, vol. 18, no. 6, 1972.

Gore, Mary Jane. "Cholesterol Test Standards Sought." *Clinical Chemistry News*, vol. 12, no. 1, January 1986.

Heiss, Gerardo, M.D., et al. "Lipoprotein-Cholesterol Distributions in Selected North American Populations: The Lipid Research Clinics Program Prevalence Study." *Circulation*, vol. 61, no. 22, February 1980.

Hoeg, Jeffrey M., M.D., et al. "An Approach to the Management of Hyperlipoproteinemia." *Journal of the American Medical Association*, vol. 255, no. 4, January 24/31, 1986.

Little, Linda. "New Test Found for Cholesterol." *Dallas Times Herald*, April 3, 1986.

O'Brien, Joseph E., M.D. "Reliability of Lipid and Lipoprotein Testing(II)." *American Journal of Cardiology*, vol. 56, 1985, p. 95.

Rippey, Robert M. "Overview: Seasonal Variations in Cholesterol." *Preventive Medicine*, vol. 10, 1981, pp. 655–59.

Warnick, G. Russell, et al. "Dextran Sulfate-Mg_2+ Precipitation Procedure for Quantitation of High-Density-Lipoprotein Cholesterol." *Selected Methods of Clinical Chemistry*, vol. 10, G.R. Cooper, ed., American Association for Clinical Chemistry, Washington D.C., 1983, pp. 91–99.

Wen, Chi-Pang, M.D., M.P.H., DR.P.H., and David S. Greenbaum, M.D. "Prevalence and Awareness of Hyperlipoproteinemia in Physicians and Their Spouses." *Research*, vol. 68, January 1976.

Chapter Nine

Blume, Elaine. "Trouble from the Tropics." *Nutrition Action Health Letter,* July/August 1986.

"Cholesterol-Free Nondairy Creamers: Compositional Conundrums and Cardiovascular Contradictions." Correspondence, *New England Journal of Medicine,* vol. 314, no. 10, 1986.

Curb, J.D., D.M. Reed, J.A. Kautz, et al. "Coffee, Caffeine, and Serum Cholesterol in Japanese Men in Hawaii." *American Journal of Epidemiology,* vol. 123, no. 4, April 1986, pp. 648–55.

"Fish Oils versus Coronary Heart Disease." *Nutrition & Health News,* vol. 3, no. 1, spring 1986.

Fisher, Marc, M.D., et al. "The Effect of Vegetarian Diets on Plasma Lipid and Platelet Levels." *Archives of Internal Medicine,* vol. 146, June 1986.

"Going for the Greens." *Newsweek,* May 19, 1986.

Grundy, Scott M., M.D., Ph.D. "Comparison of Monounsaturated Fatty Acids and Carbohydrates for Lowering Plasma Cholesterol." *New England Journal of Medicine,* vol. 314, no. 12, 1986.

Hagan, R. Donald, et al. "High Density Lipoprotein Cholesterol in Relation to Food Consumption and Running Distance." *Preventive Medicine,* vol. 12, 1983, pp. 287–95.

Jones, S.D.M., Ph.D. "Chemical Composition of Selected Cooked Beef, Steaks and Roasts." *Journal of the Canadian Dietetic Association,* vol. 46, no. 1, winter 1985.

———. "The New Composition of Red Meats." Paper presented in Vancouver, January 29 and 30, in support of Meat Month, 1986. Unpublished.

Kromhout, Daan, Ph.D., M.P.H., et al. "The Inverse Relation between Fish Consumption and 20-Year Mortality from Coronary Heart Disease." *New England Journal of Medicine,* vol. 312, no. 19, May 9, 1985.

"Nutritional Implications of Lactose and Lactase Activity." *Dairy Council Digest,* vol. 56, no. 5, September–October, 1985.

"Provisional Dietary Fiber Table." *Journal of the American Dietetic Association,* vol. 86, no. 6, June 1986.

"Shopping for Health in All the Right Places." *Dallas City,* June 1, 1986.

Touche, Amanda. "Shopping for Health in All the Right Places." *Dallas City,* June 1, 1986.

Tuomilehto, Jaakko, et al. "Factors Associated with Changes in Serum Cholesterol During a Community-Based Hypertension Programme." *Acta Medica Scandinavica*, vol. 217, no. 3, 1985, pp. 243–52.

"View and Review." *Environmental Nutritional*, vol. 9, no. 4, April 1986.

Chapter Ten

Camargo, Carlos A., Jr., et al. "The Effect of Moderate Alcohol Intake on Serum Apolipoproteins A-I and A-II." *Journal of the American Medical Association*, vol. 253, no. 19, May 17, 1985.

Dai, Wanju S., et al. "Alcohol Consumption and High Density Lipoprotein Cholesterol Concentration Among Alcoholics." *American Journal of Epidemiology*, vol. 122, no. 4, 1985.

Ernst, Nancy, M.S., R.D., et al. "The Association of Plasma High-Density Lipoprotein Cholesterol with Dietary Intake and Alcohol Consumption." *Circulation*, vol. 62, suppl. IV, November 1980, pp. 41–52.

Gordon, Tavia, and Joseph T. Doyle, M.D. "Alcohol Consumption and Its Relationship to Smoking, Weight, Blood Pressure, and Blood Lipids—The Albany Study." *Archives of Internal Medicine*, vol. 146, February 1986.

Heath, Dwight B. "In a Dither about Drinking." *The Wall Street Journal*, February 25, 1985.

Heaton, Kenneth W., M.A., M.D., F.R.C.P. "On Gallstones . . . And Why a Little Alcohol Should Help . . . And Help Blood Cholesterol, Too." *Executive Health Report*, vol. 21, no. 11, August 1985.

"Unresolved Issue: Do Drinkers Have Less Coronary Heart Disease?" Medical News, *Journal of the American Medical Association*, vol. 242, no. 25, December 21, 1979.

Chapter Eleven

Criqui, Michael H., M.D., M.P.H., et al. "Cigarette Smoking and Plasma High-Density Lipoprotein Cholesterol." *Circulation*, vol. 62, suppl. IV, November 1980, pp. 70–76.

"Quit Smoking—Or Suffer Low Blood HDL Levels." Medical
    News, *Journal of the American Medical Association*, vol.
    239, no. 8, February 20, 1978.
Tuomilehto, Jaakko, et al. "Long-Term Effects of Cessation of
    Smoking on Body Weight, Blood Pressure and Serum
    Cholesterol in the Middle-Aged Population with High Blood
    Pressure." *Addictive Behaviors*, vol. 11, 1986, pp. 1–9.

Chapter Twelve

Berg, A., et al. "Lipoprotein-Cholesterol in Well-Trained Ath-
    letes." *International Journal of Sports Medicine*, vol. 1,
    1980, pp. 137–38.
———. "HDL-Cholesterol (HDL-C) Changes During and After
    Intensive Long-lasting Exercise." *International Journal of
    Sports Medicine*, vol. 2, 1981, pp. 121–23.
Brownell, Kelly D., Ph.D., et al. "Changes in Plasma Lipid and
    Lipoprotein Levels in Men and Women After a Program of
    Moderate Exercise." *Circulation*, vol. 65, no. 3, 1982.
Carlson, Lars A., and Folke Mossfeldt. "Acute Effects of Pro-
    longed, Heavy Exercise on the Concentration of Plasma
    Lipids and Lipoproteins in Man." *Acta Physiologica Scandi-
    navica*, vol. 62, 1964, pp. 51–59.
Carlson, L.A., M.D., and B. Pernow, M.D. "Studies on Blood
    Lipids During Exercise." *Journal of Laboratory and Clini-
    cal Medicine*, vol. 53, no. 6, June 1959.
Cooper, Kenneth H., M.D. "Physical Training Programs for
    Mass Scale Use: Effects on Cardiovascular Disease—Facts
    and Theories." *Annals of Clinical Research*, vol. 14, suppl.
    34, 1982, pp. 25–32.
Crouse, Stephen F., Ph.D., et al. "Zinc Ingestion and Lipopro-
    tein Values in Sedentary and Endurance-Trained Men."
    Journal of the American Medical Association, vol. 252, no.
    6, August 10, 1984.
Cowan, George O., MB, FRCP, RAMC. "Influence of Exer-
    cise on High-Density Lipoproteins." *American Journal of
    Cardiology*, vol. 52, no. 4, August 22, 1983.
Erkelens, Willem D., M.D., et al. "High-Density Lipoprotein-
    Cholesterol in Survivors of Myocardial Infarction." *Journal
    of the American Medical Association*, vol. 242, no. 20,
    November 16, 1979.

Hagan, R.D., Ph.D., and L.R. Gettman, Ph.D. "Maximal Aerobic Power, Body Fat, and Serum Lipoproteins in Male Distance Runners." *Journal of Cardiac Rehabilitation*, vol. 3, no. 5, May 1983.

————. "High Density Lipoprotein Cholesterol in Relation to Food Consumption and Running Distance." *Preventive Medicine*, vol. 12, 1983, pp. 287–95.

Hartung, Harley G., Ph.D. "Diet and Exercise in the Regulation of Plasma Lipids and Lipoproteins in Patients at Risk of Coronary Disease." *Sports Medicine*, vol. 1, 1984, pp. 413–18.

————, et al. "Effects of Marathon Running, Jogging, and Diet on Coronary Risk Factors in Middle-Aged Men." *Preventive Medicine*, vol. 10, 1981, pp. 316–23.

————, and William G. Squires, Ph.D. "Exercise and HDL Cholesterol in Middle-Aged Men." *Physician and Sportsmedicine*, vol. 8, no. 1, January 1980.

Haskell, William L., Ph.D., et al. "Strenuous Physical Activity, Treadmill Exercise Test Performance and Plasma High-Density Lipoprotein Cholesterol." *Circulation*, vol. 62, suppl. IV, 1980.

Huttunen, Jussi K., M.D., et al. "Effect of Moderate Physical Exercise on Serum Lipoproteins." *Circulation*, vol. 60, no. 6, December 1979.

Kahrs, S.J., M.S., et al. "Effect of Exercise Training and Diet Modification on Serum Lipids and Lipoproteins in Coronary Artery Disease Patients Treated with Thiazides." *American Journal of Cardiology*, vol. 8, no. 12, 1985, pp. 636–40.

Malinow, M.R., and A. Perley. "The Effect of Physical Exercise on Cholesterol Degradation in Man." *Journal of Atherosclerosis Research*, vol. 10, 1969, pp. 107–11.

Nikkila, Esko A., et al. "Effect of Physical Inactivity on Plasma Lipoproteins: Decrease of High-Density Lipoproteins and Apolipoprotein A-I in Immobilized Patients." Abstracts, *Circulation*, vol. 62, suppl. III, October 1980.

"Relationship between Baseline Risk Factors and Coronary Heart Disease and Total Mortality in the Multiple Risk Factor Intervention Trial." *Preventive Medicine*, vol. 15, 1986, pp. 254–73.

"Runners Score with Good Cholesterol." *The Health Letter*, vol. 13, no. 1, January 12, 1979.

Simko, V., and R.E. Kelley. "Physical Exercise Modifies the Effect of High Cholesterol-Sucrose Feeding in the Rat." *European Journal of Applied Physiology*, vol. 40, 1979, pp. 145–53.

Streja, Dan, M.D., and David Mymin, M.D. "Moderate Exercise and High-Density-Lipoprotein-Cholesterol." *Journal of the American Medical Association*, vol. 242, no. 20, November 16, 1979.

Tran, Zung Vu, et al. "The Effects of Exercise on Blood Lipids and Lipoproteins: A Meta-Analysis of Studies." *Medicine and Science in Sports and Exercise*, vol. 15, no. 5, 1983, pp. 393–402.

Valimaki, I., et al. "Exercise Performance and Serum Lipids in Relation to Physical Activity in Schoolchildren." *International Journal of Sports Medicine*, vol. 1, 1980, pp. 132–36.

Wood, Peter D., et al. "Plasma Lipoprotein Distributions in Male and Female Runners." *Annals New York Academy of Sciences*, vol. 301, 1977, pp. 748–63.

———. "Increased Exercise Level and Plasma Lipoprotein Concentrations: A One-Year, Randomized, Controlled Study in Sedentary, Middle-Aged Men." *Metabolism*, vol. 32, no. 1, January 1983.

The Year Book of Sports Medicine 1979. Year Book Medical Publishers, Inc., 1979.

Chapter Thirteen

Alberts, A.W., et al. "Mevinolin: A Highly Potent Competitive Inhibitor of Hydroxy Methylglutaryl-Coenzyme A Reductase and a Cholesterol-Lowering Agent." *Proceedings of the National Academy of Sciences* (USA), vol. 77, 1980, pp. 3957–61.

Ames, Richard P., M.D., and Peter Hill, Ph.D. "Elevation of Serum Lipid Levels During Diuretic Therapy of Hypertension." *American Journal of Medicine*, vol. 61, November 1976.

Bishop, Jerry E. "Merck Cholesterol-Lowering Medicine Enhanced by Upjohn Drug, Study Says." *The Wall Street Journal*, January 2, 1987.

Blakeslee, Sandra. "Laser Is Designed to Clean Arteries." *The New York Times*, January 29, 1985.

"Coronary Drug Project Research Group: Clofibrate and Niacin in Coronary Heart Disease." *Journal of the American Medical Association*, vol. 231, 1975, pp. 360–81.

Davignon, Jean, M.D. "Medical Management of Hyperlipidemia and the Role of Probucol." *American Journal of Cardiology*, vol. 57, June 27, 1986, pp. 22H–28H.

Dujovne, Carlos A., M.D., et al. "Controlled Studies of the Efficacy and Safety of Combined Probucol-Colestipol Therapy." *American Journal of Cardiology*, vol. 57, June 27, 1986, pp. 36H–42H.

"Effect of Cholestyramine on Low-Density Lipoprotein." Letters to the Editor, *New England Journal of Medicine*, vol. 303, no. 16, October 16, 1980.

Glueck, Charles J., M.D. "Influence of Lipid Regulating Drugs on High-Density Lipoprotein Cholesterol." *Perspectives in Lipid Disorders*, vol. 1, no. 3, October 1983.

Goldman, Anne I., Ph.D., et al. "Serum Lipoprotein Levels during Chlorthalidone Therapy." *Journal of the American Medical Association*, vol. 244, no. 15, October 10, 1980.

Hoeg, Jeffrey M., M.D., et al. "An Approach to the Management of Hyperlipoproteinemia." *Journal of the American Medical Association*, vol. 255, no. 4, January 24/31, 1986.

Illingworth, L.D. "Fish Oils Reduce Postprandial Lipemia." *Circulation*, vol. 74, suppl. II, 1986, p. 33.

Kesaniemi, Y. Antero, M.D., and Scott M. Grundy, M.D., Ph.D. "Influence of Gemfibrozil and Clofibrate on Metabolism of Cholesterol and Plasma Triglycerides in Man." *Journal of the American Medical Association*, vol. 251, no. 17, May 4, 1984.

"Lipid Abstracts." *The Royal Society of Medicine*, vol. 7, no. 4, 1983.

Miettinen, Tatu A., M.D., et al. "Long-Term Use of Probucol in the Multifactorial Primary Prevention of Vascular Disease." *American Journal of Cardiology*, vol. 57, June 27, 1986, pp. 49H–54H.

"Profile of Currently Used Lipid-Lowering Agents." Parke-Davis, Warner-Lambert Company, 1986.

Reeder, Guy S., M.D., et al. "Is Percutaneous Coronary Angioplasty Less Expensive Than Bypass Surgery?" *New England Journal of Medicine*, vol. 311, no. 18, November 1, 1984.

"The Relationship of Reduction in Incidence of Coronary Heart Disease to Cholesterol Lowering—The Lipid Research Clinics Coronary Primary Prevention Trial Results: II." *Journal of the American Medical Association*, vol. 251, 1984, pp. 365–74.

Rothschild, Jonathan, M.A. "These Nutrients Can Keep You from Dying of Heart Disease." *Health Quarterly*, February 1983.

"Update on Mevinolin." *Nutrition Letter*, University of Texas Health Science Center at Dallas, January 1986.

Vogelberg, K.H., et al. "Effects of Neomycin Sulphate Alone and in Combination with D-Thyroxine on Serum Lipoproteins in Hypercholesterolaemic Subjects." *European Journal of Clinical Pharmacology*, vol. 22, 1982, pp. 33–38.

Wallace, Robert B., M.D., et al. "Alterations of Plasma High-Density Lipoprotein Cholesterol Levels Associated with Consumption of Selected Medications." *Circulation*, vol. 62, suppl. IV, November, 1980.

Wilcox, H.G., et al. "Effects of Thyroid Status on Plasma High Density Lipoproteins (HDL)." Abstracts, *Circulation*, vol. 62, suppl. III, October 1980.

Chapter Fourteen

Curb, J. David, et al. "Coffee, Caffeine, and Serum Cholesterol in Japanese Men in Hawaii." *American Journal of Epidemiology*, vol. 123, 1986, pp. 648–55.

"Coffee and Cholesterol." Correspondence, *New England Journal of Medicine*, vol. 309, no. 20, November 17, 1983.

"Coffee and Serum Cholesterol." Short Reports, *British Medical Journal*, vol. 288, June 30, 1984.

Forde, H., et al. "The Tromso Heart Study; Coffee Consumption and Serum Lipid Concentrations in Men with Hypercholesterolaemia: A Randomised Intervention Study." *British Medical Journal*, vol. 290, March 23, 1985.

Haffner, Steven M., et al. "Coffee Consumption, Diet, and Lipids." *American Journal of Epidemiology*, vol. 122, no. 1, July 1985.

Heyden, Siegfried, M.D., et al. "The Combined Effect of Smoking and Coffee Drinking on LDL and HDL Cholesterol." *Circulation*, vol. 60, no. 1, 1979.

Kark, J.D., et al. "Coffee, Tea, and Plasma Cholesterol: The Jerusalem Lipid Research Clinic Prevalence Study." *British Medical Journal*, vol. 291, September 1985.

Mathias, Susan, et al. "Coffee, Plasma Cholesterol, and Lipoproteins." *American Journal of Epidemiology*, vol. 121, no. 6, 1985.

Shirlow, Megan J., and Colin D. Mathers. "Caffeine Consumption and Serum Cholesterol Levels." *International Journal of Epidemiology*, vol. 13, no. 4, 1984.

Thelle, Dag S., M.D., et al. "The Tromso Heart Study—Does Coffee Raise Serum Cholesterol?" *New England Journal of Medicine*, vol. 308, no. 24, June 16, 1983.

"Too Much Java Tied to Heart Ills." *Daily News*, September 17, 1986.

Williams, Paul T., et al. "Coffee Intake and Elevated Cholesterol and Apolipoprotein B Levels in Men." *Journal of the American Medical Association*, vol. 253, no. 10, March 8, 1985.

Chapter Fifteen

"Dietary Omega-3 Fatty Acids in Health and Disease." *Nutrition Research Newsletter*, vol. 4, no. 12, December 1985, pp. 133–40.

"Fish, Fatty Acids, and Human Health." Editorials, *New England Journal of Medicine*, vol. 312, no. 19, May 9, 1985.

"Fish Ingestion Beneficial for Preventing Coronary Heart Disease." *Internal Medicine Alert*, vol. 7, no. 9, May 15, 1985.

Fish Nutrition. Published by North Atlantic Seafood Association.

"Fish Oils versus Coronary Heart Disease." *Nutrition & Health News*, vol. 3, no. 1, spring 1986.

Hepburn, Frank N., et al. "Provisional Tables on the Content of Omega-3 Fatty Acids and Other Fat Components of Selected Foods." *Journal of the American Dietetic Association*, vol. 86, no. 6, June 1986.

Knapp, Howard R., M.D., Ph.D., et al. "In Vivo Indexes of Platelet and Vascular Function During Fish-Oil Administration in Patients with Atherosclerosis." *New England Journal of Medicine*, vol. 314, no. 15, April 10, 1986.

Kromhout, Daan, Ph.D., M.P.H., et al. "The Inverse Relation Between Fish Consumption and 20-Year Mortality from Coronary Heart Disease." *New England Journal of Medicine*, vol. 312, no. 19, May 9, 1985.

Lee, Tak H., M.D., et al. "Effect of Dietary Enrichment with Eicosapentaenoic and Docosahexaenoic Acids on in Vitro Neutrophil and Monocyte Leukotriene Generation and Neutrophil Function." *New England Journal of Medicine*, vol. 312, no. 19, May 9, 1985.

"The MaxEPA Story in a Nutshell." Kal Self-Education Series, Makers of KAL, Inc.

"Omega-3, A Fish Story to Take to Heart." *Better Homes and Gardens*, June 1986.

Phillipson, Beverley E., M.D., et al. "Reduction of Plasma Lipids, Lipoproteins, and Apoproteins by Dietary Fish Oils in Patients with Hypertriglyceridemia." *New England Journal of Medicine*, vol. 312, no. 19, May 9, 1985.

Chapter Sixteen

Brownell, Kelly D., Ph.D., and Albert J. Stunkard, M.D. "Differential Changes in Plasma High-Density Lipoprotein-Cholesterol Levels in Obese Men and Women During Weight Reduction." *Archives of Internal Medicine*, vol. 141, August 1981.

Hagan, R. Donald, et al. "High Density Lipoprotein Cholesterol in Relation to Food Consumption and Running Distance." *Preventive Medicine*, vol. 12, 1983, pp. 287–95.

Nichols, Allen B., M.D., et al. "Independence of Serum Lipid Levels and Dietary Habits—The Tecumseh Study." *Journal of the American Medical Association*, vol. 236, no. 17, October 25, 1976.

Tran, Zung Vu, Ph.D., and Arthur Weltman, Ph.D. "Differential Effects of Exercise on Serum Lipid and Lipoprotein Levels Seen with Changes in Body Weight." *Journal of the American Medical Association*, vol. 254, no. 7, August 16, 1985.

Chapter Seventeen

Chapman, John M., et al. "Relationships of Stress, Tranquilizers, and Serum Cholesterol Levels in a Sample Population Under Study for Coronary Heart Disease." *American Journal of Epidemiology*, vol. 83, no. 3, 1966.

Clark, Dale A., et al. "Serum Cholesterol Levels in Selected Air Force Cadets Compared with Levels in the West Point Study." *Aviation, Space, and Environmental Medicine*, January 1980.

Flynn, Margaret A., Ph.D., et al. "Eggs, Serum Lipids, Emotional Stress, and Blood Pressure in Medical Students." *Archives of Environmental Health*, p. 90.

Herd, J. Alan, M.D. "Neuroendocrine Factors." *Masters in Cardiology*, vol. 2, no. 1, August 1984.

Kasl, Stanislav V., Ph.D., et al. "Changes in Serum Uric Acid and Cholesterol Levels in Men Undergoing Job Loss." *Journal of the American Medical Association*, vol. 206, no. 7, November 11, 1968.

Kirkeby, O.J., et al. "Serum Cholesterol and Thyroxine in Young Women During Mental Stress." *Experimental and Clinical Endocrinology*, vol. 83, no. 3, 1984, pp. 361–63.

Martinsen, K., et al. "Intrapartum Stress Lowers the Concentration of High Density Lipoprotein Cholesterol in Cord Plasma." *European Journal of Clinical Investigation*, vol. 11, 1981, pp. 351–54.

Rahe, LCDR Richard H., M.C., U.S.N., and CDR Ransom J. Arthur, M.C., U.S.N. "Stressful Underwater Demolition Training." *Journal of the American Medical Association*, vol. 202, no. 11, December 11, 1967.

Rahe, Richard H., et al. "Serum Uric Acid, Cholesterol, and Psychological Moods Throughout Stressful Naval Training." *Aviation, Space, and Environmental Medicine*, August 1976.

Stark, Christine, Cornell Cooperative Extension. "Not All Bran is Created Equal." *Homemakers News*, March 1986, Sullivan County Cooperative Extension Service Association.

Symbas, Panagiotis, M.D., et al. "Surgical Stress and Its Effects on Serum Cholesterol." *Surgery*, vol. 61, no. 2, February 1967, pp. 221–27.

"This Month's Master." *Masters in Cardiology*, vol. 2, no. 1, August 1984.

Thomas, Caroline Bedell, et al. "Youthful Hypercholesteremia: Its Associated Characteristics and Role in Premature Myocardial Infarction." *Johns Hopkins Medical Journal*, vol. 136, 1975, pp. 193–208.

Thomas, Paula D., R.N., M.S., et al. "Effect of Social Support on Stress-Related Changes in Cholesterol Level, Uric Acid Level, and Immune Function in an Elderly Sample." *American Journal of Psychiatry*, vol. 142, no. 6, June 1985, pp. 735–37.

Troxler, R.G., M.D., and H.A. Schwertner, B.S., Ph.D. "Cholesterol, Stress, Lifestyle, and Coronary Heart Disease." *Aviation, Space, and Environmental Medicine*, July 1985.

Yastrebtsova, N.L., and L.V. Simutenko. "Investigation of the Role of Prolonged Emotional Stress in the Genesis of Hypercholesteremia and Hypertension." Paper read at the 24th All-Union Conference on Problems in Higher Nervous Activity, Moscow, June 1974, Plenum Publishing Corporation, 1979.

Chapter Eighteen

"Research Report on Rise of Plasma LDL with Age." *Nutrition Letter*, University of Texas Health Science Center at Dallas, July/August, 1986.

Chapter Nineteen

Adams, Lucile L., Ph.D., et al. "Sex Differences in High-Density Lipoprotein Cholesterol and Subfractions Among Young Black Adults." *Preventive Medicine*, vol. 15, 1986, pp. 118–26.

Cooper, Richard, M.D., et al. "High-Density Lipoprotein Cholesterol and Angiographic Coronary Artery Disease in Black Patients." *American Heart Journal*, vol. 110, 1985, p. 1006.

Dai, Wanju, M.D., et al. "Plasma Testosterone and High Density Lipoprotein Cholesterol." Presented at the American Heart Association Meeting, Dallas, Texas, November 16, 1981. Unpublished.

Follick, Michael J., Ph.D., et al. "Contrasting Short- and Long-Term Effects of Weight Loss on Lipoprotein Levels." *Archives of Internal Medicine*, vol. 144, August 1984.

Gordon, Tavia, et al. "Lipoproteins, Cardiovascular Disease, and Death." *Archives of Internal Medicine*, vol. 141, August 1981.

Morgan, Don W., M.S., et al. "HDL-C Concentrations in Weight-Trained, Endurance-Trained, and Sedentary Females." *Physician and Sportsmedicine*, vol. 14, no. 3, March 1986.

" 'Pill' Use Again Linked to Changes in Blood Lipid Levels." Medical News, *Journal of the American Medical Association*, vol. 239, no. 8, February 20, 1978.

Tyroler, H.A., M.D., et al. "Plasma High-Density Lipoprotein Cholesterol Comparisons in Black and White Populations." *Circulation*, vol. 62, suppl. IV, 1980.

Chapter Twenty

Anderson, James W., M.D., and Janet T. Clark, R.D. "Soluble Dietary Fiber: Metabolic and Physiologic Considerations." *Contemporary Nutrition*, vol. 11, no. 9, 1986.

"Bran Reduces Cholesterol Saturation of Bile." Medical News, *Journal of the American Medical Association*, vol. 241, no. 11, March 16, 1979.

"Diet to Prevent Heart Attacks and Strokes." *Health Letter*, vol. 14, no. 4, February 22, 1980.

Mazer, Eileen. "The Miracle Food that Pampers Your Heart and Peps Up Your Life." *Prevention*, March 1983.

"New Research on Oats Verifies Ability to Reduce Cholesterol." Release from Consumer Affairs Center, Quaker Oats Company, June, 1986.

"The Oat Report." *Runner's World*, April 1985.

Palumbo, P.J., M.D., et al. "High Fiber Diet in Hyperlipidemia." *Journal of the American Medical Association*, vol. 240, no. 3, July 21, 1978.

Van Horn, Linda V., Ph.D., R.D., et al. "Serum Lipid Response to Oat Product Intake with a Fat-Modified Diet." *Journal of the American Dietetic Association*, vol. 86, no. 6, June 1986.

Chapter Twenty-one

"An 'Ideal' Serum Cholesterol Level?" Medical News, *Journal of the American Medical Association*, vol. 241, no. 19, May 11, 1979.

Beaglehole, Robert, M.D., et al. "Plasma High-Density Lipoprotein Cholesterol in Children and Young Adults." *Circulation*, vol. 62, suppl. IV, 1980.

Berenson, G.S., et al. "Plasma Glucose and Insulin Levels in Relation to Cardiovascular Risk Factors in Children from a Biracial Population—The Bogalusa Heart Study." *Journal of Chronic Diseases*, vol. 34, 1981, pp. 379–91.

Bilheimer, David W., M.D., et al. "Liver Transplantation to Provide Low-Density-Lipoprotein Receptors and Lower Plasma Cholesterol in a Child with Homozygous Familial Hypercholesterolemia." *New England Journal of Medicine*, vol. 311, no. 26, December 27, 1984.

Brody, Jane E. "Personal Health." *The New York Times*, October 29, 1986.

"Cholesterol and Children." *Journal of the American Medical Association*, vol. 256, no. 20, November 28, 1986.

Cuthbert, Jennifer A., M.B., B.S., et al. "Detection of Familial Hypercholesterolemia by Assaying Functional Low-Density-Lipoprotein Receptors on Lymphocytes." *New England Journal of Medicine*, vol. 314, no. 14, April 3, 1986.

East, Cara, M.D., et al. "Normal Cholesterol Levels with Lovastatin (Mevinolin) Therapy in a Child with Homozygous Familial Hypercholesterolemia Following Liver Transplantation." *Journal of the American Medical Association*, vol. 256, no. 20, November 28, 1986.

Edelson, Edward. "Kids & Low-Fat Diets: Experts Can't Agree." *New York Daily News*, September 8, 1986.

Freedman, David S., Ph.D., et al. "Relationship of Changes in Obesity to Serum Lipid and Lipoprotein Changes in Childhood and Adolescence." *Journal of the American Medical Association*, vol. 254, no. 4, July 26, 1985.

Frerichs, Ralph R., et al. "Serum Lipids and Lipoproteins at Birth in a Biracial Population: The Bogalusa Heart Study." *Pediatric Research*, vol. 12, 1978, pp. 858–63.

"Growth Study." *Insight*, September 8, 1986.

Harrell, Ann. " 'Cholesterol Kids' Treated at UTHSCD." *Nutrition & Health News*, vol. 3, no. 3, winter 1986.

"Lowering Blood Cholesterol to Prevent Heart Disease." Consensus Conference, *Journal of the American Medical Association*, vol. 253, no. 14, April 12, 1985.

Moll, Patricia P., Ph.D., et al. "Total Cholesterol and Lipoproteins in School Children: Prediction of Coronary Heart Disease in Adult Relatives." *Circulation*, vol. 67, no. 1, 1983.

Reed, Terry, Ph.D., M.P.H., et al. "Young Adult Cholesterol as a Predictor of Familial Ischemic Heart Disease." *Preventive Medicine*, vol. 15, 1986, pp. 292–303.

Van Stiphout, Willy-Anne H.J., M.D., et al. "Distributions and Determinants of Total and High-Density Lipoprotein Cholesterol in Dutch Children and Young Adults." *Preventive Medicine*, vol. 14, 1985, pp. 169–80.

Williams, Roger R., M.D., et al. "Evidence that Men with Familial Hypercholesterolemia Can Avoid Early Coronary Death." *Journal of the American Medical Association*, vol. 255, no. 2, January 10, 1986.

Chapter Twenty-two

"Cholesterol and Noncardiovascular Mortality." *Journal of the American Medical Association*, vol. 244, no. 1, July 4, 1980.

"Cholesterol Hits Below the Belt." *New York Daily News*, December 26, 1986.

"Colon Cancer and Blood-Cholesterol." *Lancet*, June 1974.

"Lowering Cholesterol May Be Hazardous to Health." *Nutrition Research Newsletter*, February 1985.

Mannes, Gerd Alexander, M.D., et al. "Relation Between the Frequency of Colorectal Adenoma and the Serum Cholesterol Level." *New England Journal of Medicine*, vol. 315, no. 26, December 25, 1986.

Neugut, Alfred I., M.D., Ph.D., et al. "Serum Cholesterol Levels in Adenomatous Polyps and Cancer of the Colon." *Journal of the American Medical Association*, vol. 255, no. 3, January 17, 1986.

Sidney, Stephen, et al. "Serum Cholesterol and Large Bowel Cancer." *American Journal of Epidemiology*, vol. 124, no. 1, 1986, pp. 33–38.

Spitz, Margaret R., M.D., M.P.H. "Cholesterol and Cancer Relationship." *Cancer Bulletin*, vol. 37, no. 3, 1985.

Tornberg, Sven A., M.D., et al. "Risks of the Colon and Rectum in Relation to Serum Cholesterol and Beta-Lipoprotein." *New England Journal of Medicine*, vol. 315, no. 26, December 25, 1986.

Chapter Twenty-three

Cumberland, D.C., et al. "Percutaneous Laser Thermal Angioplasty: Initial Clinical Results with a Laser Probe in Total Peripheral Artery Occlusions." *Lancet*, June 28, 1986.

"More Evidence That Coronary Artery Disease Is Reversible." *Health Letter*, vol. 15, no. 7, April 11, 1980.

APPENDIX I

Calorie, Fat, and Cholesterol Content of Commonly Used Foods

Caloric Value (Kcal), Fat and Cholesterol Content of Commonly Used Foods*

Food	Amounts	Kcal	(gm) Fat	(mg) Cholesterol
APPLE				
Raw	1 medium	70	trace (tr)	0
Baked, with sugar	1 medium	120	tr	13
Brown Betty	½ cup	175	4	20
Juice or cider	½ cup	60	tr	0
Pie (see PIES)				
Applesauce, canned sweetened	½ cup	115	tr	0
canned unsweetened	½ cup	50	tr	0
APRICOT				
Fresh	3 small	55	tr	0
Canned in syrup	½ cup or 4 medium halves	110	tr	0
Dried, stewed with sugar	½ cup or 8 medium halves	135	tr	0
Nectar	½ cup	70	tr	0
ASPARAGUS, cooked	½ cup	15	tr	0
AVOCADO, raw	½ medium	185	19	0

*Data from B. K. Watt and A. L. Merrill, *Composition of Foods—Raw, Processed and Prepared*, U.S. Department of Agriculture, Washington, D.C. 1963; *Nutritive Value of Foods*, Home and Garden Bulletin no. 72, rev., U.S. Department of Agriculture, Washington, D.C., 1971.

Food	Amounts	Kcal	(gm) Fat	(mg) Cholesterol
BACON				
Broiled or fried	2 slices, cooked crisp	90	8	14
Canadian, cooked	3 slices, cooked crisp (1.5 ounces)	100	12	20
BANANA, raw	1 medium, 6 inches long	100	tr	0
BEANS				
Sprouts, mung, cooked	½ cup	18	tr	0
raw	1 cup	25	tr	0
Green snap, cooked	½ cup	15	tr	0
Green lima, cooked	½ cup	130	tr	0
Baby green lima, cooked	½ cup	100	tr	0
Red kidney, canned	½ cup	115	1	0
White, canned with tomato sauce, without pork	½ cup	155	3	0
White, canned with tomato sauce, with pork	½ cup	155	3	3
Lentils (see LENTILS)				
BEEF				
Corned, canned	3 ounces	185	10	56
Corned hash, canned	½ cup	155	10	23
Dried or chipped	2 ounces (4 thin slices)	115	4	38
Ground, broiled	3 ounces (1 patty, 3 inch diameter)	245	17	60
Heart, braised	3 ounces	160	5	235
Liver, fried	2 ounces	130	6	250
Meat loaf, baked	1 slice	240	17	45
Potpie	1 pie, 4½ inch diameter	560	33	41
Pot roast, cooked	3 ounces	245	16	70
Roast, cooked	3 ounces	165	7	60
Steak, lean (sirloin), broiled	3 ounces	178	9	77
Steak, regular (rib eye), broiled	3 ounces	330	30	80
Stroganoff, cooked	½ cup	250	18	65
Stew	1 cup	245	11	72
Tongue, braised	3 ounces	210	14	120
BEETS, cooked	½ cup	28	tr	0
BEVERAGES				
Carbonated, soft drinks	12 ounces (1 can)	150	0	0

Food	Amounts	Kcal	(gm) Fat	(mg) Cholesterol
BEVERAGES (cont'd)				
Club soda	12 ounces	0	0	0
Ginger Ale	12 ounces (1 can)	110	0	0
BISCUITS, baking powder	1 biscuit, 2 inch diameter	105	5	2
BLACKBERRIES, raw	½ cup	45	1	0
BLUEBERRIES, raw	½ cup	45	1	0
BOLOGNA, beef	2 ounces (2 slices)	146	13	26
BOUILLON CUBES	1 cube	5	tr	0
BREAD				
Boston brown	1 slice, 3 × ¾ inch	100	1	1
Cracked wheat	1 slice	65	1	1
French or Vienna	1 slice, 3 inches	60	1	0
Italian	1 slice, 3 inches	55	tr	1
Light or dark rye	1 slice	60	tr	1
Pumpernickel	1 slice	85	0	1
Raisin	1 slice	65	1	1
White	1 slice	70	1	1
Whole wheat	1 slice	60	1	1
Crumbs	¼ cup	98	1	1
BROCCOLI, cooked	½ cup	20	1	0
raw	1 cup	20	1	0
BRUSSELS SPROUTS, cooked	½ cup (5 medium)	28	1	0
BUNS (see ROLLS)				
BUTTER	1 tablespoon	100	12	31
CABBAGE				
Cooked	½ cup	15	tr	0
Raw	½ cup	10	tr	0
CAKE				
Angel food, without icing	1 slice (12 slices/ cake)	135	tr	0
Boston cream pie	1 slice (12 slices/ cake)	210	6	53
Coffee cake, with icing	1 slice, 3 × 3 × 1¼ inches	260	11	30
Plain cupcakes, with icing	1	130	5	54
Plain cupcakes, without icing	1	90	3	47
Chocolate cake, 2 layer, with chocolate or vanilla icing	1 slice (16 slices/ cake)	235	9	29
Fruitcake	1 slice (30 slices/ loaf)	55	2	7

Food	Amounts	Kcal	(gm) Fat	(mg) Cholesterol
CAKE (cont'd)				
Pound, without icing	1 slice (1 ounce)	140	9	30
Sponge, wihout icing	1 slice (12 slices/ cake)	195	4	162
White cake, 2 layer, with chocolate or vanilla icing	1 slice (16 slices/ cake)	250	8	31
CANDY				
Caramels	4 small	115	3	2
Plain chocolate	1 ounce	150	9	3
Chocolate with almonds	1.8 ounces	265	19	7
Chocolate creams	1 ounce (2 pieces)	110	4	4
Chocolate fudge	1 ounce (1 inch square)	115	4	5
Hard	1 ounce (6 pieces)	110	tr	0
Peanut brittle	1 ounce (1 piece)	125	4	2
CANTALOUPE	½ melon	60	tr	0
CARROTS				
raw	1 or ½ cup grated	20	tr	0
cooked	½ cup	23	tr	0
CATSUP, Tomato	1 tablespoon	18	tr	0
CAULIFLOWER, cooked	½ cup	13	tr	0
raw	1 cup	13	tr	0
CELERY, raw	1 stalk or ½ cup	8	tr	0
cooked	1 cup	16	tr	0
CEREALS				
Bran flakes, 40% bran	1 ounce (¾ cup)	80	1	0
Cooked, all types	⅔ cup	87	1	0
Corn flakes	1 ounce (1⅓ cup)	130	tr	0
Puffed Rice	1 ounce (2 cups)	120	tr	0
Rice flakes	1 ounce (1 cup)	115	tr	0
Wheat flakes	1 ounce (1 cup)	105	tr	0
Shredded Wheat	1 ounce (1 biscuit or ½ cup)	90	1	0
CHEESE				
Blue (roquefort type)	1 ounce	105	9	21
Brie	1 ounce	95	8	28
Cheddar (American)	1 ounce	115	10	30
Cheddar (American), grated	1 tablespoon	30	2	8
Cottage, creamed (4% fat)	½ cup	120	5	17
Cottage, low-fat (2% fat)	½ cup	100	2	8
Cream	1 tablespoon	45	6	17

Food	Amounts	Kcal	(gm) Fat	(mg) Cholesterol
CHEESE (cont'd)				
Mozzarella, part-skim	1 ounce	80	5	16
Swiss (domestic)	1 ounce	105	8	35
Sauce	¼ cup	110	9	43
Souffle	¾ cup	200	16	132
CHEESECAKE	1 slice (10 slices/ cake)	400	23	114
CHERRIES, raw sweet	1 cup	80	tr	0
CHICK PEAS, dry raw (garbanzos)	½ cup	380	5	0
CHICKEN				
Broiled or baked	3 ounces, without bone or skin	115	2	66
Canned	3 ounces (⅓ cup) deboned	170	10	77
Creamed	½ cup	222	12	93
Breast, fried	3 ounces (½ breast) with bone	155	5	55
Drumstick, fried	1 with bone	90	4	43
Potpie, baked	1 pie, 4¼ inch diameter	535	31	13
CHILI				
Con carne with beans, canned	¾ cup	250	11	25
Con carne without beans, canned	¾ cup	383	29	30
Sauce	1 tablespoon	20	tr	0
CHOCOLATE				
Bitter	1 ounce (1 square)	145	15	0
Candy (see CANDY)				
Flavored milk drink	1 cup (made with skim milk)	190	6	8
Morsels	30 morsels or 1½ tablespoons	80	4	1
Syrup	2 tablespoons	80	tr	2
CHOP SUEY, cooked	¾ cup	325	20	32
COCOA, beverage	¾ cup (made with milk)	176	8	26
COCONUT				
Dried, shredded, sweetened	¼ cup	85	6	0
Fresh shredded	¼ cup	113	12	0

Food	Amounts	Kcal	(gm) Fat	(mg) Cholesterol
COLE SLAW, with cabbage	½ cup	50	4	4
COOKIES				
Brownies	1 piece, 2 × 2 × ½ inch	145	9	22
Chocolate chip	1 cookie, 2 inch diameter	60	3	6
Coconut bar chews	1 cookie, 2 inch diameter	55	2	6
Oatmeal with raisins and nuts	1 cookie, 2 inch diameter	65	4	4
Sugar, plain	1 cookie, 2½ inch diameter	40	2	7
CORN				
Sweet, cooked	1 ear, 5 inches long	70	1	0
Canned	½ cup	85	1	0
Grits, cooked	⅔ cup	85	tr	0
Muffins	1 muffin, 2½ inch diameter	125	4	2
Cornmeal, dry	1 cup, white or yellow	500	2	0
CRACKERS				
Graham, plain	2 squares	55	1	8
Saltines	2 crackers	35	1	6
CRANBERRY				
Juice	½ cup	85	tr	0
Sauce, canned	¼ cup	85	tr	0
CREAM				
Light cream	1 tablespoon	30	3	10
Half-and-half	1 tablespoon	20	2	6
Heavy, whipping	1 tablespoon, unwhipped	55	6	24
CREAMER (imitation cream)	1 teaspoon powder	10	1	0
CUCUMBER, raw	½	5	tr	0
CUSTARD, baked	½ cup	143	7	133
DATES, pitted	8 or ¼ cup	123	tr	4
DESSERT TOPPING, whipped	2 tablespoons (low-calorie, with nonfat dry milk)	17	0	0
DOUGHNUTS, cake-type	1	125	6	26
EGG				
Raw, boiled, or poached	1 whole egg	80	6	252
White	1 egg white	15	tr	0

Food	Amounts	Kcal	(gm) Fat	(mg) Cholesterol
EGG (cont'd)				
Yolk	1 egg yolk	60	5	252
Fried	1 egg, cooked in 1 teaspoon fat	115	10	265
Scrambled	1 egg (milk and fat added)	110	8	267
Eggnog	½ cup	335	19	73
ENDIVE, curly, raw	½ cup	10	tr	0
FARINA, cooked	⅔ cup	70	tr	0
FATS				
Cooking, lard	1 tablespoon	115	13	12
Cooking, vegetable	1 tablespoon	110	13	0
FIGS				
Dried	1 large	60	tr	0
Fresh, raw	3 small	90	tr	0
FISH				
Bluefish, baked	3 ounces	135	4	60
Codfish (dried)	½ cup	190	2	42
Clams, raw	3 ounces	65	1	42
Clams, canned	½ cup (3 medium)	80	2	50
Crab, fresh	3 ounces	80	2	85
Crab, canned	½ cup	100	2	85
Fish sticks, breaded, cooked	5 sticks, each 4 × 1 × ½ inches	200	10	80
Flounder, baked	3 ounces	85	1	59
Haddock, pan-fried	3 ounces	140	5	51
Lobster, cooked	3 ounces (½ cup)	90	1	70
Mackerel, baked	3 ounces	210	14	77
Oysters, raw	½ cup (8-10 oysters)	80	2	60
Oyster stew with milk	1 cup with 3-4 oysters	200	12	30
Perch, pan-fried	3 ounces	195	11	51
Salmon, red, cooked	3 ounces	140	5	60
Salmon, pink, canned	3 ounces (½ cup)	120	5	34
Salmon loaf	4 ounces (1 slice)	235	10	72
Sardines, canned in oil	3 ounces	175	7	85
Shad, baked	3 ounces	170	10	51
Shrimp	3 ounces (½ cup)	100	1	128
Sole, baked	3 ounces	85	1	59
Trout, baked	3 ounces	85	1	59

Food	Amounts	Kcal	(gm) Fat	(mg) Cholesterol
FISH (cont'd)				
Tuna, white, oil-packed	3 ounces (½ cup)	170	7	55
Tuna, white, water-packed	3 ounces (½ cup)	120	1	55
Tuna salad (see SALAD, TUNAFISH)	½ cup	25	18	42
FRANKFURTER	1 frankfurter	170	15	29
FRENCH TOAST, fried	1 slice	180	12	135
FRUIT COCKTAIL, canned in syrup	½ cup	98	tr	0
GELATIN				
Plain, dry	1 tablespoon (1 envelope)	25	tr	0
Dessert, plain, prepared	½ cup	70	0	0
GINGERBREAD	1 slice (2½ inch square)	175	4	0
GRAPEFRUIT				
White or pink, raw	½ medium	45	tr	0
Canned, in syrup	½ cup	88	tr	0
Juice, unsweetened	½ cup	50	tr	0
GRAPES				
Raw	1 cup	110	tr	0
Juice	½ cup	83	tr	0
GREENS				
Collards, cooked	½ cup	28	1	0
Dandelion, cooked	½ cup	30	1	0
Kale, cooked	½ cup	15	1	0
Mustard, cooked	½ cup	18	1	0
Spinach, cooked	½ cup	20	1	0
Turnip, cooked	½ cup	15	tr	0
GUAVAS, raw	1	50	tr	0
HAM				
Boiled	3 ounces	200	15	77
Cured, roasted	3 ounces	245	19	77
Luncheon, deviled, canned	2 tablespoons	165	14	28
HONEY	1 tablespoon	65	0	0
ICE CREAM				
Ice cream (10% fat)	½ cup	145	9	39
Ice cream, rich (16% fat)	½ cup	180	12	44
Ice cream, specialty (22% fat)	½ cup	300	23	153
ICE MILK	½ cup	100	4	13
JAMS, jellies, preserves	1 tablespoon	55	tr	0

Food	Amounts	Kcal	(gm) Fat	(mg) Cholesterol
LAMB				
Chop, cooked	3 ounces, without bone, fat-trimmed	185	9	80
Leg, roasted	3 ounces, without bone, fat-trimmed	160	6	75
LEMON JUICE	1 tablespoon	5	tr	0
LEMONADE, sweetened	1 cup	110	tr	0
LENTILS, all types, cooked	½ cup	120	tr	0
LETTUCE, all types	1 cup	10	tr	0
LIME JUICE	¼ cup	15	tr	0
LIVER				
Beef, fried	2 ounces	130	6	250
Calf, fried	2.5 ounces	230	15	324
Chicken, fried	3 ounces (3 medium)	235	15	634
Pork, fried	2.5 ounces	225	15	307
MACARONI				
Cooked	¾ cup	115	1	0
Macaroni and cheese, baked	¾ cup	325	17	32
MANGOES, raw	1 medium	90	0	0
MARGARINE	1 tablespoon	100	12	0
MARSHMALLOWS	1 large	25	0	0
MILK				
Dry skim (nonfat)	¼ cup powder	61	tr	3
Dry whole	¼ cup powder	129	7	25
Evaporated, canned	½ cup, undiluted and unsweetened	173	10	39
Low-fat (2% fat)	1 cup	120	5	17
Skim or buttermilk (made with skim milk)	1 cup	90	tr	5
Whole (4% fat)	1 cup	160	9	33
Malted, plain	1½ cup	368	15	49
Milkshake, chocolate	1½ cup	420	18	37
MOLASSES				
Cane, blackstrap	1 tablespoon	45	0	0
Cane, light	1 tablespoon	50	0	0
MUFFIN, plain	1 muffin, 2¾ inch diameter	120	4	2
MUSHROOMS, canned	½ cup	20	tr	0
raw	10 small	28	0	0

Food	Amounts	Kcal	(gm) Fat	(mg) Cholesterol
NOODLES, egg, cooked	¾ cup	150	2	43
NUTS				
Almonds	¼ cup	213	19	0
Cashews, roasted	¼ cup	196	16	0
Peanuts, roasted	¼ cup	210	18	0
Pecan halves	¼ cup	185	19	0
Walnut halves	¼ cup	163	16	0
OATMEAL OR ROLLED OATS, cooked	⅔ cup	87	1	0
OILS, salad or cooking, all types	1 tablespoon	125	14	0
OKRA, cooked	4 medium	13	tr	0
OLIVES				
Green	4 medium or 3 large	15	2	0
Black	2 large	37	2	0
ONION				
raw	1 medium	40	2	0
cooked	½ cup	30	tr	0
ORANGE				
Fresh	1 medium	65	tr	0
Juice	½ cup	60	tr	0
PANCAKE, wheat or white	1 medium, 5 inch diameter	60	2	16
PAPAYAS, raw	½ cup	35	tr	0
PARSLEY, raw	1 tablespoon chopped	tr	tr	0
PARSNIPS, cooked	½ cup	50	1	0
PEACHES				
Canned in syrup	½ cup	100	tr	0
Canned in water	½ cup	40	tr	0
Fresh or frozen	1 small or ½ cup	35	tr	0
PEANUT BUTTER	2 tablespoons	190	16	0
PEARS				
Canned in syrup	2 medium halves or ½ cup	90	tr	0
Fresh	1 medium	100	1	0
PEAS				
Cowpeas or blackeyed peas, cooked	½ cup	95	1	0
Green, cooked	½ cup	58	1	0

Food	Amounts	Kcal	(gm) Fat	(mg) Cholesterol
PEAS (cont'd)				
Split, cooked	½ cup	145	1	0
PEPPER				
Green, stuffed with meat	1 medium, cooked	200	14	34
Fresh, green or red	1 medium without stem and seeds	15	tr	0
PERSIMMONS, fresh	1 fruit, 2½ inch diameter	75	tr	0
PICKLE				
Relish	1 tablespoon	20	tr	0
Dill	1 large	10	tr	0
PIE (9 inch diameter)				
Apple	1 slice (8 slices/ pie)	300	13	36
Cherry	⅛ pie	300	13	12
Custard	⅛ pie	250	12	120
Lemon meringue	⅛ pie	270	10	97
Mince	⅛ pie	320	14	14
Pumpkin	⅛ pie	240	15	70
PINEAPPLE				
Canned in syrup	2 small slices or ½ cup	90	tr	0
Fresh	½ cup	38	tr	0
Juice, unsweetened	½ cup	68	tr	0
PIZZA (cheese)	⅛ of 14 inch diameter pie	185	6	31
PLANTAIN, fresh, green	1 baking banana, 6 inches long	135	0	0
PLUMS				
Canned, in syrup	½ cup or 3 small plums	100	tr	0
Raw	1 plum	25	tr	0
POPCORN, popped	1 cup (oil added)	40	2	0
PORK				
Pork chop, cooked	3 ounces, fat-trimmed, w/out bone	260	21	90
Roast, cooked	3 ounces	225	24	59
POTATO				
Potato chips	10 medium	115	8	0
Baked or boiled	1 medium	90	tr	0

Food	Amounts	Kcal	(gm) Fat	(mg) Cholesterol
POTATO (cont'd)				
French fried	10 pieces	155	7	11
Mashed	½ cup (milk and butter added)	95	4	15
PRETZELS	5, 3⅛ inch sticks	10	tr	0
PRUNES				
Dried, cooked with sugar	5 medium	160	tr	0
Juice	½ cup	100	tr	0
PUDDING				
Chocolate blanc mange	½ cup	190	8	12
Cornstarch	½ cup	140	5	18
Rice with raisins	½ cup	300	8	15
Tapioca	½ cup	140	5	8
RADISHES, raw	4 small	5	tr	0
RAISINS, seedless	1 tablespoon	30	tr	0
RASPBERRIES, raw, red	½ cup	35	1	0
RHUBARB, cooked with sugar	½ cup	190	tr	0
RICE, cooked, all varieties	¾ cup	140	tr	0
ROLLS				
Bagel (egg)	1 roll, 3 inch diameter	165	2	85
Barbecue bun	1 bun, 3½ inch diameter	120	2	1
Hard	1 large round	160	2	1
Plain, white	1 small dinner roll	85	2	1
Cinnamon	1 roll	135	4	30
RUTABAGAS, cooked	½ cup	25	tr	0
SALAD				
Chicken	½ cup, with mayonnaise	280	19	36
Egg	½ cup, with mayonnaise	190	18	262
Fresh fruit	½ cup, with French dressing	130	6	1
Jellied, vegetable	½ cup, no dressing	70	0	0
Lettuce	1 cup, with French dressing	80	6	2
Potato	½ cup, with mayonnaise	185	12	37

Food	Amounts	Kcal	(gm) Fat	(mg) Cholesterol
SALAD (cont'd)				
Tomato aspic	½ cup, no dressing	45	0	0
Tuna fish	½ cup, with mayonnaise	250	18	42
SALAD DRESSING				
Blue cheese	1 tablespoon	75	8	9
French	1 tablespoon	65	6	16
Low-calorie, oil free	2 tablespoons	17	0	2
Mayonnaise	1 tablespoon	100	11	10
Thousand Island	1 tablespoon	80	8	5
SAUCE				
Chocolate	2 tablespoons	75	4	2
Custard	2 tablespoons (low-calorie, with nonfat dry milk)	45	1	16
Hard	1 tablespoon	90	6	20
Hollandaise (mock)	2 tablespoons	75	7	84
Lemon	2 tablespoons	40	1	35
SAUERKRAUT, canned	½ cup	25	tr	0
SAUSAGE				
Liverwurst	2 ounces	150	12	198
Pork, cooked	2 small patties or links	125	11	26
Vienna	1 canned, 2 inches long	40	3	11
SHERBET, orange	½ cup	130	1	7
SYRUP, table blends	1 tablespoon, light and dark	60	0	0
SOUP				
Bean with pork, canned	1 cup	170	6	10
Beef broth, bouillon, consommé, canned	1 cup	30	0	0
Chicken noodle, canned	1 cup	65	2	6
Clam chowder, canned	1 cup	85	3	38
Cream of vegetable (e.g., tomato, mushroom), canned	1 cup	135	10	31
Gumbo	1 cup	140	1	0
Lentil	1 cup	140	1	0

Food	Amounts	Kcal	(gm) Fat	(mg) Cholesterol
SOUP (cont'd)				
Minestrone, canned	1 cup	105	3	2
Tomato, canned	1 cup	90	3	5
Vegetable, canned	1 cup	80	2	0
SPAGHETTI				
Cooked	¾ cup	115	1	
In tomato sauce, with cheese	¾ cup	200	7	21
In tomato sauce, with meat balls	¾ cup	250	9	56
SPINACH (see GREENS)				
SQUASH, summer, cooked	½ cup	15	tr	0
STRAWBERRIES, raw	½ cup	30	1	0
SUGAR				
Brown	1 tablespoon	50	0	0
Granulated	1 tablespoon	40	0	0
Lump	1 cube	25	0	0
Powdered	1 tablespoon	30	0	0
SWEET POTATO				
Baked	1 medium	155	1	0
Candied	1 medium	295	6	0
TANGERINE	1 medium	40	tr	0
TARTAR SAUCE (see SALAD DRESSING, mayonnaise)				
TOAST, melba	1 slice	20	tr	0
TOMATO				
Catsup	1 tablespoon	15	tr	0
Juice, canned	½ cup	23	tr	0
Canned	½ cup	25	1	0
Raw	1 medium	40	tr	0
TOPPING, whipped	1 tablespoon	10	1	3
TORTILLAS	1 tortilla, 5 inch diameter	50	1	0
TURKEY				
with skin	3 ounces	180	8	70
without skin	3 ounces	150	4	65
TURNIP				
Greens (see GREENS)				
Cooked	½ cup	18	tr	0

Food	Amounts	Kcal	(gm) Fat	(mg) Cholesterol
VEAL				
Cutlet, breaded (wiener schnitzel)	4.8 ounces	315	21	122
Cutlet, broiled	3 ounces	185	9	77
Roast, cooked	3 ounces	230	14	77
VINEGAR	1 tablespoon	2	0	0
WAFFLES	1 waffle, 7 inch diameter	210	7	54
WATERMELON, raw	1 wedge or 1 cup	115	1	0
WELSH RAREBIT	½ cup	330	26	114
WHEAT FLOUR				
White	1 cup	420	1	0
Whole wheat	1 cup	400	2	0
Wheat germ	2 tablespoons	30	1	0
WHITE SAUCE	¼ cup	110	8	8
YEAST				
Brewers, dry	1 tablespoon	25	tr	0
Compressed	1 ounce cake	25	tr	0
Dry active	4 packages (1 ounce each)	80	tr	0
YOGURT, plain, low-fat	1 cup	125	4	15

APPENDIX II

Calorie, Fat, Cholesterol, and Sodium Content of Common Fast Foods

	CALORIES	FAT (g)	CHOL* (mg)	Na* (mg)
BURGER KING				
Whopper Sandwich	670	38	–	975
Whopper Sandwich w/cheese	760	45	–	1260
Double Beef Whopper	890	53	–	1015
Double Beef Whopper w/cheese	980	61	–	1295
Whopper Junior Sandwich	370	18	–	545
Whopper Junior w/cheese	410	21	–	685
Hamburger	310	12	–	560
Cheeseburger	360	16	–	705
Bacon Double Cheeseburger	600	35	–	985
Veal Parmagiana	580	27	–	805
Ham & Cheese Sandwich	550	30	–	1550
Chicken Sandwich	690	42	–	775
Whaler Sandwich	540	24	–	745
Whaler Sandwich w/cheese	590	28	–	885
Regular French Fries	210	11	–	230
Regular Onion Rings	270	16	–	450
Apple Pie	330	14	–	385
Chocolate Shake	340	10	–	280
Vanilla Shake	340	11	–	320
Whole Milk	150	9	–	110
Medium Pepsi-Cola	131	–	–	8
Medium Diet Pepsi	7	–	–	52

*CHOL = Cholesterol
*Na = Sodium
– = Data Not Available

	CALORIES	FAT (g)	CHOL* (mg)	Na* (mg)
WENDY'S				
Single Hamburger	350	18	65	410
w/cheese	420	24	80	670
Double Hamburger	560	34	125	575
w/cheese	630	40	140	835
Triple Hamburger	780	47	170	630
w/cheese	920	59	200	1150
Chili	260	8	30	1070
French Fries	280	14	15	95
Chicken Sandwich	370	12	55	545
w/cheese	440	18	70	805
Taco Salad	390	18	40	1100
Frosty	400	14	50	220
Hot Stuffed Baked Potatoes				
Potato (no toppings, 8.8 oz.)	250	2	0	60
Sour Cream/Chives	460	24	15	230
Cheese	590	34	22	450
Chili & Cheese	510	20	22	610
Bacon & Cheese	570	30	22	1180
Broccoli & Cheese	500	25	22	430
Stroganoff & Sour Cream	490	21	43	910
Chicken ala King	350	6	20	820

PIZZA HUT (serving size-2 slices of medium 13" pizza: 4 servings per pizza)

	CALORIES	FAT (g)	CHOL* (mg)	Na* (mg)
THIN 'N CRISPY				
Standard Cheese	340	11	22	900
Superstyle Cheese	410	14	30	1100
Standard Pepperoni	370	15	27	1000
Superstyle Pepperoni	430	19	34	1200
Standard Pork w/Mushroom	380	14	35	1200
Superstyle Pork w/Mushroom	450	19	40	1400
Supreme	400	17	13	1200
Super Supreme	520	26	44	1500
THICK 'N CHEWY				
Standard Cheese	390	10	18	800
Superstyle Cheese	450	14	21	1000
Standard Pepperoni	450	16	21	900
Superstyle Pepperoni	490	20	24	1200
Standard Pork w/Mushroom	430	14	21	1000
Superstyle Pork w/Mushroom	500	18	21	1200
Supreme	480	18	24	1000
Super Supreme	590	26	38	1400

	CALORIES	FAT (g)	CHOL* (mg)	Na* (mg)
JACK IN THE BOX				
Hamburger	276	12	29	521
Cheeseburger	323	15	42	749
Jumbo Jack Hamburger	485	26	63	905
Jumbo Jack Hamburger w/cheese	630	35	110	1665
Bacon Cheeseburger Supreme	724	46	70	1307
Swiss and Bacon Burger	643	43	100	1354
Moby Jack Sandwich	444	25	47	820
Breakfast Jack Sandwich	307	13	203	871
Hot Ham & Cheese Supreme	497	24	74	1705
Hot Beef & Cheese Supreme	580	34	71	1501
Pita Pocket Supreme	284	8	43	953
Club Supreme	451	27	60	1323
Chicken Supreme	601	36	60	1582
Regular Taco	191	11	21	406
Super Taco	288	17	37	765
Cheese Nachos	571	35	37	1154
Supreme Nachos	718	40	55	1782
Taco Salad	377	24	102	1436
Chef Salad	253	13	110	707
Chicken Salad	470	35	104	685
Shrimp Salad	116	1	139	460
Chicken Strips Dinner	689	30	100	1316
Shrimp Dinner	731	37	157	1510
Sirloin Steak Dinner	699	27	969	1216
Croissant Supreme	547	40	178	1053
Sausage Croissant	584	43	187	1012
Bacon Croissant	480	34	194	935
Ham Croissant	447	31	166	848
French Fries	221	12	8	164
Onion Rings	382	23	27	407
Apple Turnover	410	24	15	350
Pancake Breakfast	630	27	85	1670
Scrambled Eggs Breakfast	720	44	260	1110
Vanilla Shake — Calif., Ark., Tx., Washington	320	6	25	230
Strawberry Shake — Calif., Ark., Tx., Washington	320	7	25	240
Chocolate Shake — Calif., Ark., Tx., Washington	330	7	25	270
Vanilla Shake	340	9	35	265
Strawberry Shake	380	10	35	270
Chocolate Shake	360	10	35	295
Croissants	347	23	–	–

	CALORIES	FAT (g)	CHOL* (mg)	Na* (mg)
JACK IN THE BOX (cont'd)				
Garlic Roll (1)	300	13	–	–
Kaiser Roll (1)	165	1	–	–
Tortilla Chips (1 oz.)	130	6	–	–
Pancakes (4 oz.)	210	2	–	–
ARBY'S				
Roast Beef	350	15	45	880
Beef 'N Cheddar	440	19	46	1370
Super Roast Beef	620	28	85	1420
Junior Roast Beef	220	9	35	530
Ham 'N Cheese	484	21	70	1745
Turkey Deluxe	510	24	70	1220
Club Sandwich	560	30	100	1610
Bac'n Cheddar Deluxe	560	34	80	1375
French Dip	386	12	55	1111
Roast Beef Deluxe	486	23	59	1288
Arby's Sub	484	21	76	1766
Chicken Breast Sandwich	584	28	56	1323
Potato Cakes (2)	190	9	–	476
French Fries	216	12	–	39
Arby's Sauce (1 oz.)	30	0	0	325
Horsey Sauce (1 oz.)	100	10	15	350
Apple Turnover	310	21	–	240
Cherry Turnover	320	20	–	254
Blueberry Turnover	340	20	–	255
Vanilla Shake	330	11	35	275
Chocolate Shake	370	10	30	290
Jamocha Shake	400	9	30	265
McDONALD'S				
Big Mac	563	38	86	1010
Cheeseburger	307	14	37	767
Hamburger	255	10	25	520
Quarter Pounder	424	22	67	735
Quarter Pounder w/cheese	524	31	96	1236
Filet-O-Fish	432	25	47	781
Regular Fries	220	12	9	109
McChicken	475	27	59	990
Chicken McNuggets	332	19	79	523
McFeast	435	31	76	878
McRib (onion & pickle)	461	44	52	1020
Egg McMuffin	327	15	229	885

	CALORIES	FAT (g)	CHOL* (mg)	Na* (mg)
McDONALD'S (cont'd)				
English Muffin w/butter	186	5	13	318
Hotcakes w/butter & syrup	500	10	47	1070
Sausage (pork)	206	19	43	615
Scrambled Eggs	180	13	349	205
Hashbrown Potatoes	125	7	7	325
Ham Biscuit	422	21	31	1949
Sausage Biscuit	582	40	48	1380
Apple Pie	253	14	12	398
Cherry Pie	260	14	13	427
McDonaldland Cookies	308	11	10	358
Chocolate Chip Cookies	342	16	18	313
Chocolate Shake	383	9	30	300
Strawberry Shake	362	9	32	207
Vanilla Shake	352	8	31	201
Hot Fudge Sundae	310	11	18	175
Caramel Sundae	328	10	26	195
Strawberry Sundae	289	9	20	96
Cones	185	5	24	109
KENTUCKY FRIED CHICKEN				
ORIGINAL RECIPE CHICKEN				
Wing	136	9	55	302
Drumstick	117	7	63	207
Side Breast	199	12	70	558
Thigh	257	18	109	566
Keel	236	12	87	631
EXTRA CRISPY CHICKEN				
Wing	201	14	59	312
Drumstick	155	9	66	263
Side Breast	286	18	65	564
Thigh	343	23	109	549
Keel	297	16	79	584
Chicken Breast Filet Sandwich	436	23	43	2732
Kentucky Fries	184	7	0	434
Mashed Potatoes	64	1	0	268
Gravy	23	2	0	57
Cole Slaw	121	8	7	225
Rolls	61	1	1	118
Corn (5.5 inch ear)	169	3	0	11
CHURCH'S FRIED CHICKEN				
White Chicken Portion	327	23	–	498

	CALORIES	FAT (g)	CHOL* (mg)	Na* (mg)
CHURCH'S FRIED CHICKEN (cont'd)				
Dark Chicken Portion	305	21	–	475
Dinner Roll	83	1.6	–	–
French Fries	256	12.8	–	–
Corn on the Cob	165	3.3	–	–
Pecan Pie	367	19.5	–	–
Apple Pie	300	18.6	–	–
Cole Slaw	83	7	–	–
DAIRY QUEEN				
Single Hamburger	360	16	45	630
w/cheese	410	20	50	790
Double Hamburger	530	28	85	660
w/cheese	650	37	95	980
Triple Hamburger	710	45	135	690
w/cheese	820	50	145	1010
Hot Dog	280	16	45	830
w/chili	320	20	55	985
w/cheese	330	21	55	990
Super Hot Dog	520	27	80	1365
w/chili	570	32	100	1595
w/cheese	580	34	100	1605
Fish Sandwich	400	17	50	875
w/cheese	440	21	60	1035
Chicken Sandwich	640	41	75	870
French Fries	200	10	10	115
large	320	16	15	185
Onion Rings	280	16	15	140
DQ Cone, small	140	4	10	45
regular	240	7	15	80
large	340	10	25	115
DQ Dip Cone, small	190	9	10	55
regular	340	16	20	100
large	510	24	30	145
DQ Sundae, small	190	4	10	75
regular	310	8	20	120
large	440	10	30	165
DQ Malt, small chocolate	520	13	35	180
regular	760	18	50	260
large	1060	25	70	360
Shake, small	490	13	35	180
regular	710	19	50	260
large	990	26	70	360

	CALORIES	FAT (g)	CHOL* (mg)	Na* (mg)
DAIRY QUEEN (cont'd)				
"Mr. Misty," small	190	0	0	0
regular	250	0	0	0
large	340	0	0	0
DQ Float	410	7	20	85
DQ Banana Split	540	11	30	150
DQ Parfait	430	8	30	140
DQ Freeze	500	12	30	180
Mr. Misty Freeze	500	12	30	140
Mr. Misty Float	390	7	20	95
"Dilly" Bar	210	13	10	50
DQ Sandwich	140	4	5	40
Mr. Misty Kiss	70	0	0	0
Buster Bar	390	29	10	175
Hot Fudge Brownie Delight	600	25	20	225
Peanut Buster Parfait	740	34	30	140
"Double Delight"	490	20	25	250
Strawberry Shortcake	540	11	25	215
LONG JOHN SILVER'S				
Fish w/Batter (2 pc.)	366	22	–	–
Fish w/Batter (3 pc.)	549	32	–	–
Treasure Chest	506	33	–	–
Chicken Planks (4 pc.)	457	23	–	–
Peg Legs w/Batter (5 pc.)	350	28	–	–
Ocean Scallops (6 pc.)	283	13	–	–
Shrimp w/Batter (6 pc.)	268	13	–	–
Breaded Oysters (6 pc.)	441	19	–	–
Breaded Clams (5 oz.)	617	34	–	–
Fish Sandwich	337	31	–	–
French Fries	288	16	–	–
Cole Slaw	138	8	–	–
Corn on the Cob (1 ear)	176	4	–	–
Hushpuppies (3)	153	7	–	–
Clam Chowder (8 oz.)	107	3	–	–
TACO BELL				
Bean Burrito	343	12	–	272
Beef Burrito	466	21	–	327
Beefy Tostada	331	18	–	138
Bellbeefer	221	7	–	231
Bellbeefer w/cheese	278	12	–	330
Burrito Supreme	457	22	–	367

	CALORIES	FAT (g)	CHOL* (mg)	Na* (mg)
TACO BELL (cont'd)				
Combination Burrito	404	16	–	300
Enchirito	454	21	–	1175
Pintos 'N Cheese	168	5	–	102
Taco	192	11	–	79
Tostada	156	11	–	101
Taco Supreme	237	15	–	–
Taco Bellgrande	410	26	–	–
Taco Light	170	26	–	–
HARDEE'S				
Hamburger	305	13	–	682
Cheeseburger	335	17	–	789
Big Deluxe	546	26	77	1083
¼ lb. Cheeseburger	506	25	61	1950
Roast Beef Sandwich	376	17	57	1030
Big Roast Beef	418	19	60	1770
Hot Dog	346	22	42	744
Hot Ham & Cheese	376	15	59	1067
Big Fish Sandwich	514	26	41	314
Chicken Filet	510	26	57	360
Bacon Cheeseburger	686	42	295	1074
Biscuit	275	13	3	650
Sausage Biscuit	413	26	29	864
Steak Biscuit	419	23	34	804
Ham Biscuit	350	17	29	1415
Fried Egg (1 med.)	108	9	264	169
Bacon & Egg Biscuit	405	26	305	823
French Fries (small)	239	13	4	121
French Fries (large)	381	21	6	192
Apple Turnover	282	14	5	–
Milkshake	391	10	42	–
BEVERAGES				
Coffee	2	tr	–	2
Tea	2	tr	–	–
Orange juice	82	tr	–	2
Chocolate Milk	213	9	–	118
Skim Milk	88	tr	–	127
Whole Milk	159	9	27	122
Coca-Cola	96	0	–	20
Fanta Ginger Ale	84	0	–	30
Fanta Grape	114	0	–	21

	CALORIES	FAT (g)	CHOL* (mg)	Na* (mg)
BEVERAGES (cont'd)				
Fanta Orange	117	0	–	21
Fanta Root Beer	103	0	–	23
Mr. Pibb	95	0	–	23
Mr. Pibb w/o sugar	1	0	–	37
Sprite	95	0	–	42
Sprite w/o sugar	3	0	–	42
Tab	tr	0	–	30
Fresca	2	0	–	38
EXTRAS				
DRESSINGS				
Blue Cheese (4 Tbsp.)	210	18	–	735
Buttermilk (4 Tbsp.)	290	29	–	555
French, reduced calorie (4 Tbsp.)	140	6	–	480
1000 Island (4 Tbsp.)	250	24	–	560
Ketchup (2 Tbsp.)	10	0	–	99
Grape Jelly	38	0	–	3
Table Syrup	121	0	–	6
Coffeemate packets (1)	17	1	–	6

Fat Composition of Commonly Used Foods

Fat Composition of Commonly Used Foods

FOODS	Amount

DAIRY AND EGG PRODUCTS

Cheese:
American	1 oz
Blue	1 oz
Camembert	1 oz
Cheddar	1 oz

Cottage:

Creamed, 4% fat:
Large curd	1 cup
Small curd	1 cup
Lowfat, 1% fat	1 cup
Uncreamed, dry curd, less than ½% fat	1 cup
Cream	1 oz
Mozzarella, made with part skim milk	1 oz
Muenster	1 oz
Parmesan, grated	1 tbsp[2]
Ricotta, made with part skim milk	1 oz
Swiss	1 oz

[1]Trace.
[2]Tablespoon.
[3]Average of available data.
[4]Major sources of cholesterol are eggs and butter.
[5]Major sources of cholesterol are milk and butter.
[6]Major source of cholesterol is eggs.
[7]Major source of cholesterol is animal shortening.
[8]Source of cholesterol is milk solids.
[9]Source of cholesterol is cheese.
[10]Source of cholesterol is tallow.
N.A. = data not available.

Source: Provisional Table on the Fatty Acid and Cholesterol Content of Selected Foods, United States Department of Agriculture, Human Nutrition Information Service, Washington: United States Government Printing Office, June 1984.

Total Calories	Calories from Fat gm	Total Fat gm	Fatty acids			Cholesterol mg
			Saturated gm	Monounsaturated gm	Polyunsaturated gm	
106	78	8.9	5.6	2.5	0.3	27
100	72	8.2	5.3	2.2	0.2	21
85	61	6.9	4.3	2.0	0.2	20
114	83	9.4	6.0	2.7	0.3	30
232	89	10.1	6.4	2.9	0.3	34
217	84	9.5	6.0	2.7	0.3	31
164	20	2.3	1.5	0.7	0.1	10
123	5	0.6	0.4	0.2	Tr[1]	10
99	87	9.9	6.2	2.8	0.4	31
72	40	4.5	2.9	1.3	0.1	16
104	75	8.5	5.4	2.5	0.2	27
23	13	1.5	1.0	0.4	Tr	4
39	19	2.2	1.4	0.7	0.1	9
107	69	7.8	5.0	2.1	0.3	26

FOODS	Amount
Cream, sweet:	
Half-and-half (cream: and milk)	1 tbsp
Light, coffee, or table	1 tbsp
Heavy, whipping, unwhipped	1 tbsp
Cream, sour, cultured	1 tbsp
Cream products, imitation (made with vegetable fat):	
Coffee whitener:	
Liquid, frozen (contains coconut or palm kernel oil)	1 tbsp
Powdered (contains coconut or palm kernel oil)	1 tbsp
Dessert toppings (nondairy):	
Powdered, made with whole milk	1 tbsp
Pressurized	1 tbsp
Milk, fluid:	
Whole, 3.3% fat	1 cup
Lowfat, 2% fat	1 cup
Lowfat, 1% fat	1 cup
Nonfat, skim	1 cup
Buttermilk, cultured	1 cup
Milk beverages:	
Eggnog	1 cup
Shakes, thick, vanilla	1 container
Milk desserts, frozen:	
Ice cream:	
Regular (about 10% fat)	1 cup
Rich (about 16% fat)	1 cup
Ice milk:	
Hardened (about 4.3% fat)	1 cup
Soft serve (about 2.6% fat)	1 cup
Sherbet (about 2% fat)	1 cup
Yogurt:	
Made with lowfat milk	8 oz
Made with nonfat milk	8 oz
Made with whole milk	8 oz
Eggs, large:	
Hard cooked, shell removed	1 egg
Fried in butter	1 egg
Scrambled (milk added) in butter. Also omelet.	1 egg

FATS, OILS, AND RELATED PRODUCTS

Fats (solid at room temperature):	
Butter	1 tbsp
Lard	1 tbsp
Shortening (animal and vegetable fat)	1 tbsp
Shortening (vegetable)	1 tbsp

Total Calories	Calories from Fat gm	Total Fat gm	Fatty acids			Cholesterol mg
			Saturated gm	Monounsaturated gm	Polyunsaturated gm	
20	15	1.7	1.1	0.5	0.1	6
29	25	2.9	1.8	0.8	0.1	10
52	49	5.6	3.5	1.6	0.2	21
26	22	2.5	1.6	0.7	0.1	5
20	13	1.5	1.4	Tr	Tr	0
33	19	2.1	1.8	Tr	Tr	0
8	4	0.5	0.4	Tr	Tr	Tr
11	8	0.9	0.8	0.1	Tr	0
150	72	8.2	5.1	2.4	0.3	33
125	41	4.7	2.9	1.4	0.2	18
104	21	2.4	1.5	0.7	0.1	10
90	5	0.6	0.4	0.2	Tr	5
99	19	2.2	1.3	0.6	0.1	9
342	167	19.0	11.3	5.7	0.9	149
350	84	9.5	5.9	2.7	0.4	37
269	126	14.3	8.9	4.1	0.5	59
349	208	23.7	14.7	6.8	0.9	88
184	49	5.6	3.5	1.6	0.2	18
223	40	4.6	2.9	1.3	0.2	13
270	33	3.8	2.4	1.1	0.1	14
194	25	2.8	1.8	0.8	0.1	11
127	4	0.4	0.3	0.1	Tr	4
139	65	7.4	4.8	2.0	0.2	29
79	51	5.6	1.7	2.2	0.7	274
94	66	7.2	2.7	2.7	0.8	279
107	72	8.0	3.2	2.9	0.8	282
102	102	11.4	7.1	3.3	0.4	31
116	116	12.8	5.0	5.8	1.4	12
115	115	12.8	5.2	5.7	1.4	7
113	113	12.8	3.2	5.7	3.3	0

FOODS

	Amount
Fats (cont'd)	
Tallow, edible	1 tbsp
Margarine, regular (at least 80% fat):	
Stick:	
Corn oil	1 tbsp
Soybean oil	1 tbsp
Tub:	
Corn oil	1 tbsp
Soybean oil	1 tbsp
Margarine, diet (about 40% fat), tub[3]	1 tbsp
Oils (liquid at room temperature):	
Coconut	1 tbsp
Corn	1 tbsp
Olive	1 tbsp
Palm	1 tbsp
Palm kernel	1 tbsp
Peanut	1 tbsp
Safflower	1 tbsp
Soybean oil (partially hydrogenated)	1 tbsp
Soybean-cottonseed oil blend (partially hydrogenated)	1 tbsp
Sunflower	1 tbsp
Related products:	
Mayonnaise	1 tbsp
Light mayonnaise	1 tbsp
Peanut butter	1 tbsp
Salad Dressings:	
Russian	1 tbsp
French	1 tbsp
Ranch	1 tbsp
Low-calorie Italian	1 tbsp
Italian	1 tbsp
Blue cheese	1 tbsp
Mayonnaise-type	1 tbsp
Thousand Island	1 tbsp

FISH, SHELLFISH, MEAT, POULTRY, AND RELATED PRODUCTS

Fish:	
Cooked:	
Flounder or sole (a lean fish) baked	3 oz
Salmon, red (a fatty fish) baked	3 oz
Canned:	
Salmon, pink, water pack	3 oz
Sardines, Atlantic, oil pack	3 oz
Tuna, chunk light, oil pack	3 oz

Total Calories	Calories from Fat gm	Total Fat gm	Fatty acids			Cholesterol mg
			Saturated gm	Monounsaturated gm	Polyunsaturated gm	
116	116	12.8	6.4	5.3	0.5	14
102	102	11.4	2.0	5.5	3.4	0
102	102	11.4	2.4	5.4	3.0	0
102	102	11.4	2.0	4.5	4.4	0
102	102	11.4	1.8	5.1	3.9	0
50	50	5.7	1.2	2.4	2.1	0
117	117	13.6	11.8	0.8	0.2	0
120	120	13.6	1.7	3.3	8.0	0
119	119	13.5	1.8	9.9	1.1	0
120	120	13.6	6.7	5.0	1.3	0
117	117	13.6	11.1	1.5	0.2	0
119	119	13.5	2.3	6.2	4.3	0
120	120	13.6	1.2	1.6	10.1	0
120	120	13.6	2.0	5.9	5.1	0
120	120	13.6	2.4	4.0	6.5	0
120	120	13.6	1.4	2.7	8.9	0
99	99	11.0	1.6	3.1	5.7	8
40	36	4.0	N.A.	N.A.	N.A.	6
95	73	8.3	1.7	3.8	2.4	0
75	70	7.8	1.1	1.8	4.5	0
65	60	6.4	1.5	1.2	3.4	2
50	45	5.0	0.9	1.3	2.9	4
16	15	1.5	0.2	0.3	0.9	1
70	65	7	1.0	1.7	4.1	–
80	70	8	1.5	1.9	4.3	9
60	45	5	0.7	1.3	2.6	4
60	55	6	0.9	1.3	3.1	5
82	9	1.0	0.3	0.2	0.4	59
140	49	5.4	1.2	2.4	1.4	60
120	45	5.0	0.9	1.5	2.1	34
173	85	9.4	2.1	3.7	2.9	85
167	63	7.0	1.4	1.9	3.1	55

FOODS

	Amount
Fish: (cont'd)	
Tuna, chunk light, water pack	3 oz
Shellfish:	
Raw:	
Clams, unspecified	3 oz
Oysters, Eastern	3 oz
Canned:	
Crabmeat	3 oz
Shrimp, dry pack	3 oz
Meat:	
Beef:	
Eye of round, lean only, roasted	3 oz
Rib roast, lean and fat, roasted	3 oz
Ground beef, cooked, well done	3 oz
Pork:	
Ham, roasted	3 oz
Bacon, fried crisp	2 slices
Lamb, loin chop:	
Lean only	3 oz
Lean and fat	3 oz
Veal cutlet (1 cutlet)	3 oz
Poultry:	
Chicken:	
Dark meat, baked without skin	3 oz
Light meat, baked without skin	3 oz
Dark meat, fried with skin	3 oz
Light meat, fried with skin	3 oz
Related products:	
Beef liver, fried	3 oz
Frankfurters (beef)	1 frank
Bologna (beef and pork)	1 slice
Salami, cooked (beef and pork)	1 slice
Braunschweiger	1 slice

MISCELLANEOUS ITEMS
(with ingredients of animal origin as sources of cholesterol)

	Amount
Beef pot pie	1 piece
Beef stew	1 cup
Chicken pot pie	1 piece
Chicken a la king	1 cup
Chili with beef	1 cup
Cakes:	
Pound	1 slice
White, 2 layer with chocolate icing[5]	1 piece

| Total Calories | Calories from Fat gm | Total Fat gm | Fatty acids | | | Cholesterol mg |
			Saturated gm	Monounsaturated gm	Polyunsaturated gm	
95	4	1.0	N.A.	N.A.	N.A.	60
65	13	1.4	0.3	0.3	0.3	42
56	14	1.5	0.5	0.2	0.5	42
86	19	2.1	0.3	0.5	0.8	85
99	8	0.9	0.2	0.2	0.4	128
156	53	5.9	2.4	2.7	0.2	56
330	254	28.2	11.7	13.6	1.0	70
244	141	15.6	7.6	8.5	0.7	88
187	85	9.4	3.2	4.2	1.1	80
73	56	6.2	2.2	3.0	0.7	11
183	77	8.5	3.5	3.2	0.5	80
250	153	17.0	7.7	6.8	1.0	82
185	85	9.4	4.0	4.0	0.4	86
174	75	8.3	2.3	3.0	1.9	79
147	34	3.8	1.1	1.3	0.8	72
242	130	14.4	3.9	5.7	3.3	78
209	93	10.3	2.8	4.1	2.3	74
195	81	9.0	2.5	3.6	1.3	372
184	152	16.8	6.8	8.2	0.7	27
89	72	8.0	3.0	3.8	0.7	16
71	51	5.7	2.3	2.6	0.6	18
102	82	9.1	3.1	4.2	1.1	44
515	275	30.5	7.9	12.9	7.4	42
220	95	10.5	4.4	4.5	0.5	72
545	282	31.3	10.3	15.5	6.6	56
470	320	35.5	12.9	13.4	6.2	220
340	141	15.6	5.8	7.2	1.0	28
160	88	10.0	5.9	3.0	0.6	68
250	68	7.7	3.0	2.9	1.3	3

FOODS

	Amount
Cakes: (cont'd)	
Yellow, 2 layer with chocolate icing[6]	1 piece
Cookies:	
Brownies, with chocolate icing[4]	1 brownie
Chocolate chip[6]	4 cookies
Vanilla wafers[6]	10 cookies
Crackers:	
Graham	2 crackers
Saltines[7]	4 crackers
Cupcakes, with chocolate icing[4]	1 cupcake
Doughnuts, cake type[6]	1 doughnut
Doughnuts, yeast-leavened[6]	1 doughnut
Chocolate, milk (20% milk solids)[8]	1 oz
Pizza with cheese[9]	1 sector
Potatoes, french-fried (fried in edible tallow)[10]	10 strips

Total Calories	Calories from Fat gm	Total Fat gm	Fatty acids			Cholesterol mg
			Saturated gm	Monounsaturated gm	Polyunsaturated gm	
235	70	7.9	3.0	3.0	1.4	36
105	47	5.3	2.0	2.3	0.7	13
205	105	12.0	3.5	4.6	3.2	21
185	59	6.7	1.7	2.8	1.7	25
55	11	1.3	0.3	0.5	0.4	0
50	9	1.0	0.4	0.4	0.2	3
130	41	4.6	2.0	1.7	0.7	15
100	42	4.7	1.2	1.2	2.0	10
205	118	13.4	3.3	5.8	3.5	13
145	80	9.0	5.4	3.0	0.3	5
145	35	4.0	2.1	1.2	0.5	13
158	75	8.3	3.4	4.0	0.5	6

ABOUT THE AUTHOR

KENNETH H. COOPER, M.D., M.P.H., received his M.D. degree from the University of Oklahoma School of Medicine, and his M.P.H. degree from the Harvard University School of Public Health. A recipient of many awards and honors, he is the author of *Aerobics,* the landmark book that coined that term and started America running. Dr. Cooper is founder of the Cooper Clinic and director of the Aerobics Center in Dallas, Texas, and an acknowledged world leader in health and fitness. His exclusive aerobics system is used by many military organizations throughout the world including both the U.S. Navy and Air Force. His other bestselling books include: *The New Aerobics for Women* (with Mildred Cooper), *The Aerobics Way, The New Aerobics, The Aerobics Program for Total Well-Being* and *Running Without Fear.*

INDEX

RECIPE INDEX

Laboratory Form

Note to Patient:

Write your name, address and zip code on the reverse side of this card, and affix a stamp. Then, after a 12- to 14-hour fast, take the card to a qualified laboratory for your blood test. Ask those performing the blood test to fill in the information below and return this card to you. If any of your blood values place you in a risk range higher than the 25th percentile "Excellent Protection" category indicated on p. 53 of Dr. Kenneth H. Cooper's Preventive Medicine Program: *Controlling Cholesterol*, follow the appropriate recommendations and programs described in that book. The final interpretation of the results of the blood test should be made by your physician.

Note to Blood Laboratory:

Please fill in the information required in the blank spaces below, and return this card to the address on the reverse side.

1. Total Cholesterol: _____ mg/dl
2. LDL Cholesterol: _____ mg/dl
3. HDL Cholesterol: _____ mg/dl
4. Triglycerides: _____ mg/dl
5. Total Cholesterol/HDL Ratio _____

Laboratory Form

Note to Patient:

Write your name, address and zip code on the reverse side of this card, and affix a stamp. Then, after a 12- to 14-hour fast, take the card to a qualified laboratory for your blood test. Ask those performing the blood test to fill in the information below and return this card to you. If any of your blood values place you in a risk range higher than the 25th percentile "Excellent Protection" category indicated on p. 53 of Dr. Kenneth H. Cooper's Preventive Medicine Program: *Controlling Cholesterol*, follow the appropriate recommendations and programs described in that book. The final interpretation of the results of the blood test should be made by your physician.

Note to Blood Laboratory:

Please fill in the information required in the blank spaces below, and return this card to the address on the reverse side.

1. Total Cholesterol: _____ mg/dl
2. LDL Cholesterol: _____ mg/dl
3. HDL Cholesterol: _____ mg/dl
4. Triglycerides: _____ mg/dl
5. Total Cholesterol/HDL Ratio _____

NUTRITIONAL AND EXERCISE EVALUATION WITH THE COOPER CLINIC

Your daily diet is a key determinant of your overall health, fitness, and energy. Sensible eating can help prevent or manage many health problems, including heart disease, obesity, hypertension, diabetes, ulcers, digestive problems, and colon cancer. Moreover, eating right adds to your sense of well-being. This analysis of your eating patterns will help to evaluate and enhance your present diet, for your best health.

PLEASE BE ACCURATE AND THOROUGH in completing this 3-day food record so that your NUTRITIONAL EVALUATION will be valuable to you. READ ALL INSTRUCTIONS AND EXAMPLES BEFORE YOU BEGIN. All data on page 1 must be completed before we can enter your food and exercise data.

We will send you the NUTRITIONAL EVALUATION of your diet within two weeks.

Mail this record and $20 (payable to the "Cooper Clinic") to the Cooper Clinic, Nutrition Program, 12200 Preston Rd., Dallas, Texas 75230.

CLINIC USE ONLY
Date _____
I.D. # _____

PLEASE COMPLETE EACH ITEM BELOW FOR COMPLETE AND ACCURATE ANALYSIS:

FULL NAME _____
      Last   First   Middle

TITLE (Circle One) Mr. Mrs. Ms. Miss Dr. Rev.

STREET ADDRESS _____

CITY _____ STATE _____ ZIP _____

SOCIAL SECURITY # _____ AGE _____

PHONE # (hm) _____ (wk) _____

PRESENT WEIGHT _____ DESIRED WEIGHT _____

HEIGHT _____ inches   % BODY FAT _____
                                         (if available)

SEX F ____ M ____

If FEMALE, are you pregnant or lactating? _____
                                    (No or P or L)

Are you currently following a weight loss diet? Yes ____ No ____

WEEKLY EXERCISE RECORD

RECORD THE **TOTAL** NUMBER OF **MINUTES/WEEK** YOU REGULARLY DO THESE ACTIVITIES.

Sample Exercise Record

		Min/Week Walking/Jogging
1	_____	5.2 mph (11:30 min/mi.)
2	_____	5.5 mph (11 min/mi.)
3	_150_	6 mph (10 min/mi.)
4	_____	6.5 mph (9 min/mi.)
9	_____	7 mph (8:30 min/mi.)
40	_____	Aerobic Dancing
76	_____	Archery
73	_____	Baseball
71	_90_	Basketball
75	_____	Bowling
41	_____	Calisthenics

_____ No regular exercise

		Min/Week Walking/Jogging				**Min/Week** Walking/Jogging
15	_____	3 mph (20 min/mi.)		38	_____	Cycling (outdoor-racing)
14	_____	3.5 mph (17 min/mi.)		35	_____	Cycling (stationary)
16	_____	4 mph (15 min/mi.)		36	_____	Cycling (Schwinn
17	_____	4.4 mph (13:30 min/mi.)				Aerodyne) bike load = 2.5
18	_____	5 mph (12 min/mi.)		50	_____	Downhill Skiing
1	_____	5.2 mph (11:30 min/mi.)		77	_____	Golf (no cart)
2	_____	5.5 mph (11 min/mi.)				90-120 min
3	_____	6 mph (10 min/mi.)		79	_____	Golf (with cart)
4	_____	6.5 mph (9 min/mi.)				90-120 min
9	_____	7 mph (8:30 min/mi.)		80	_____	Horseback riding
5	_____	7.5 mph (8 min/mi.)		70	_____	Racquetball/Handball/
10	_____	8 mph (7:30 min/mi.)				Squash
6	_____	8.5 mph (7 min/mi.)		90	_____	Rope Skipping
7	_____	10 mph (6 min/mi.)		85	_____	Rowing (sculling or
8	_____	11 mph (5:30 min/mi.)				machine
				72	_____	Softball
40	_____	Aerobic Dancing		20	_____	Swimming 30 yd./min
76	_____	Archery				(60 min/mi.)
73	_____	Baseball		21	_____	Swimming 39 yd./min
71	_____	Basketball				(45 min/mi.)
75	_____	Bowling		60	_____	Tennis (singles)
41	_____	Calisthenics		61	_____	Tennis (doubles)
30	_____	Cycling (outdoor)		12	_____	Treadmill
		9.4 mph (6.4 min/mi.)		74	_____	Volleyball
31	_____	Cycling (outdoor)		78	_____	Weight Lifting/
		5.5 mph (11 min/mi.)				Training

OTHER ACTIVITIES

_____ _____

_____ _____

_____ _____

FOOD RECORD INSTRUCTIONS

1. <u>Record everything</u> you eat for 3 days — meals, snacks, beverages, etc. Record <u>immediately</u> after eating for best recall. INCLUDE:

PREPARATION	baked . . . broiled . . . fried . . . breaded . . . buttered . . . sauteed . . . creamed . . . broiled . . . any other
EXTRAS	butter/margarine (or diet marg.) . . . sour cream . . . mustard/catsup . . . salad dressing (or low-calorie) & what kind . . . salt . . . pepper. . . mayonnaise (or low-calorie) . . . gravies . . . sauces . . . jelly . . . etc.!
BEVERAGES	water . . . beer (lite or regular) . . . wine . . . liquor . . . lemonade . . . soft drinks (regular or diet) . . . coffee or tea (with cream/sugar) . . . milk (½%, 2%, whole) . . . Gatorade

2. Include <u>2 weekdays + 1 weekend day</u>,' — these should be <u>typical eating days</u> and not necessarily consecutive days! Specify meals as breakfast, lunch, dinner, or snack.

3. List portions <u>accurately</u> — this is ESSENTIAL! Sample portions: 1 cup, 1 tsp., 1 Tbsp., 4 oz., 2 slices

SAMPLE FOOD RECORD

TIME & MEAL	WHERE	FOOD	SERVING SIZE AMOUNT
6pm Dinner	Home Dining Room	Chicken breast-baked; no sauce	4 oz.
		Baked potato with;	1 medium
		margarine	2 pats
		cheese sauce	¼ cup
		Broccoli ; steamed	½ cup
		Apple ; fresh	1 large
		Dinner roll ; no margarine	1 small
		2% milk	8 oz.

TYPICAL PORTIONS

Meat, Poultry, Fish
3 oz. = size of palm of a lady's hand (don't count fingers!)
         = amount in a sandwich
         = amount in a quarter pound hamburger (cooked)
         = chicken breast (3″ across)
6 oz. = restaurant chicken breast (6″ across)
         = common luncheon or cafeteria portion
8 oz. = common evening restaurant portion

Cheese
1 oz. = 1 slice on sandwich or hamburger
         = 1″ cube or 1 wedge airplane serving
½ cup = 1 scoop cottage cheese

Salads
1 cup = dinner salad;   2-4 cups = salad bar

Potato
1 small = 2½″ long   1 large = 5″ long = restaurant portion
1 med. = 4″ long   1 huge = 6″ long = meal-in-one potato

Vegetables
½ cup = cafeteria or restaurant portion
        = coleslaw or beans at a BBQ restaurant

Fats
1 tsp. margarine/butter = 1 pat
1 Tbsp. mayonnaise = typical amount on sandwiches
2 Tbsp. dressing = typical amount on a dinner salad
              = 1 small ladle (restaurant)
              = ½ large ladle (restaurant)

Beverages
4 oz. (½ cup) = typical juice portion
8 oz. (1 cup) = common milk portion
4 oz. = small glass of wine
12 oz. = 1 can of beer or soft drink
1½ oz. = 1 jigger per alcoholic drink

Snacks
chips — 10   choc. cake with frosting — 1 slice
pretzels — 5 (3 ring)   oatmeal cookies — 2 medium
peanuts — 20 whole (salted) donut — 1 medium
pizza — ½ of 13″; or 4 slices apple pie — ⅛ of 9″ pie

Casseroles & Sandwiches
Chicken Divan (1 cup) = chicken, broccoli, cheese, chicken soup,
                        mayo, croutons
      Hamburger = 6 oz. meat, 1 slice cheese, lettuce, tomato,
                    1 bun, 1 Tbsp. mayo, 1 Tbsp. catsup
     Ham Sandwich = 3 oz. ham, 1 Tbsp. mayo, 2 slices whole-wheat
                    bread, 1 dill pickle, 2 slices tomato, lettuce

WEEKDAY 1

TIME & MEAL	WHERE	FOOD	SERVING SIZE AMOUNT
		PLEASE PUT ONE FOOD PER LINE!	

WEEKDAY 2

TIME & MEAL	WHERE	FOOD	SERVING SIZE AMOUNT
		PLEASE PUT ONE FOOD PER LINE!	

<u>WEEKEND</u> DAY 3

TIME & MEAL	WHERE	FOOD	SERVING SIZE AMOUNT
		PLEASE PUT ONE FOOD PER LINE!	